Child Health Psychology
(PGPS-113)

Pergamon Titles of Related Interest

DiMatteo/DiNicola ACHIEVING PATIENT COMPLIANCE:
The Psychology of the Medical Practitioner's Role
Morris/Kratochwill PRACTICE OF THERAPY WITH CHILDREN:
A Textbook of Methods
Morris/Kratochwill TREATING CHILDREN'S FEARS AND PHOBIAS:
A Behavioral Approach
Rachman CONTRIBUTIONS TO MEDICAL PSYCHOLOGY,
Volumes 1 and 2
Schwartz/Johnson PSYCHOPATHOLOGY OF CHILDHOOD:
A Clinical-Experimental Approach

Related Journals*

ANALYSIS AND INTERVENTION IN DEVELOPMENTAL
DISABILITIES
APPLIED RESEARCH IN MENTAL RETARDATION
JOURNAL OF CHILD PSYCHOLOGY & PSYCHIATRY
JOURNAL OF PSYCHOSOMATIC RESEARCH
SOCIAL SCIENCE & MEDICINE

*Free specimen copies available upon request.

PERGAMON GENERAL PSYCHOLOGY SERIES

EDITORS

Arnold P. Goldstein, *Syracuse University*
Leonard Krasner, *SUNY at Stony Brook*

Child Health Psychology
Concepts and Issues

Paul Karoly
University of Cincinnati

John J. Steffen
University of Cincinnati

Donald J. O'Grady
Children's Hospital, Cincinnati

PERGAMON PRESS
New York   Oxford   Toronto   Sydney   Paris   Frankfurt

RJ
47.5
.C443
1982

Pergamon Press Offices:

U.S.A.	Pergamon Press Inc., Maxwell House, Fairview Park, Elmsford, New York 10523, U.S.A.
U.K.	Pergamon Press Ltd., Headington Hill Hall, Oxford OX3 0BW, England
CANADA	Pergamon Press Canada Ltd., Suite 104, 150 Consumers Road, Willowdale, Ontario M2J 1P9, Canada
AUSTRALIA	Pergamon Press (Aust.) Pty. Ltd., P.O. Box 544, Potts Point, NSW 2011, Australia
FRANCE	Pergamon Press SARL, 24 rue des Ecoles, 75240 Paris, Cedex 05, France
FEDERAL REPUBLIC OF GERMANY	Pergamon Press GmbH, Hammerweg 6 6242 Kronberg/Taunus, Federal Republic of Germany

Copyright © 1982 Pergamon Press Inc.
Library of Congress Cataloging in Publication Data

Main entry under title:

Child health psychology.

    (Pergamon general psychology series ; 113)
    Bibliography: p.
    Includes indexes.
    1. Pediatrics--Psychological aspects.
2. Child psychology. 3. Medicine and psychology.
I. Karoly, Paul. II. Steffen, John. III. O'Grady,
Donald J. IV. Series. [DNLM: 1. Child psychology.
2. Pediatrics. WS 105 C534]
RJ47.5.C443   1982   618.92'8   82-7486
ISBN 0-08-029368-9   AACR2

Printed in the United States of America

*This book is fondly dedicated to our col-
league Will Seeman, empiricist, hu-
manist, and intellectual free spirit, who
would certainly not be offended by the
open-ended, unfinished domain of inquiry that is health psychology.*

Contents

Preface

The surge of popular and professional interest in the field of "behavioral medicine" or "health psychology" belies the fact that what psychology and medicine are currently experiencing is a process of *rediscovery*. Recognition of the basic integrity of human adaptation, the wholeness of the human experience, the bidirectional nature of the mind-body and behavior-environment transactions can be traced to the ancient Greeks. And while some may mark the official birth of the new behavioral medicine with the 1977 Yale Conference (Schwartz & Weiss, 1978), the period of incubation began in the 1950s with the pioneering work of Hans Selye (1956), Franz Alexander (1950), and George Engel (1962).

Despite the existence of numerous conceptual precedents, however, there can be no doubt that the present "infectious" interest in psychological applications in health and disease derives primarily from the building of a *technological bridge* to medicine. Beginning with the perhaps overstated claims of biofeedback advocates, the procedures associated with the experimental analysis of behavior (operant psychology) began to find their way into the clinical armamentarium of both physicians and psychologists working in medical settings (cf. Gentry & Matarazzo, 1981). Today professional journals, clinical training programs, and a growing number of textbooks are appearing, built solely upon the principles of learning and the empirical methods for assessing and altering behavior that most readily apply to health-related disorders.

Pediatric implementation of behavioral procedures has been an integral part of the reemergence of psychology in medicine, extending well beyond the more or less traditional emphasis upon developmental problems like enuresis and encopresis to such areas as asthma, diabetes, hospital fears, chronic pain, and medical noncompliance (cf. Melamed & Siegel, 1980).

Without minimizing the importance of viable techniques for behavioral assessment and modification, the position can be taken that the current deemphasis of theory may ultimately stunt the growth of psychology's liaison with medicine. Knowing *why* is as essential as knowing *how*—perhaps even more important in an emergent discipline. And as far as children's health problems are concerned, it is unlikely that a downward extension of adult-oriented procedures will adequately address the unique aspects of childhood growth and development as they are affected by disease, physical trauma, and stress. As Tefft and Simeonsson (1979) have noted:

> The first "comprehensive" encyclopedia of pediatric psychology (Wright, Schaefer, & Solomons, 1978) consists of diagnostic and treatment considerations for over 100 individual pediatric problems. With the exception of a brief introductory chapter, there is no effort to explore the history, conceptual framework, or professional issues in pediatric psychology [p. 564].

The purpose of the present volume is to provide the student or professional in psychology, medicine, or nursing with a working knowledge of basic assumptions, theories, and issues underlying the practice of child health psychology. While our volume is not intended as a textbook (since the field is too young to have achieved textbookish consensus), we feel that the topics selected for inclusion offer a broad sampling of fundamental material.

Chapter 1 introduces the reader to the realities and complexities of child psychology practiced within a medical setting. As the author, Dennis Drotar, points out, "many psychologists begin their work in pediatric settings with a largely traditional training background," and the same can be said of other health professionals (nurses, social workers, and so forth). Drotar provides a thorough guide to the hospital culture, the avenues for interdisciplinary cooperation, work-related stresses, and the medical models within which physicians currently function. No amount of technical expertise will ever translate into patient service if the nonmedical practitioner is forced to move like a "stranger in a strange land." Chapter 1 is, therefore, an essential conceptual road map for the would-be health professional who plans on working in a hospital or clinic environment.

Chapter 2 is an attempt to place childhood illness in a life-span adaptational perspective in order to illustrate the potential conceptual and clinical advantages that accrue to an approach that emphasizes continuity (rather than episodic disruptions), health (rather than disease), multiple causation (rather than unilateral determinants), the social context (rather than just the biological), and a relativistic view of competence (in contrast to disciplinary attempts to define it in absolute terms). In addition to outlining an organizational framework for "developmental pediatrics," Karoly draws from a cross section of the child development literature in order to underscore the adaptive resources that may derive from the emergent self-knowledge, interpersonal skill repertoires, self-regulatory mechanisms, and information-processing capacities of children and adolescents.

Surprisingly little has been written in behavioral medicine texts or journals about children's emergent understanding of their health and illness. In Chapter 3, Jordan and O'Grady pull together a disparate literature on health beliefs, their nature, development, and assessment, and the putative relationship between beliefs and actual health or illness behavior(s).

A necessary component of any child health curriculum is epidemiology, particularly dealing with the course of childhood disease. Lewis and Craft present an information-packed yet thoroughly entertaining introduction to epidemiological concepts in Chapter 4. The methods of epidemiological exploration are similar to those of the master detective. Using the strange and exotic malady kuru as their vehicle, the authors take the reader on an adventure whose twists and possibilities would have challenged the great Sherlock Holmes. In fact the solution of the kuru puzzle in the mid-1970s earned epidemiologist Carlton Gadjusek a Nobel Prize.

In the next chapter Edward Christophersen reviews the numerous methodological issues that are often neglected by pediatric researchers. Whether the reader plans to conduct research or simply "consume" the ever-expanding literature, the discussion in Chapter 5 will prove extremely helpful.

Perhaps no area of child health dysfunction research has been as productive yet inaccessible to the average practitioner as pediatric neuropsychology, the study of brain-behavior relationships in childhood. In Chapter 6 Wilkening and Golden explain the basic tools of neuropsychological investigation, the research on specific disorders, and the development of a comprehensive theoretical approach. Included is a discussion of the popular Halstead-Reitan assessment procedure and sections devoted to an explication of head trauma, central nervous system infections, leukemia, and aphasia in children. The authors also discuss the controversial Luria-Nebraska neuropsychological battery.

Chapter 7 offers an excellent accounting of what is and isn't known about medicine's most basic and pervasive symptom—pain. While much has been written about the pain experience in adults, children's pain remains relatively unexplored (certainly *under*explored). J. Gerald Beales, an active British investigator, goes beyond "impression and assumption" and presents an in-depth and firsthand analysis of children's pain experiences, the effect of parental perceptions on children's pain, the effects of learning, age as it relates to pain sensation and adaptation, cognitive controls over the pain experience, and the methods and issues associated with accurate pain assessment. Beales concludes with an appraisal of pain management procedures for children with acute or chronic conditions.

Another fundamental concept in pediatric psychology is the designation of "high risk." In Chapter 8 Tiffany Field, one of the country's leading investigators of infants who have experienced reproductive or early caretaking casualties, explores the nature of the complex interaction between adults and so-called high-risk infants. For the most part, investigators have been content to classify and "track" high risk populations or to presume high risk status and intervene in the absence of careful assessment. Field offers intriguing data on high-risk mother-infant dyadic interaction and suggests a possible link between maternal activity and infant behavior, heart rate, and blood pressure. Most important from a clinical standpoint is the possible alteration of infant cardiovascular response through planned changes in maternal activity levels.

Because the subject of children's activity level has been linked to learning disorders and to potential academic and social incompetence in later life, the next chapter, dealing with "hyperactivity," seeks to sort through the varied etiological proposals currently in vogue. Donald Kanter organizes the findings on the causal significance of genetics, pre-, peri-, or postnatal trauma, lead, salicylates, radiation, biochemical imbalances, and social and cultural factors in childhood hyperactivity and suggests future integrative directions.

The final basic concept to be discussed (in Chapter 10) may be the least understood and potentially the most cost-effective avenue for clinical intervention in the health disorders of children. Addrisi and Handy, coordinators of the country's largest grant-supported project for this purpose, discuss early mental health screening and intervention in the public schools. The reader will be introduced to the ideas of secondary prevention, mass screening, and competence training and to the fundamental short- and long-term issues and problems associated with working in a public school setting.

Taken together, the chapters in this volume provide a much-needed conceptual grounding for an evolving discipline. Even if ten years hence the field of child health psychology has been all but totally transformed, the ideas in this book will have played a key role in the process of growth that is the essence of science and of enlightened application.

REFERENCES

Alexander, F. *Psychosomatic medicine: Its principles and applications.* New York: Norton, 1950.

Engel, G. L. *Psychological development in health and disease.* Philadelphia: W. B. Saunders, 1962.

Gentry, W. D., & Matarazzo, J. D. Medical psychology: Three decades of growth and development. In C. K. Prokop & L. A. Bradley (Eds.), *Medical psychology: Contributions to behavioral medicine.* New York: Academic Press, 1981.

Melamed, B. G., & Siegel, L. J. *Behavioral medicine: Practical applications in health care.* New York: Springer, 1980.

Schwartz, G. E., & Weiss, S. M. Yale conference on behavioral medicine: A proposed definition and statement of goals. *Journal of Behavioral Medicine,* 1978, **1**, 3–12.

Selye, H. *The stress of life.* New York: McGraw-Hill, 1956.

Tefft, B. M., & Simeonsson, R. J. Psychology and the creation of health care settings. *Professional Psychology,* 1979, **10**, 558–570.

Acknowledgments

The editors wish to acknowledge the assistance of several "behind the scenes" persons whose efforts on behalf of this volume have been considerable. Our editor at Pergamon, Jerry Frank, has provided consistent encouragement and support at all stages of production, along with a unique brand of gentle and constructive criticism. In Cincinnati, two facilitators of this volume's birth deserve special mention. Diane Kopriwa, as usual, managed to type much of the manuscript (correcting misspellings and awkward phrases along the way) while handling two dozen other chores with equal skill. And Robert Stutz, in his role as head of the Department of Psychology, managed to make it possible for us to work productively and efficiently on this project in an atmosphere of economic belt-tightening (where the editing of books too often seems like a luxury no one can afford). As the funniest psychologist since Bob Newhart, Bob also kept us laughing all the way. Finally, to our patient wives and families, we give our love and, eventually, our royalty checks.

1

The Child Psychologist in the Medical System

Dennis Drotar

In recent years opportunities for research and clinical practice in medical settings for psychologists trained to work with children have dramatically expanded. Psychologists now collaborate with physicians in a wide range of hospital facilities, including ambulatory settings (Botinelli, 1975; Schroeder, 1979; Smith, Rome, & Freedheim, 1967), specialized centers for the treatment of chronic illnesses (Koocher, Sourkes, & Keane, 1979), and hospital wards (Drotar, 1976a,b,c; Toback, Russo, & Gururaj, 1975). Pediatric hospitals have a number of special advantages as work environments for psychologists: rewarding features of such settings include varied and challenging patient populations which range from infants through young adults, opportunities for health-oriented preventive intervention, and work with clinical populations that involve complex interrelationships between physical status and behavior (Wright, 1979). The opportunity to collaborate with other professional disciplines and apply psychological knowledge to their work environment provides another important challenge. Many psychologists find the rich mix of clinical work, consultation, and research with pediatric populations quite compatible with their professional development.

Now that increasing numbers of psychologists are making a career commitment to work in pediatric settings (Nathan, Lubin, Matarazzo, & Persely, 1979), the psychologist's role in the medical setting, most especially the nature of collaboration with physicians, deserves special scrutiny. My experience in a university-based pediatric hospital (Drotar, 1976b; Drotar, 1977a) has strongly underscored the need to understand the way psychologist-physician transactions are influenced by the structure, organization, and culture of medical settings. The ideas presented here have been forged from a ten-year experience with children, families, and professional staff at Rainbow Babies' and Children's Hospital, which is a referral center for northeastern Ohio and a major teaching hospital for Case Western Reserve University School of Medicine. Serving patients from a large geographic area, this hospital has a 220-bed

1

inpatient service and an ambulatory care service for large numbers of middle-class and poverty-level families in areas proximate to Cleveland. In this setting, the psychologists form a division of psychology within a large, highly specialized Department of Pediatrics that includes over 60 full-time faculty pediatricians. Although this exposition of the child psychologist's role and functioning within a medical setting is shaped by experiences most characteristic of complex, university-based centers, the reader should recognize the potential applicability of this discussion to other medically based professional environments.

PREPARATION FOR PSYCHOLOGICAL PRACTICE IN PEDIATRIC HOSPITAL SETTINGS

Despite an increasing number of innovations in graduate and clinical training in health psychology, behavioral medicine, and pediatric psychology (Drotar, 1978; Matarazzo, 1980; Olbrisch and Sechrest, 1979; Ottinger & Roberts, 1980; Stone, 1979; Tuma, 1975), many psychologists begin their work in pediatric settings with a largely traditional training background in clinical psychology, which may be supplemented by practicum, internship, or postdoctoral training experiences in pediatric settings. Currently pediatric psychology is not included as part of the graduate curriculum in most programs. Moreover, since the majority of pediatric psychology practitioners are not active in graduate training, most psychologists are not exposed to professional opportunities in pediatric psychology until later in their careers. Health care psychologists' difficulties in learning their trade are further complicated by a lack of agreement concerning the specialized knowledge and clinical techniques that are most appropriate for their professional development.

Despite these obstacles, traditionally trained child psychologists will find many of their clinical and research skills potentially applicable to pediatric settings, particularly if such skills are enhanced by intensive experience in pediatric hospitals and a thorough exposure to child developmental theory and research. For example, there is a range of clinical procedures, particularly with children and families in psychosocial crises, that are potentially applicable to the complex clinical problems encountered in a pediatric setting. Diagnostic experience with a variety of childhood adjustment problems is needed to help pediatric colleagues make recommendations for psychosocial treatment. Psychotherapeutic skills with children and families are also quite applicable to the clinical interventions required by pediatric populations (Johnson, 1979). Since pediatric populations provide fertile opportunities for research, particularly in areas related to chronic and psychosomatic illness, neuropsychology, or developmental disorders, prior familiarity with psychological research with children is a special asset. Finally, clinical experiences that require psychologists to translate their knowledge into information that can be applied by other professional disciplines are especially compatible with work in general medical settings.

On the other hand, the psychologist who wishes to pursue a career in a medical setting should *not* assume that traditional training provides sufficient preparation to function effectively in a pediatric hospital. Specialized training is needed because the psychologist who works within a pediatric facility must confront a work environment and an institutional structure quite unlike that encountered in graduate school or in clinical training in community mental health and psychiatric settings. Clinical work and research in pediatric settings require special perspectives that can only be gained by intensive exposure to the workings of pediatric hospitals (Tefft & Simeonsson, 1979). Pediatric hospitals house complex, highly specialized and varied clinical populations that tax the knowledge and experience of traditionally trained psychologists. Moreover, since each medical setting is characterized by different areas of faculty expertise and levels of program development, health care psychologists will often learn much of their craft through a trial-by-fire approach in a given setting (Gabinet & Friedson, 1980).

Yet despite wide individual variation across pediatric facilities, there are commonalities in patient populations and clinical methods. For example, problems involving chronic physical illnesses, psychosomatic problems, functionally based pain, neurological conditions, behavior problems of infancy and early childhood, and developmental disorders are encountered with greater than average frequency in pediatric facilities. In our setting, for instance, almost half of the total requests for psychological consultations during our psychology division's first three years concerned questions of intellectual deficits associated with a large variety of problems such as language disabilities, chronic illness, psychosocial deprivation, and congenital anomalies. Nearly one-third of all referrals concerned management of patients with chronic illness and related adjustment problems, or acute medical or psychosocial crises such as child abuse, accidents, and burns. A smaller group, which included less than 10 percent of total referrals, included children referred for primary behavior disorders (Drotar, 1977a). Such complex patient populations require the psychologist to become familiar with a range of clinical techniques and knowledge of child development far outstripping that required by other settings that provide mental health services for children. For example, on hospital wards psychologists are asked to evaluate such disparate problems as disruptive behavior, poor compliance with treatment regimens, severe anxiety or depression, problematic adaptation to school or family, and preparation for hospitalization or surgery (Johnson, 1979). Moreover, the primary behavioral disorders encountered in pediatric settings range from the milder adjustment problems identified in the context of primary health care to severe psychosocial problems such as suicidal behavior or anorexia nervosa that necessitate admission to pediatric hospitals. These problems lend themselves to a range of therapeutic modalities including short-term structured reality-based approaches, behaviorally oriented interventions, parent guidance, and family approaches, as well as longer-term treatment (Johnson, 1979; Power & Del Orto, 1980). Although mastery of each and every one of these techniques is not possible, the psychologist in a pediatric setting must be sufficiently conversant in a number of therapeutic approaches to allow effective clinical function. Since pediatric hospitals treat a variety of infants and preschoolers at special risk owing to abuse and neglect, familiarity with the clinical methods employed with this age group is especially advantageous. However, clinical work with infants and young children requires experience with specialized assessment tools such as the Bayley Scale (Bayley, 1967), and with observational methods involving a transactional approach to the study of clinical problems (Rexford, Sander, & Shapiro, 1976; Sameroff, 1975) that are not emphasized in many clinical training programs.

Clinical problems commonly referred to psychologists in the pediatric setting often reflect a complex interplay between organic and environmental influences. For this reason, familiarity with specialized techniques for the assessment of children with physical handicaps and neurological or sensory impairments is especially useful. Psychologists in pediatric settings are also asked to evaluate the relative contribution of psychological influences to psychosomatic problems such as asthma or diabetes, to help differentiate between psychological and organic influences in somatic symptoms such as pain or seizures, or to evaluate the factors involved in a chronically ill child's psychological adaptation to the disease or compliance with physical treatment regimens. Since every physical disease has a unique natural history, set of treatment regimens, and stresses that must be thoroughly understood in order to appraise maladaptive versus adaptive adjustment, the psychologist must learn about various physical diseases, their treatment regimens, and the special impact of physical disease and treatment on child and family functioning (Pless & Pinkerton, 1975). Because chronic physical illnesses are not unitary categories, but complex conditions that include a number of subgroups differing in symptoms, prognosis, or severity, experience with children of different ages with a variety of illnesses is very helpful.

To best facilitate work with children and families who face stressful life circumstances, the clinician in a pediatric setting needs to construe clinical problems in ways that depart from psychopathology-based concepts. For example, a coping and adaptation framework that considers how the child's behavior is functionally related to the unique circumstances associated with chronic illnesses or other life stresses is especially well suited to certain pediatric populations (Lazarus, Averill, & Opton, 1974; Lazarus & Launier, 1978). Finally, since many pediatric hospitals are located in large urban centers, psychologists who work in such settings must become conversant with the special stress-related problems of the urban poor.

Psychologists in pediatric settings must also grapple wth ethically troubling problems that cannot easily be solved, even with the most sensitive of clinical interventions (Drotar, 1976c; Fox & Swazey, 1978; Katz & Capron, 1975). The compelling human problems encountered in pediatric settings, such as physical trauma, child abuse and neglect, or chronic life-threatening illnesses, also engender feelings of stress and helplessness in medical and nursing staff, who may nevertheless expect the psychologist to be unflappable in the face of troubling human situations. For this reason, psychologists in health care settings must have or develop the capacity to work calmly with stress-related problems in a way that is helpful not only to child and family but to medical and nursing staff. For this reason, one of the psychologist's most important skills involves the ability to translate psychological knowledge into *concrete plans* that can potentially benefit the staff's work and/or the child's problem. Since each of these parties' needs may be at odds with one another, the psychologist's transactions with patients and staff should include a high level of sensitivity and diplomacy.

Psychologists who work within a medical setting must acquire the skill to translate and communicate their knowledge in ways that can be effectively accepted by other professional disciplines. To accomplish this, a successful psychological consultant must understand the difficulties encountered by physicians and other professionals in their work, command and show respect for pediatric colleagues, and appreciate yet work within the confines of the hospital's unique organizational problems. Effective consultation in pediatric settings is not restricted to a patient-centered approach (Caplan, 1970) but involves a *process* consultation that focuses on transactions with staff and includes conjoint planning and education (Koocher, Sourkes, & Keane, 1979; Stabler, 1979). Such consultation skills cannot be learned apart from detailed attention to the various forces that affect psychologist-physician transactions, to which we now turn.

LEARNING THE HOSPITAL CULTURE

Failure to appreciate the unique culture of the hospital may lead to a series of frustrating encounters for the psychologist, which in turn can result in unwitting participation in enterprises that undermine professional autonomy and contribute to maladaptive functioning (Tefft & Simeonsson, 1979). The psychologist's task as a consultant is further complicated by the fact that the initial "contract," or, more aptly, the understanding with the pediatric staff concerning the psychologist's role, is often not highly structured. For example, the psychologist may be hired to provide "service" to the hospital or establish a "program" of psychology (Drotar, 1976b). Moreover, since physicians may not have a complete understanding of psychologist's potential role(s), they may not be able to provide meaningful direction to role clarification. Although this lack of specific role definition has the clear advantage of encouraging autonomy, it can also be confusing and hence counterproductive to the psychologist's efforts. To facilitate their potential role, psychologists in medical settings must take the initiative in learning about hospital culture. Attending formal conferences, joining staff on medical rounds, and being informally present in hospital wards and clinics are fruitful ways of learning about the hospital culture. The psychologist's physical presence also communicates visibility, availability, and hence interest in the medical and nursing staff's activities. The informal exchanges that are facilitated by physical presence help pediatric staff become familiar with the psychologist's style, values, and interests (Geist, 1977). Even more important, such contacts provide the psychologist with an opportunity to discover people who may have a special interest in psychological issues and thus may be congenial collaborators in patient care or research endeavors.

Psychologists in a pediatric setting establish their presence through informal contacts with staff and gain their credibility through demonstration of effective action, i.e., clinical assessments and interventions that prove helpful to children and families and to medical and nursing staff. In the action-oriented medical setting, the psychologist's willingness to become involved with children and families and facilitate effective case dispositions is highly prized by medical staff. In fact, physicians' requests for psychological consultation often include an unstated "test" of the psychologist's competence and interest in their patients. Thus it is not uncommon for initial referrals for psychological consultation to be among the physician's most difficult, complex, or "hateful" patients (Groves, 1978). In the interests of fostering relationships with the pediatric staff, it is often wise to respond to such initial consultation requests even if they are poorly framed, ambiguous, or unreasonably emergent. In the initial phases of consultation, a lack of personal familiarity with the psychologist may lead physicians to have a secretary call the consultant or to send a formal written request. Later, as the consultant becomes established in the setting and gains credibility, referrals for psychological consultation can be actively clarified with greater consistency (Drotar, Benjamin, Chwast, Litt, & Vajner, 1982). Since such requests can be the beginning of a more personalized relationship, it is advantageous to follow them up with a personal meeting that includes further clarification and data gathering concerning the referral (Stabler, 1979). Interested data gathering, supportive empathizing with the patient's predicament, and specification of what the psychologist can realistically provide can generally shape a more adaptive use of psychological consultation.

THE IMPACT OF HOSPITAL CULTURE ON THE COLLABORATIVE PROCESS

It is usually not difficult to generate pediatric interest in psychological services. In fact, before long most psychologists in pediatric settings will find themselves immersed in the setting with more than enough work to do. Over a period of time the psychologist must come to terms with a variety of special problems that may affect their day to day functioning and long-term goals.

Physical Space and Time

With few exceptions (Ack, 1974), most pediatric hospital environments are not designed in accord with the child or the family's emotional needs. Physical space is limited, and children and their families spend time on crowded wards or in congested, noisy clinics. The close proximity of rooms, the lack of soundproofing, and frequent interruptions may constrain patient-physician transactions as well as psychological consultation by depriving children and family of the privacy necessary to introduce and explore sensitive psychological issues (Drotar et al., 1982).

Different professional disciplines negotiate the hospital context according to different rules. For example, nurses are expected to remain on hospital divisions at all times and thus have closest contact with child and family. Although pediatric interns and residents are assigned to manage wards, they have freer rein to leave the physical space of the division. Faculty physicians may not be physically located in a ward or clinic setting and thus can come and go at times of their own convenience. In hospital settings, most of the action concerning patient care takes place in close physical proximity to the ward or clinic. For this reason, physicians and nurses are accustomed to having consultants come to the division or clinic to see their patients and come to expect the psychologist's presence or quick response to their request. However, since psychologists are generally deployed in a number of different wards or clinics, it is very difficult to maintain a salient physical presence in a given setting without compromising one's work with children and families.

In addition to these physical constraints, medical diagnosis and treatment takes place within a severely compressed time span. Physicians see large numbers of patients each day and are mandated to solve each clinical problem quickly. Such time pressures can affect pediatricians' expectations of the psychologist's functioning. For example, physicians who are accustomed to working with many patients over a short period of time usually underestimate the time involved in psychologists' contacts with children and families. Moreover, they may fail to recognize that meaningful psychological intervention takes place in a series of extended contacts rather than in a discrete contact. Although the enterprising psychologist will accommodate to the time pressures inherent in hospital culture by working more quickly than is usually necessary in other settings, capitulating to time pressures by working as rapidly as physicians might wish is not always in the children's or families' best interest. For example, on inpatient divisions it is not uncommon for a child to be referred when hospital discharge is near, thus posing an unreasonable obstacle to the quality of the assessment. Yet if some explanation is provided, medical staff can be convinced to provide additional time for psychological assessment, particularly if they perceive psychological consultation as important to the child's care.

The Hospital as an Interdisciplinary Organization

To facilitate patient care, pediatric medical facilities require the cooperative interaction of a number of disciplines, each of which includes staff and trainees. In pediatric hospitals pediatricians, nurses, dietitians, laboratory technicians, physical and occupational therapists, social workers, psychologists, psychiatrists, teachers, and child life workers all may contribute in various ways to children's care. The complex organizational structure of pediatric hospitals encompasses these different professions as well as subspecialties within them, an elaborate system of specialized tasks, and a large number of people with diverse backgrounds (Georgeopoulous & Mann, 1979). Since lines of authority and communication are structured along disciplinary lines rather than with regard to patient care functions, the coordination of effort required by patient care is inevitably disrupted. the sheer number of professional disciplines, each with its own responsibilities, language, perspectives, and physical location, means that they cannot easily be molded into a cohesive unit with a single purpose. Moreover, specialization in professional functions can dilute physicians' personal responsibility by relieving them of direct, continuing accountability for patient care (Mechanic, 1972). Such dispersion of responsibility can profoundly affect the quality of care provided to child and family. The array of professional disciplines is often quite confusing to families, who may receive discrepant information from different persons. Moreover, each professional discipline may be privy to only a portion of the information that is available concerning the child's medical condition, adjustment, or family functioning. These features of hospital organization are not only stressful to families but make special demands on the psychologist. Since a sound psychological assessment usually involves an understanding the child's adjustment in the context of the child's transactions with other professional disciplines, psychologists face a formidable task in gathering relevant information concerning the staff's observations of the child and integrating their interventions with that of other professional disciplines. Maintaining adequate communication among professionals and family is extremely difficult in an action-oriented hospital environment where the physician who has the authority and responsibility for the patient's care may be unavailable for periods of time. The sheer presence of many professional disciplines also does not insure that someone will assume responsibility for maintaining personal contact with child and family or for planning necessary psychosocial intervention (Naylor & Mattson, 1973). Maintaining continuous and personal contact with children and families is particularly problematic in cases that require chronic medical or psychosocial intervention (Mechanic, 1972). Because of the fragmentation of effort inherent in the hospital culture, psychologists must take care that their consultation is not used as a substitute for physicians' responsibilities in managing cases, giving information, or providing emotional support.

In the interdisciplinary world of the medical setting, it is very important that psychologists recognize and value the potential contributions of other disciplines. However, since there is little precedent for such collaboration, competition for turf and territory can easily develop among the psychologist and other mental-health-related disciplines such as social work and psychiatry. This kind of competition, which is so counterproductive to patient care, is easily triggered. For example, in difficult clinical situations, it is not uncommon for pediatricians to split the functioning of mental health disciplines by asking for more than one discipline to see a child or family. Yet if the mental health disciplines are divided in their efforts, they cannot mount a unified response to an individual clinical problem or address problematic aspects of the hospital system. A unified effort among the psychosocial disciplines also encourages adaptive pediatric utilization of mental health services. Moreover, close interdisciplinary collaboration is absolutely necessary to the success of comprehensive care programs where the demands of patient care prevent any single professional discipline from meeting the psychosocial needs of child, family, or staff (Drotar & Ganofsky, 1976).

Work-Related Stress

Professionals in hospital settings operate under a high level of stress that results in a considerable interpersonal burden (Axelrod, 1979; Cartwright, 1979). Physicians and nurses must witness great suffering which they cannot assuage, work within the limitations and uncertainties of medical knowledge (Fox, 1979), and relate to a range of children and families who experience physical pain and psychological stress. Further, since the volume of work cannot be easily controlled, staff can feel overwhelmed and hence not in control of their work. Physicians and nurses are confronted with emergencies and a seemingly never-ending flood of clinic visits and hospital admissions. Moreover, pediatric faculty members face the added demands of teaching, research, and writing, which can pull them in a variety of different directions and engender chronic feelings that they are not meeting expectations (Axelrod, 1979). Physicians are charged with the next-to-impossible responsibility of accomplishing an effective diagnosis and treatment in each and every case. Such work-related stress has a number of special implications for the psychologist's functioning: pressure to "do something" may lead physicians to request psychological consultation because they expect the psychologist to accomplish a task that they feel either unable or unprepared to do. Moreover, such feelings of helplessness may also color the staff's appraisal of human problems. For example, in an effort to get help from a psychologist to resolve a clinical dilemma, the staff may misconstrue normal human reactions to stress as psychopathology. To be most effective, the psychologist must recognize when requests for psychological consultation are colored by the staff's feelings of helplessness or anxiety about a stressful situation. Since the medical staff does not easily either recognize the impact of work-related stress or feel permission to experience them, psychological referrals can be couched in misleading requests to change patients and their families, as in the following example:

> Jill, a nineteen-year-old patient with cystic fibrosis, was referred for treatment of anxiety which was described by the pediatric house staff as pathological. Closer examination of this young woman's problem indicated that she was reacting quite realistically to her imminently terminal condition, which stressed the entire staff on the division. In meeting with the staff, it became apparent that they were upset by her condition but could not admit to themselves just how sick she really was.

In highly confined and emotionally charged hospital environments such as the neonatal intensive care nursery (Drotar, 1976a), it is common for staff and families' transactions with one another to reach the boiling point and necessitate a consultation, as in the following vignette:

> The angry, agitated response of the parents of a very sick premature who had been on the respirator for two months troubled the staff, who were highly upset about the family's expression of open resentment toward the staff. The family wanted a new doctor and "their own" nurse who would care for their child. In turn, the staff was angered and frustrated by this request. However, as the discussion continued, it became clear that the family's response was characterized not only by anger but also by attachment to the staff: the parents had brought gifts for the nurses, flowers for the nursery, and made positive relationships to various staff members. As the staff reviewed their observations, they saw that there was a realistic basis to the parents' anxiety and anger over their infant's condition, which remained critical over a long period of time. The parents' difficult but realistic questions concerning the child's present condition and his future development intensified the staff's anxiety. Communications with the parents were also strained by the fact that many different staff members were involved in the child's care, but few were known by the family or had communicated with the parents concerning the child's prognosis.

In this intensive care unit and others like it, the treatment of infants takes place in the context of palpable uncertainty concerning the quality of the child's future development (Duff & Campbell, 1973). Moreover, the hectic work life of the medical and nursing staff leaves little opportunity to reflect on the personal impact of clinical decisions concerning the child's treatment and the staff's personal reactions to these situations. Psychologists who work in medical settings are by no means immune to such troubling feelings and cannot help but be touched and, at times, severely stressed by the poignant struggles of children, families, and staff.

THE IMPACT OF DIFFERING PROFESSIONAL TRADITIONS ON COLLABORATION

Psychologists must appreciate the vast differences in training backgrounds, values, and perspectives between they and their physician colleagues. Although physicians and psychologists share common interests in certain clinical and research problems, significant differences in professional perspective allow no easy rapprochement. However, if the sources of these differences are appreciated, it may be easier for psychologists to understand their physician colleagues and engage in more productive transactions with them.

The Acute Illness Model

In pediatric hospitals, much of patient care is conducted according to an acute care model of illness involving rapid diagnosis, institution of treatment, and remission of symptoms. In this model, intense concentration is given to present rather than past problems and to disease-related rather than developmental problems. Moreover, since illness is localizable inside the child, medical attention is inevitably directed toward diagnosis of individual problems rather than a consideration of the child's transactions in life contexts, such as family, school, or community (Hobbs, 1975). Clinical problems that clash with this model of care are not easily accommodated. For example, chronic illnesses or psychosocial problems frequently require prolonged assessment and intervention that takes place over a period of time. In addition, behavioral problems generally do not remit within a short time frame and involve an attention to broader contexts such as family and community that is quite foreign to the emphasis on disease. Such problems are especially frustrating to physicians because they do not fit a narrow disease model (Engel, 1977) and hence cannot be treated rapidly or easily (Duff, Rowe, & Anderson, 1972). Once such problems are identified as psychosocial rather than medical, some physicians lose interest in them because they feel the problem no longer falls within the framework of their perceived expertise. In other clinical situations, application of the acute care model to a wide variety of symptoms and conditions that are not strictly diseases, such as functionally based pain, child neglect, and developmental problems, can lead to naive or unreasonably rapid clinical dispositions that do not address the complexity of these problems.

The hospital's focus on acute care also has a number of impressive consequences on patient-centered psychological consultation. When psychologists are asked to consult on a problem, they may be expected to accomplish a narrowly construed "diagnosis." Moreover, the physcan may expect that the information obtained in a psychological consultation will fit within the framework of an acute infectious disease in the sense that it leads to a rapid, concrete treatment. Thus the psychologist often faces the difficult task of informing pediatric colleagues of the impossibility of their requests. In addition, an acute disease-related orientation may be quite frustrating to the psychologist who is more interested in health-oriented or preventive approaches to children's problems (Tefft & Simeonsson, 1979). Since public health topics such as nutrition, growth, and development have long been underemphasized in pediatric education and practice (Haggerty, Roghmann, & Pless, 1975; Knowles, 1977; Task Force on Pediatric Education, 1975), psychologists must use their influence to help the medical staff recognize the potential value of a broader biopsychosocial approach to the understanding of child and family problems (Engel, 1977).

In medical settings complex psychosocial problems may be construed as medical problems, thus posing obstacles to effective intervention. For example, the diagnosis and treatment of such disparate problems as hyperactivity and child abuse and neglect (Conrad, 1975; Newberger & Bourne, 1978) may fall under the medical purview even though this can lead to inefficient case dispositions. In our setting, existing patterns of medical care for infants hospitalized for poor weight gain owing to environmental factors (Hannaway, 1970) provided a prime illustration of the limitations of medical diagnosis and treatment directed toward a complex psychosocial problem. Despite the fact that failure to thrive is a common pediatric condition that is often associated with family stress (Drotar, Malone, & Negray, 1979), in many centers the hospitalization of failure-to-thrive infants remains oriented toward the physical diagnosis rather than the psychosocial aspects of this problem (Drotar, Malone, Negray, & Dunnstedt, in press). Once purely physical causes for this condition are ruled out, there is pressure to have the child discharged home because the child does not have a physical disease that is seen to warrant continued hospitalization. Family influences are generally not explored during the hospitalization, and treatment planning efforts are minimal (Drotar, Malone, et al., in press). As a consequence, many such children are discharged without addressing the problems that may have given rise to their poor weight gain. It seems that the disappointing long-term psychological outcomes for children that have been diagnosed with failure to thrive as infants (Hufton & Oates, 1977) may be at least partially attributable to the fact that traditional hospital-based care does not consider the family transactional context of this problem (Drotar et al., 1979). In our setting psychologists were asked to function within this model of care by evaluating the individual child's cognitive development, even though such requests often came too late in the hospital admission to allow a comprehensive evaluation and resulted in frustrating consultative experiences.

The acute, infectious disease model also has significant implications for patient-physician interaction. In the case of an infectious disease, treatments are prescribed for and applied to a patient who is directed to take them. In contrast, psychosocial diagnosis and treatment are transactional in nature, requiring more active give-and-take between child, family, and professional caregiver. In addition, children may be involved in psychological intervention over a period of time extending well beyond the time spent in the hospital. Unfortunately, the transactional nature of the physician's dealings with child and family is not often recognized as a legitimate area of inquiry. The physician may wish to establish the diagnosis of a psychological problem and then apply a given treatment which the child or family is expected to follow. When a child or family is unwilling or unable to do so, they may be labeled uncooperative, in need of education, or having a serious emotional problem (Meyer & Mendelson, 1961). It is often very difficult for physicians to recognize how children's and families' expectations can legitimately clash with their own views and to appreciate the impact of their own behavior on their data gathering in medical visits. For example, pediatricians may ignore parents' questions about their children's development (Korsch & Morris, 1968) or avoid the child's requests for information about his or her condition (Raimbault, Cachin, Limal, Elincheff, & Rappaport, 1975). The psychologist who feels that a family needs greater or more clearly outlined information from the physician about medical diagnosis or treatment, more personal contact, or increased continuity of care faces a dilemma concerning how to best communicate this information to the physician without alienating him or her. Such consultation dilemmas are particularly difficult if the physician expects the psychologist to "fix" the child or family's problem but not tamper with the physician's approach to the family.

Medical Authority and Responsibility

The tradition of medical authority also poses knotty problems for collaboration between psychologists and physicians, both of whom are accustomed to a high degree of professional autonomy. In medical settings psychologists function in unfamiliar surroundings in which their authority is not clearly sanctioned. Moreover, the lines of authority and responsibility among the nonmedical professional disciplines are not clearly demarcated. On the other hand, throughout their training physicians have been accustomed to directing the care of patients and the functions of other professions and encouraged to consider themselves as an elite group with a unique position and responsibilities (Freidson, 1970). Physicians are not only expected to carry out very difficult responsibilities, but are sanctioned by society as experts who can define their own province of functioning, as well as those of other professions (Freidson,

1970). However, the level of authority and expertise that is culturally sanctioned for physicians may not always be warranted by their training. For example, physicians must master knowledge concerning a variety of subjects and apply this knowledge in a variety of different activities for which they often receive little training or supervision.

Pediatric training is particularly limited in its focus on interactions with child or family, appraisal of psychosocial problems, or management of chronic illness (Haggerty, Roghmann, & Pless, 1975). Moreover, since physicians' training is highly dependent on the clinical problems that come into the hospital, they may be trained intensively with regard to some clinical problems but have relatively little expertise with others. Although all physicians must grapple with uncertainties about their own knowledge and about the state of medical knowledge in general, acculturation in their professional role may lead them to handle these uncertainties by behaving as if they possess knowledge they do not in fact have (Fox, 1979). With regard to psychosocial problems, the physician's assumption of unilateral authority for case management can disrupt effective interdisciplinary collaboration. In such instances, differing perspectives between psychologists and physicians concerning patient care decisions can cause clashes. Psychologists' commitment to their professional autonomy and expertise concerning children's problems generates inevitable conflicts over clinical decision making. For example, some physicians want the psychological consultant to function in a prescribed way and not to question aspects of the hospital context or the physician's functioning. Some physicians are most satisfied with a psychological consultant who provides information that fits with their own way of thinking and enhances their status or expert position. Since physicians are accustomed to being responsible for a child's care and ordering consultations from other medical specialties to help them with problems, they may assume that their requests for psychological consultations are always warranted. On the other hand, psychologists may wish to retain the right to determine the manner in which their services are used, as in the following hypothetical example:

> During a physical exam, a physician notes that a child is developmentally delayed and requests formal psychological testing. A close review of the history indicates that the child had recently been tested in school, which, in the psychologist's view, renders the physician's request for testing superfluous. However, the physician may press this further if he or she does not trust the testing because it was not done by the hospital staff. If the psychologist acquiesces to the demand and does the assessment, the family is subjected to a needless testing. On the other hand, if the psychologist does not do the testing, the physician may see him or her as uncooperative.

Such binds can only be resolved through honest, open interchange that includes the possibility of disagreement, accommodation, and mutual learning (Stabler, 1979).

Since physicians are accustomed to working with professionals who assist rather than replace the physician in tasks of diagnosis and treatment (Freidson, 1970), they must gradually learn about psychologists' unique skills, style of working, and independence. In order to survive in a medical setting, psychologists must retain the right to control their professional functioning and to refuse requests from physicians that are not judged to be in their professional interests. In many situations the painful art of saying no can actually lead to more adaptive interdisciplinary collaboration. For example, as our clinical services were accepted by the pediatric staff, we were asked to evaluate an increasing number of children from an ever-widening group of subspecialists, as well as provide intervention for these problems. The rapid expansion of medical subspecialties associated with new treatment programs in ambulatory care, childhood cancer, renal failure, and gastrointestinal disease brought new patient populations, each with complex psychosocial needs, to our hospital. Service problems were raised not only by the sheer numbers of patients but by inconsistent or superficial planning for psychological supports for highly stressed children and families. Decisions about allocation of services were also complicated by the lack of clarity in the definition of the psychologists' positions. In our setting, psychologists were hired as general consultants for the Department of Pediatrics rather than as consultants to a particular pediatric subspecialty. As a consequence, some physicians came to perceive the psychologists as their own, expected special service for their patients, and did not appreciate the time constraints posed by a burgeoning number of referrals. Moreover, each pediatric subspecialty operated independently and had differing expectations of the psychologists. Although certain patient care needs were met by expanding our staff, we seriously questioned the wisdom of providing clinical services to each and every patient group because of the consequent fragmentation of effort and dilution of the quality of psychological service. For this reason, our division began to refuse certain referrals and encouraged pediatricians to refer an increasing number of children to mental health practitioners in the community (Drotar, Malone et al., in press).

Although psychologists in medical settings must inevitably set priorities with regard to clinical activities to protect their own interests, this kind of autonomy may frustrate pediatric colleagues who are themselves under extraordinary work pressures that cannot easily be abandoned (Axelrod, 1979). The art of saying no must be handled with some diplomacy to avoid the perception that one is simply withholding services. Pediatricians cannot easily understand why they should send their referrals elsewhere when they have consulting psychologists close at hand, and may perceive the services offered by psychologists in hospital settings as the only available mental health services. For this reason, as part of my ongoing collaborative efforts we have found it useful to clarify our own limitations in regard to time, interests, and ability with physician colleagues. It is also helpful to develop guidelines concerning pediatric referrals that should receive priority for psychological consultation. For example, the physician's willingness to become involved in conjoint medical and psychosocial care following a psychological consultation is a demonstration of a mutual commitment that should be respected. Moreover, the psychological problems of chronically ill children or children with neurological problems that necessitate periodic and conjoint medical and psychological follow-up in a hospital setting also warrant being given priority for psychological consultation. Finally, the psychologist's own interest and expertise in specialized clinical populations also should be considered in setting priorities for service and research.

Physicians who need a psychologist usually are struggling with difficult patient populations that they believe would benefit from a psychologist's involvement. However, the mere fact that physicians perceive a need for a psychologist does not ensure that they have a cogent idea concerning the psychologist's role or that collaboration will facilitate the psychologist's professional development. For example, some physicians may want the psychologist to provide service for their patients or function according to a prescribed role as a tester, but not to participate in broader decision or policymaking concerning services. My experience has led me to place special value on those collaborations in which my input can lead to programmatic changes in the overall organization of care, or collaborative research, and hence to greater benefit for larger numbers of children and their families (Drotar, Ganofsky, Makker, & DeMaio, in press).

Medical Action and Psychological Consultation

Medicine is an applied professional discipline that emphasizes concrete, practical solutions to difficult human problems. For this reason, a physician's clinical experience commands a primary emphasis and respect in the hospital culture (Freidson, 1970). The ability to act and act quickly is another hallmark of clinical practice in a hospital setting. By accommodating to this action orientation, psychologists can learn to quickly translate their knowledge into practical solutions. On the other hand, since concrete action may not be appropriate to each and every clinical situation, the psychologist should be prepared to question an action orientation when it proves maladaptive.

Physicians' expectations concerning the psychologist's functioning are heavily influenced by their prior experiences with medical consultations. For example, many physicians perceive psychologists as diagnostic experts similar to medical consultants who may apply tests to answer a clinical dilemma. Pediatricians often expect that psychological evaluation will inevitably generate quantifiable information in the same way that other medical consultations involve laboratory tests. Moreover, some physicians assume that testing is appropriate in all psychological consultations, or that it is intrinsically therapeutic (Chwast, 1980). At times, referrals for narrowly construed testing may represent physicians' attempts to distance themselves from their feelings about a difficult clinical problem, or from more generalized problems in the system of medical care (Drotar, Benjamin, et al., 1982). For example, initial requests for consultation to our comprehensive care program for children with end-stage renal failure who were undergoing dialysis and transplantation seemed to reflect the staff's uncertainty about the new and ethically troubling treatment of transplantation. We were asked to evaluate the psychological adjustment of children with severe renal disease to determine who would be a "good" candidate for transplantation. Such requests were impossible to answer considering the state of knowledge of this problem, were ethically troubling, and did not address the compelling needs of each and every child in this particular patient group for psychosocial support (Drotar & Ganofsky, 1976; Sachs, 1978). In the interests of furthering collaboration with physicians whom we respected, we initially complied with these requests as best we could. Over time, our clinical experiences with children and families eventually helped create changes in services to facilitate psychosocial support for all children with renal failure, not just those who were highly stressed.

Other commonly encountered misunderstandings are triggered by the physician's expectation that the psychologist can and should intervene in any problem situation that is deemed an emotional, developmental, or mental health problem. Since relatively few mental health professionals work in the hospital context, overburdened physicians understandably hope that psychological services will always address the diversity of their patients' needs for emotional support and information about their disease. However, psychological consultation can be maladaptive if it substitutes for the physician's continuous involvement with families at times of medical crisis. Situations involving chronic life-threatening illness represent a case in point: a chronically ill child who experiences a severe physical crisis or faces imminent death is more in need of continuous contact and understanding from familiar persons such as family and physicians than "treatment" from a psychologist, which can be experienced as stigmatizing. In such situations, the physician's understandable wish to help a highly stressed child may unwittingly lead to a premature application of a psychological treatment which the child perceives as an indictment (Drotar & Chwast, 1978).

MAKING ADAPTIVE ACCOMMODATIONS TO THE MEDICAL SYSTEM

Psychologists must achieve a delicate balance among accommodation to the demands of the medical setting, concern with the needs of children, parents, and professional staff, and attention to their own professional development.

Certain strategies of accommodation, such as being available or visible, that encourage physicians to utilize psychological services can be a double-edged sword. For example, the psychologist's informal availability may lead physicians to feel that the consultant can and should be available at a moment's notice for any request. For this reason, a response to individual clinical problems must be tempered by close attention to the overriding question of the psychologist's role in the setting. As psychologists develop a sensitivity to the structure of the hospital system, they will begin to construe their functioning in terms of its potential effects on various professional groups. To accomplish this psychologists must recognize how different professionals in the setting relate to one another, how various factors in the setting interfere with group efforts concerning patient care, and how one might intervene with larger groups in the setting to enhance their work with children and families.

Group-Oriented Approaches to Consultation

The fragmentation of professional effort that is part and parcel of a large medical center is one of the most pervasive and compelling problems that can be addressed through a group consultation format. In pediatric hospitals, professional effort is fragmented in a variety of ways. The paucity of contexts for different professional disciplines to discuss their work as a group poses an important obstacle to coordinated patient care. For example, pediatricians and nurses have their own rounds. Each pediatric subspecialty also meets to discuss issues specific to the patient groups served by that specialty. On the other hand, there are few functional links among either the various professional disciplines or among subspecialists in the same discipline.

Psychologists may be helpful to staff by facilitating contexts for staff to meet together to address patient care problems. In our own work, we have found a group-oriented consultation format, in which various staff meet regularly to discuss management of psychosocial problems, to be a cogent approach to certain systems problems. Such groups may take very different forms, depending on the work environment and the nature of the clinical problems encountered there. For example, on our adolescent division interdisciplinary group meetings with nursing, child life, social service, and pediatrics staff, including interns, residents, and medical students, have been quite useful. Such conferences take a good bit of preparation. To arrange the conference, we meet with the head nurse the week prior to the conference to discuss cases that might be presented and to learn about special circumstances in the division that might be affecting staff and patients. It is also useful to inquire about emergent, life-threatening problems, work demands, and staff conflicts in the division for that week. The conference itself begins with a brief history by the physician or nurse who has made a request to discuss the case.

After the presentation of the history, input is obtained from other staff. If the psychology staff has already seen the patient or family, these impressions are presented along with didactic input about this particular case. At the same time, the staff's input and conjoint problem solving are strongly encouraged. As the staff shares concerns and provides further information, an attempt is made to clarify staff feelings or clinical dilemmas, suggest avenues for working with patients and their families, and present alternatives for a disposition. During the next week the case may be discussed along with follow-up information so that the effectiveness of the staff's interventions can be reviewed. Providing staff with information concerning families' progress following hospitalization is a particularly helpful intervention because staff rarely have the experience of following patients once they return home. Working in a pediatric inpatient division entails close, intensive contact with families during the hospitalization, followed by a total break in contact. As a consequence, medical and nursing staff relate almost exclusively to children who are in the throes of medical crises and rarely have the gratifying experience of seeing children in their life contexts. Moreover, since children are discharged as soon as they are physically well, the staff does not have an opportunity to appreciate their own successes or determine whether and how their psychosocial interventions have been helpful to children and families.

The free-ranging discussions in interdisciplinary group meetings will sometimes involve role conflicts with nursing and house staff (Bates, 1970), disagreements between house staff and senior staff, or generalized frustrations about the work environment. The intent of these discussions is not to stimulate the staff's helplessness or to further create conflict, but to address underlying work-related problems that relate to patient care. Our experience has been that when the staff is able to recognize some of their general work-related strains they are less likely to attribute psychopathology to children and families, as is shown in the following case vignette:

At one meeting, the staff raised the problem of a fourteen-year-old girl with sickle-cell anemia who seemed to be asking for more than the average amount of pain medication. The staff wondered whether these requests were emotionally based and a sign of her significant psychological disturbance. The adolescent's mother was dissatisfied with the room arrangements and quite vocal about her unhappiness. This girl had not had a hospital admission in the recent past and thus was not well known to staff. It seemed that the alienation that developed between staff and family was at least partially attributable to parent and child's anxieties about being in a foreign, unfamiliar setting and the staff's own unfamiliarity with the family. As the discussion unfolded, the pediatric staff reported that they felt especially helpless in this case because they could neither make a diagnosis nor solve the presenting complaint for this adolescent. The staff didn't have objective evidence to know how much was "real" pain versus how much other factors were involved.

A related concern included the staff's fears that they would "hurt" the patient through their efforts by addicting her to pain medications if she did not have real pain. The staff felt somewhat reassured by the comment that most patients with sickle-cell used their pain medication judiciously. This patient-related discussion eventually led to disclosure of problems in other areas of the medical system, particularly the lack of consistent decision making concerning the hospital admissions of children with sickle-cell anemia. As these different sources of stress were clarified, the staff's anxieties diminished and they were able to relate more productively to child and family.

Group meetings are an especially useful way of helping the staff work with chidren, adolescents, and families whose problems engender conflictual feelings and whose care is shared by many professional disciplines. The following case illustrates how group meetings can be used to clarify the staff's understanding of a particular child's physical condition and coordinate interventions in the compelling case of a critically ill child:

A thirteen-year-old critically ill cystic fibrosis patient, Cal, was well known to the staff from his many previous hospital admissions. His physical condition had recently deteriorated and he remained gravely ill during a month-long hospital admission. Although the nursing staff knew that Cal was very ill, there was little recognition of the imminence of his death. Instead, the staff was concerned about Cal's anxious, agitated behavior and that of his family. The inconsistency of the staff's approach to Cal became apparent in the group meeting. Some staff felt that Cal should carry on with his activities as normally as possible and "not be so anxious." Others supported his verbalization of his worries that he was "going to die."

The ensuing discussion revealed that the staff's inconsistencies related to their incomplete recognition of how close to death he really was. Because he had been hospitalized numerous times before and had always recovered, many people assumed that this hospitalization would be no different. Hence Cal was initially encouraged to continue his treatments as usual, to handle his anxieties related to his illness but not to focus on the fact that he might die. However, as his condition failed to improve, it became increasingly clear to his primary physician that this admission would be his last. Although the gravity of his condition was known to his physician, some nursing and house staff were not fully aware that Cal was dying. It was only after the group recognized the closeness of his death that they were able to coordinate their efforts in a meaningful plan that would aid Cal and his family in coping with his death. For example, the staff no longer supported Cal's avoidance of the topic of death and instead helped his death fears. The nurse and physician who had the closest relationship with Cal's family took the responsibility of communication with the parents. The staff also brought the parents together to discuss their concerns about Cal and their grief over their impending loss.

Adapting Methods to Fit the Setting

The psychologist consultant will need to adapt the format of group meetings to the specific culture of the staff's work environment. For example, in the pediatric intensive care nursery, which is a highly pressurized, acute care unit in which life-and-death issues are commonplace, the staff experienced some benefit from meetings directed to discussions of physician-nurse communications problems and work-related stress, including the enormous ethical problems raised by the care of very sick infants (Drotar, 1976a). On the other hand, in another hospital division where infants were not as critically ill and the staff stresses were less compelling, the medical staff has had the time and energy to profit from a more didactic approach, in which meetings are focused on infant development, with the evaluation and observation of an infant serving as a vehicle for discussion (Drotar & Malone, 1980). The psychologist who works with a group of professional staff in a given hospital context should be prepared to flexibly adapt consultation to that particular group's needs by negotiating the content and format of the meetings with representatives of various professional disciplines. In addition, it is helpful to review the effectiveness of such meetings on an ongoing basis and revamp the format of the meetings if needed. Given the regular changes in pediatric trainees owing to rotations, the psychologist's energies are critical to keeping such meetings going. One of the major frustrations of medically related consultation is posed by the continuous turnover of interns and residents who are responsible for running the wards for a period of time but are relative transients in a given context. Given the variability in the medical staff's interests concerning psychosocial problems, the psychological consultant must be prepared for the possibility that successful meetings may be followed by less than optimal consultation experiences. Many physicians remain most concerned with their responsibility for the child's acute medical care and impatient with what they consider to be the less compelling issue of the child's psychological adjustment. Owing to a lesser emphasis on acute care and greater potential for continuity experiences for patient, physician, and psychological consultant, the ambulatory care setting is generally much more congenial for the teaching of behaviorally related topics than are inpatient units. In our ambulatory setting, it has been possible to initiate a series of didactic conferences devoted to behavioral and psychological topics that are integrated with the hospital's general medical teaching.

Psychological consultants in pediatric settings must also recognize that successful group consultation is difficult to initiate, and emerges only gradually from contacts with key staff that have developed over a long period of time. Our experience indicates that the interest of key persons such as the head nurse on the hospital division or the senior resident is critical to establish and maintain such meetings. In addition, since the heavy work demands of the setting inevitably disrupt interest in and attendance at such conferences, the consultant must be flexible in arranging a time for the meetings.

In addition to meetings that are oriented toward patient care, time-limited meetings for purposes of planning for special populations are often quite useful. For example, meetings with various pediatric subspecialties can help address some of their perceived needs for psychosocial consultation and plan services for their patient groups. Meetings can also be focused on general problems and policy formulation. For example, in our setting the dilemmas raised by critically ill adolescents led to the formation of a work group that implemented a ward atmosphere that encouraged a more open discussion of death (Drotar & Doershuk, 1979). We have also arranged impromptu group meetings to bring together the relevant participants to discuss a crisis situation and plan disposition. Finally, no matter how successful such meetings are, it should be recognized that the creation of group contexts will not solve the enormous moral and ethical problems associated with various problems in medical settings or overriding problems of hospital organization (Drotar, 1976c).

ANTICIPATING NEW DIRECTIONS: MAINTAINING AUTONOMY AND SUPPORT

In order to maintain a reasonable work environment, it is desirable for psychologists to reshape the direction of their professional responsibilities in line with their interests. To best accomplish this, psychologists must continue to redefine their roles and functions in ongoing dialogues with their pediatric colleagues. Such reshaping of professional directions can occur on many different levels. For example, in patient-related consultations, psychologists can assume responsibility for comprehensive assessment that extends beyond physicians' initial referral questions. At a more programmatic level, one can structure priorities for clinical endeavors with different patient groups or allocate energies to research or consultation activities that extend beyond patient care. In our setting, we have chosen to focus our clinical energies on patient groups of special interest and to direct our consultative efforts toward physicians who are congenial collaborators with an interest in sharing decision making. In large medical settings, selectivity in the development of a psychology service is critical to avoid diffusion of effort. Setting research or clinical priorities in accord with mutually satisfying professional partnerships with pediatricians is a promising strategy of collaboration.

It should be noted that the assumption of responsibility for program development is not compatible with every psychologist's skills or career aims. For example, some psychologists may find it more comfortable and satisfying to fit within a well-defined role that fits the physician's requests. Moreover, there are many pragmatic obstacles to a unified program of psychological services in a large medical setting. It is often difficult to choose a focus among the wealth of possibilities in patient populations and activities. Some pediatricians may feel that psychologists who specialize in research and clinical work with other patient populations are not sensitive to the needs of their particular patient group. Finally, assuming the burden of funding psychological activities is difficult and time-consuming, but quite necessary if psychologists are to freely choose their activities. Fortunately, it is possible to develop funded projects in which medical and psychological interests are mutually served. For example, many physicians are quite interested in utilizing the psychologist's potential talents as a researcher to explore questions such as the impact of chronic illness on development, the effectiveness of psychosocial intervention with pediatric populations, or the adjustment of the survivors of a chronic illness. In addition, some pediatricians may value the psychologist's potential contributions to the development of their clinical programs sufficiently to reserve funds for these services on their grants.

The psychologist's ability to develop independently areas of professional interest is a singularly important means of reducing "burnout," which is increasingly recognized as a potential problem in high stress pediatric or general medical settings (Koocher, 1980; Kushner & Asken, 1980). Psychologists in pediatric settings are called upon to work very hard, respond quickly to demands for service, and thus suspend their own needs in deference to pediatric requests. Over a long period of time the psychologist can develop the very real feeling that he or she is constantly putting out fires but not pursuing his or her own interests in depth. Physicians in medical settings are understandably oriented toward their own professional aims and do not ordinarily consider psychologists' unique professional needs. For this reason, it is very important for the psychologists who work in a pediatric setting to reserve time to reflect upon their own interests and plan projects that fit with these. Fortunately, the setting is rich enough to accommodate a broad range of interests in clinical and research activities.

Group support is another critical aid to professional growth among the psychologists who work in a medical setting. Since psychologists in large pediatric centers often work in disparate work environments within a large setting, they need a chance to get together and discuss common professional concerns and potential new directions. In our group, an informal weekly meeting serves this purpose. This structure not only encourages a sense of group unity but helps facilitate a visible, unified professional identity. Perhaps the most important function of group support is the sharing of mutual frustrations and work-related concerns, as well as planning service and consultation strategies. It is very important that psychologists feel that they can actively initiate change and are not at the mercy of the hospital's structural problems. For this reason, psychologists' ability to plan new initiatives as a group and participate in department-level planning is an important goal. Planning new programs of research and intervention that are primarily directed by psychologists not only facilitates professional autonomy but provides alternatives to medical models of care. Our response to the difficulties involved in working with the families of infants with environmentally based failure to thrive within traditional patterns of hospital-based care represents a case in point. Our clinical experiences suggest that existing hospital-based care for infants who fail to thrive should be markedly changed to emphasize outreach interventions designed to help families continue to nurture their children once they are returned home (Drotar, Malone, & Negray, 1979). We were able to organize and eventually fund a research project to study the effectiveness of family-oriented outreach intervention designed to prevent the growth and developmental problems usually associated with failure to thrive. This project provided not only a much-needed service to a disadvantaged population but also a base to study a common infant psychosocial problem. In addition, funds from this grant not only provided staffing to carry out this project but financial support to reallocate psychological services to maintain the level of services in the inpatient divisions.

The rapid expansion of medical subspecialties and programs is another feature of medical settings that requires concerted planning efforts. Although pediatric subspecialities will bring in new patient populations that require a high level of psychosocial services and consultation, the development of such programs does not necessarily proceed in concert with collaborative input from psychologists. Programs of physical treatment develop and are already in place before concerted attention is given to the psychosocial problems of a given patient population. Physicians may then ask psychologists to become involved to handle the psychological "fallout" from these programs, which can come in the form of distressed children and families. However, if psychologists do not have prospective input into a service, it may not be realistic for them to attempt to fit into such a program. This proved to be the case in regard to our division's involvement with bone marrow transplantation, a new treatment alternative that poses unusual stresses and grave ethical problems to children and families. After this program of physical treatment was already in place, the physicians wanted a psychologist to help support children who were given this procedure, but were not prepared (in our view) to make changes in their functioning to facilitate informed consent and psychological support. As a consequence, this particular collaboration did not work out and was abandoned.

Our experience strongly suggests that to achieve maximum autonomy within a large medical setting, psychologists must become active in developing and maintaining control over their own sources of funding through patient fees and research or training grants. As the need for psychological services expands, salaries for new positions are not necessarily funded by pediatric departments or hospitals. Active negotiation about the responsibilities and direction of these new positions is critical to maintain the professional integrity of psychology in a large medical setting. For this reason, ongoing attention to increasing the administrative visibility of psychology as a discipline is an important long-term goal. In our setting, psychology did not initially have a visible identity as a division within our pediatric department. As is true of many psychologists in medical school settings, our major administrative appointment was in psychiatry with a secondary appointment in pediatrics (Nathan, Lubin, Matarazzo, & Perseley, 1979). Although this arrangement was congenial in some ways, the arrangement—working in one setting but having one's administrative appointment in another department—posed a number of problems. For example, at times we felt that our professional needs were not being met in either department. Our group's special interests were often bypassed, funding arrangements were unclear to us, and faculty members in both departments did not have a clear way of communicating with our group. The formation of a Division of Pediatric Psychology that is on a similar administrative footing with pediatric subspecialties such as neurology or cardiology helped to alleviate these problems but did not necessarily ensure that our professional aims were met. Since psychologists' professional needs do not have much visibility when compared to larger programmatic considerations, such as expansion of medical services, the burden of responsibility falls to psychologists to make their needs clear to hospital and medical administrators. My impression is that medical settings offer psychologists exciting opportunities for professional development together with considerable responsibilities. As the ideas presented in this chapter indicate, clinical work, research, and consultation in medical settings is a viable career direction for child psychologists that may be beneficial to the lives of those children and families who intersect with the health care system.

REFERENCES

Ack, M. The psychological environment of a children's hospital. *Pediatric Psychology,* 1974, **2,** 3–5.

Axelrod, B. H. The chronic care specialist— "but who supports us." In O. J. Sahler (Ed.), *The child and death.* New York: C. V. Mosby, 1979.

Bates, B. Doctor and nurse: Changing roles and relations. *New England Journal of Medicine,* 1970, **283,** 129–134.

Bayley, N. *Bayley Scale of Mental Development: Manual.* New York: Psychological Corporation, 1967.

Botinelli, S. B. Establishment of an outpatient psychology screening clinic: Preliminary considerations. *Pediatric Psychology,* 1975, **3,** 10–11.

Caplan, G. *The theory and practice of mental health consultation.* New York: Basic Books, 1970.

Cartwright, L. K. Sources and effects of stress in health careers. In G. C. Stone, F. Cohen, & N. E. Adler (Eds.), *Health psychology.* San Francisco: Jossey-Bass, 1979.

Chwast, R. Personal communication. Cleveland, Ohio, 1980.

Conrad, P. The discovery of hyperkinesis: Notes on the medicalization of deviant behavior. *Social Problems,* 1975, **23,** 12–21.

Drotar, D. Death in the pediatric hospital: Psychological consultation with medical and nursing staff. *Journal of Clinical Child Psychology,* 1975, **4,** 33–35.

Drotar, D. Mental health consultation in the pediatric intensive care nursery. *International Journal of Psychiatry in Medicine,* 1976, **7,** 69–81. (a)

Drotar, D. Psychological consultation in the pediatric hospital. *Professional Psychology,* 1976, **9,** 77–83 (b)

Drotar, D. Shared dilemmas of modern medical care. Paper presented at the annual meeting of American Psychological Association, Washington, D.C., 1976. (c)

Drotar, D. Clinical psychological practice in the pediatric hospital. *Professional Psychology,* 1977, **10**, 72–80. (a)

Drotar, D. Family oriented intervention with the dying adolescent. *Journal of Pediatric Psychology,* 1977, **2**, 68–71. (b)

Drotar, D. Training psychologists to consult with pediatricians: Problems and prospects. *Journal of Clinical Child Psychology,* 1978, **7**, 57–61.

Drotar, D., Benjamin, P., Chwast, R., Litt, C. L., & Vajner, P. The role of the psychologist in pediatric inpatient and outpatient facilities. In J. Tuma (Ed.), *Handbook for the practice of pediatric psychology,* New York: Wiley, 1982.

Drotar, D., & Chwast, R. Family oriented intervention in chronic illness. Paper presented at the annual meeting of the Ohio Psychological Association, Cleveland, 1978.

Drotar, D., & Doershuk, C. F. The interdisciplinary case conference: An aid to pediatric intervention with the dying adolescent. *Archives of the Foundation of Thanatology,* 1979, **7**, 79–96.

Drotar, D., & Ganofsky, M. A. Mental health intervention with children and adolescents with end stage renal failure. *International Journal of Psychiatry in Medicine,* 1976, **7**, 181–194.

Drotar, D., Ganofsky, M.A., Makker, S., & DeMaio, D. A family oriented supportive approach to renal transplantation in children. In N. Levy (Ed.), *Psychological factors in hemodialysis and transplantation.* New York: Plenum Press, in press.

Drotar, D., & Malone, C. A. The developmental case conference as a method of teaching pediatricians about child development on an inpatient service. *Clinical Pediatrics.* 1980, **19**, 261–262.

Drotar, D., Malone, C. A., & Negray, J. Psychosocial intervention with the families of children who fail to thrive. *Child Abuse and Neglect: The International Journal.* 1979, **3**, 927–935.

Drotar, D., Malone, C. A., Negary, J., & Dennstedt, M. Psychosocial assessment and care of infants hospitalized for non-organic failure to thrive. *Journal of Clinical Child Psychology,* in press.

Duff, R. S., & Campbell, A. G. M. Moral and ethical dilemmas in the special care nursery. *New England Journal of Medicine,* 1973, **289**, 890–894.

Duff, R. S., Rowe, D. S., & Anderson, F. P. Patient care and student learning in a pediatric clinic. *Pediatrics,* 1972, **50**, 839–846.

Engel, G. L. The need for a new medical model: A challenge for biomedicine. *Science,* 1977, **196**, 127–136.

Fox, R. *Essays in medical sociology.* New York: Wiley, 1979.

Fox, R. C., & Swazey, J. P. *The courage to fail: A social view of organ transplants and dialysis.* Chicago: University of Chicago Press, 1978.

Freidson, E. *Profession of medicine.* New York: Harper & Row, 1970.

Gabinet, L., & Friedson, W. The psychologist as front-line mental health consultant in a general hospital. *Professional Psychology,* 1980, **11**, 939–945.

Geist, R. Consultation on a pediatric surgical ward: Creating an empathic climate. *American Journal of Orthopsychiatry,* 1977, **47**, 432–444.

Georgeopoulous, B. S., & Mann, F. C. The hospital as an organization. In E. G. Jaco (Ed.), *Patients, physicians and illness.* New York: Macmillan, 1979.

Groves, J. E. Taking care of the hateful patient. *New England Journal of Medicine,* 1978, **298**, 883–887.

Haggerty, R., Roghmann, K. J., & Pless, I. B. *Child health and the community.* New York: Wiley, 1975.

Hannaway, P. J. Failure to thrive—a study of 100 infants and children. *Clinical Pediatrics,* 1970, **9**, 96–99.

Hobbs, N. *The futures of children.* San Francisco: Jossey-Bass, 1975.

Hufton, I. W., & Oates, R. K. Non-organic failure to thrive: A long term follow-up. *Pediatrics,* 1977, **59,** 75–79.

Johnson, M. Mental health intervention with medically ill children: A review of the literature, 1970–77. *Journal of Pediatric Psychology,* 1979, **4,** 147–164.

Katz, J., & Capron, A. M. *Catastrophic diseases: Who decides what?* New York: Russell Sage, 1975.

Knowles, J. H. Doing better and feeling worse: Health in the United States. *Daedalus,* 1977, **106,** 1–7.

Koocher, G. P. Pediatric cancer: Psychosocial problems and the high costs of helping. *Journal of Child Clinical Psychology,* 1980, **8,** 2–5.

Koocher, G. P., Sourkes, B. M., & Keane, W. M. Pediatric oncology consultations: A generalizable model for medical settings. *Professional Psychology,* 1979, **10,** 467–474.

Korsch, B. M., & Morris, M. Gaps in doctor-patient communication: Patients' response to medical advice. *New England Journal of Medicine,* 1968, **280,** 535–540.

Kushner, K., & Asken, M. Burnout among psychologists working in primary health care settings: Potential origins and recognition of the problem. Paper presented at the annual meeting of the American Psychological Association, Montreal, 1980.

Lazarus, R. S., Averill, T. R., & Opton, E. M. The psychology of coping: Issues of research and assessment. In G. V. Coelho, D. A. Hamburg, & T. E. Adams (Eds.), *Coping and adaptation.* New York: Basic Books, 1974.

Lazarus, R., & Launier, R. Stress related transactions between person and environment. In L. W. Pervin & M. Lewis (Eds.), *Perspectives in interactional psychology.* New York: Plenum Press, 1978.

Matarazzo, J. D. Behavioral health and behavioral medicine: Frontiers for a new health psychology. *American Psychologist,* 1980, **35,** 807–817.

Mechanic, D. *Public expectations and health care.* New York: Wiley, 1972.

Meyer, E., & Mendelson, M. Psychiatric consultations with patients on medical and surgical wards: Patterns and processes. *Psychiatry,* 1961, **24,** 197–205.

Nathan, R. G., Lubin, B., Matarazzo, J. D., & Persely, G. W. Psychologists in schools of medicine—1955, 1964, and 1977. *American Psychologist,* 1979, **34,** 622–627.

Naylor, K. A., & Mattson, A. "For the sake of the children": Trials and tribulations of child psychiatry—liaison service. *Psychiatry in Medicine,* 1973, **4,** 389–402.

Newberger, E. H., & Bourne, R. The medicalization and legalization of child abuse. *American Journal of Orthopsychiatry,* 1978, **48,** 593–607.

Olbrisch, M. E., & Sechrest, L. Educating health psychologists in traditional graduate training programs. *Professional Psychology,* 1979, **10,** 589–595.

Ottinger, D. R., & Roberts, M. C. A university-based predoctoral practicum in pediatric psychology. *Professional Psychology,* 1980, **11,** 707–714.

Pless, I. B., & Pinkerton, P. *Chronic childhood disorders: Promoting patterns of adjustment.* Chicago: Year Book Medical Publishers, 1975.

Power, P. W., & Del Orto, A. E. (Eds.) *Role of the family in the rehabilitation of the physically disabled.* Baltimore: University Park Press, 1980.

Raimbault, G., Cachin, O., Limal, J. M., Elincheff, C., & Rappaport, L. Aspects of communication between patients and doctors: An analysis of the discourse in medical interviews. *Pediatrics,* 1975, **55,** 401–405.

Rexford, E., Sander, L., & Shapiro, T. *Infant psychiatry: A new synthesis.* New Haven: Yale University Press, 1976.

Sachs, M. Social psychological contributions to a legislative subcommittee on organ and tissue transplants. *American Psychologist,* 1978, **33,** 680–690.

Schroeder, C. S. Psychologists in a private pediatric practice. *Journal of Pediatric Psychology,* 1979, **4,** 5–18.

Smith, E. E., Rome, L. P., & Freedheim, D. K. The clinical psychologist in the pediatric office. *Journal of Pediatrics,* 1967, **71,** 48–51.

Sameroff, A. Transactional models in early social relations. *Human Development,* 1975, **18,** 65–79.

Stabler, B. Emerging models of psychologist-pediatrician liaison. *Journal of Pediatric Psychology,* 1979, **4,** 307–313.

Stone, G. C. A specialized doctoral program in health psychology: Considerations in its evaluation. *Professional Psychology,* 1979, **10,** 596–604.

Task Force on Pediatric Evaluation. *The future of pediatric education.* Evanston, Ill.: Author, 1978.

Tefft, B. M., & Simeonsson, R. J. Psychology and the creation of health care settings. *Professional Psychology,* 1979, **10,** 558–570.

Toback, C., Russo, R. M., & Gururaj, V. J. Pediatric psychology as practiced in a large municipal hospital setting. *Pediatric Psychology,* 1975, **3,** 10–11.

Tuma, J. Pediatric psychology? . . . Do you mean clinical child psychology? *Journal of Clinical Child Psychology,* 1975, **4,** 9–12.

Wright, L. A comprehensive program for mental health and behavioral medicine in a large children's hospital. *Professional Psychology,* 1979, **10,** 458–466.

2

Developmental Pediatrics: A Process-oriented Approach to the Analysis of Health Competence

Paul Karoly

Man does not grow up *pari passu,* but in continuous interaction with his care-takers, siblings, peers, social group, geography, and culture, all of which elicit or impair the development of his individual potentialities. At the same time, every mediating and organ system of his body has its own maturational and developmental sequence, which has been structured by genetic, nutritional, and experiential factors.

—H. Weiner (1977)

Scientific medicine has as its object the discovery of changed conditions characterizing the sick body or the individual suffering organ. Its object is also the delineation of deviations experienced by the phenomena of life under certain conditions, and finally the determination of means by which these abnormal conditions can be counteracted. This therefore presupposes the knowledge of the normal course of the phenomena of life and of the conditions under which this course is possible.

—Rudolf Virchow (1847)

Otitis media, an inflammation of the middle ear, is a high-incidence condition in young children which, in its chronic or recurrent form, often leads to conductive hearing loss. Clearly a "medical problem," otitis media also has "psychological" consequences (or *developmental sequelae*), including deficits in speech and language learning and vocal production as well as depressed intelligence test scores (Howie, 1980). Approaching this disorder from an interdisciplinary perspective is considered reasonable practice. Audiologists

29

test for it. Physicians and surgeons attempt to preserve or restore the affected child's hearing. Speech therapists, school psychologists, pediatricians, educators, and parents are all involved in assisting the child to cope with and overcome the cognitive and social handicaps that otitis media engenders.

Unfortunately, it is not always easy to assume a "divide and conquer" attitude toward children's illness and disease. Integrating points of view from the submicroscopic to the societal is an enormously difficult task for any medical professional. In fact, in many areas the biomedical perspective contends with the psychosocial, the nutritional, the genetic, and the politicoeconomic. Questions exist, for example, as to whether various "learning disabilities" are the result of impoverished environments, minimal brain damage, disordered mother-child interaction patterns, or the failure of contemporary educational practices. Many health professionals believe that infantile autism and childhood schizophrenia will eventually be "reduced" to their neurological and biochemical "essences" and treated successfully by pharmacologic or surgical means. Further, despite the existence of a Society for Pediatric Psychology and publications like the *Journal of Pediatric Psychology,* it is still unlikely that very many practicing pediatricians (at least those based somewhere *other* than in a medical school) routinely consult with psychologists, educators, and other social and behavioral scientists to help them deal with the complexities of treating children with diabetes, hemophilia, cancer, phenylketonuria, tracheotomy addiction, hyperactivity, cystic fibrosis, multiple sclerosis, and the host of more common maladies of childhood (cf. Task Force on Pediatric Education, 1978).

Thus while enthusiasm grows for the pursuit of "health care pediatric psychology" (Wright, 1979), "behavioral pediatrics" (Kenny & Clemmens, 1980), and "pediatric behavioral medicine" (Williams, Foreyt, & Goodrick, 1981), the foundations of this emerging field remain open to various interpretations and its advocates subject to the criticism of being interdisciplinary in spirit but rarely in fact. It might, therefore, be helpful to draw some key territorial distinctions in the hope of sharpening the focus on the interface of psychology and pediatric medicine.

First, *clinical child psychology* is a field which, unlike its adult-centered counterpart, developed as an adjunct to psychiatry and the child guidance movement. It has only weak historic ties to clinical medicine or to academic psychology (Santostefano, 1978). Concerned with diagnosing and treating various forms of psychopathology, clinical child psychologists often encounter syndromes with "physical manifestations" (such as eating disorders, movement disorders, stuttering, and bladder and bowel control problems) as well as "psychophysiologic" disorders (involving a primary malfunction of a bodily process for which a presumed etiologic element is psychological in nature). However, neither the developmental nor the psychobiological aspects of children's disorders have been as central to clinical child psychology as have the descriptive and the rehabilitative. As regards intervention, clinical child psychology has traditionally been concerned with health care only in secondary or indirect forms (Wright, 1979).

On the other hand, advocates of the *behavioral medicine* perspective have sought to apply the classical, operant, biofeedback, and social learning perspectives on behavior analysis to the evaluation of children's medical disorders and the design of cost-effective and reliable treatments. Whether consulting with parents to help ensure children's compliance with their medical regimen, working with children prior to their hospitalization to reduce or minimize fears associated with hospitalization and medical intervention, or working in concert with teachers, nurses, dentists, and other professionals to shape prohealth habits, the practitioner of *pediatric behavioral medicine* has been the most visible link between psychology and pediatrics in the last decade (Melamed & Siegel, 1980).

Nevertheless, despite the contributions from clinical child psychology to the resolution of the emotional and adjustive sequelae of illness and the contributions from the systematic application of learning principles to the prevention, remediation, and management of children's psychophysiologic problems, the hoped-for integration of developmental psychology and pediatric medicine (cf. Engel, 1962; Richmond, 1967) has been slow in arriving. The descriptive and clinical focus on common childhood diseases has obvious conceptual merit. Yet the deficiency-based (pathology-oriented) models of medicine and psychology have contributed little to our appreciation of how the developing mind and the developing body interrelate, and of how illnesses (from infectious disease to bodily injury) influence and are influenced by the processes of physical, social, and cognitive maturation.

Modern medicine has devoted comparatively little attention to the study of the natural history of disease, in adults or children, while psychology's historical perspective has traditionally been carved in rather large chunks—including developmental milestones and psychosocial crises. From the perspective of contemporary developmental psychology, however, the child with a diagnosed illness is not just a *product* (the interaction of "being four years old" and "having the mumps") or just a *problem* (e.g., an unwilling recipient of a vaccination). Rather the sick child can be viewed in *process* terms—that is, as a person with emergent cognitive, instrumental, and expressive competencies trying to make sense of a specific biopsychosocial deviation (or deviations) from the norm. Knowing that the client is a child per se does not aid the clinician, for there are "as many different types of children as there are people defining what a child is" (Denzin, 1977, p. 17). And of course knowing the medical diagnosis tells the clinician nothing about the child's mode of coping, the mechanisms that set the stage for the particular illness, or the interpersonal and psychological factors that may improve or worsen the prognosis.

The integration of child development and pediatric medicine obviously

requires metatheories, concepts, methodologies, facilitative political structures, and professional training opportunities that are, as yet, unavailable or in
nascent form. In an editorial appearing in the inaugural issue of the *Journal of
Developmental and Behavioral Pediatrics,* physician George W. Brown (1980)
inquired into the nature of the challenge that the study of psychology and
pediatrics posed, and pointed out that

> the range of topics involving developmental pediatrics begins in the arcane com-
> plexities of cellular differentiation in embryogenesis, through antenatal genetic
> diagnosis, to neonatology, maternal-infant attachments, language development,
> motor skill acquisition, pre-school temperament and behavior, academic progress,
> and through adolescents' self-image, Piagetian formal cognitive stages, sexual
> maturation, socialization and entry into the responsibility and privileges of adult-
> hood [p. 3].

Thus the purpose of the present chapter is necessarily limited. It is my intent
to place childhood illness in a life-span adaptational context in order to
depathologize it. The presentation is conceptual rather than data-based. Starting from the broad descriptive framework illustrated in figure 2.1, I believe it is
appropriate to argue that the relationship between physical illness (factor f)
and adaptive resiliency is best understood in a larger developmental and
interactional context that includes (but is not limited to) factors a through g.
Such a viewpoint may eventually provide the necessary empirical foundation
for intervention approaches that are now based largely on clinical lore and
discrete (problem-specific) theorizing. Similarly, in view of the calls for a
reformulation of the *disease model* of medicine (e.g., Engel, 1977; Weiner,
1977), a thorough integration of child development and personality concepts
with pediatrics would aid in the efforts to graft a historical arm onto the
functionalist body of modern medical science. In fact, Dupue, Monroe, and
Shackman (1979) have suggested that a comprehensive theory of disease
should incorporate three main foci: (1) predisposition to disease, (2) initiation
of disease, and (3) mediation processes. It is with respect to the third of these
that the present analysis would seem most relevant.

In view of the fact that most research on the relationship between illness and
"psychological development" has employed cross-sectional rather than some
form of sequential (longitudinal) methodology (cf. Wohlwill, 1973), there is
little that can now be said of patterned changes in children's coping with illness
over time. Even more critical than the neglect of factor g as it interacts with the
other elements of the equation (for we must recognize how costly such research
would be) is the paucity of studies on the differential impact of illness (at any
given age) as a function of elements a through e (and their interaction). But
even in this arena, the failure to clarify seemingly obvious relationships could be
simply explained on the basis of the traditional separation between the con-

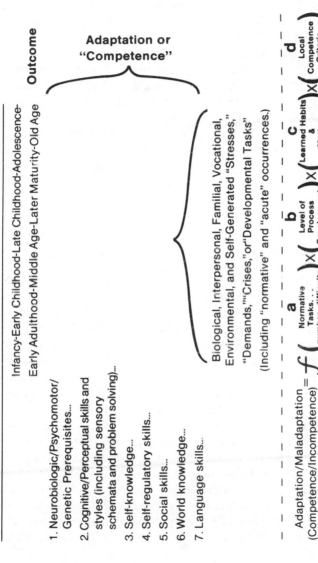

Fig. 2.1. A clinical-developmental framework for human adaptation.

cerns of the applied child clinician (hospital-based) and those of the developmentalist (who has typically examined memory, language, problem solving, and the like in the "sterile" laboratory context). Therefore, because a supportive empirical literature is lacking, the sole objective of the present chapter is to serve as a bridge between two fields, pediatrics and child development, currently trying valiantly to find each other. It is hoped that some of the assertions to be offered will be read as hypotheses worthy of experimental testing.

After providing a rationale for each of the factors in the so-called "clinical-developmental framework" (figure 2.1), I shall focus upon the developmental processes labeled 2, 3, 4, and 5. The fundamental neurophysiological aspects of growth and development (process 1) and the linguistic aspects (process 7) are perhaps the least in need of explication to students and professionals in medicine, nursing, rehabilitation, or psychology. Perhaps the most critical aspect of "world knowledge" (process 6) for children with various forms of illness is their conceptualization of disease and its meaning (e.g., health beliefs)—a topic covered in depth by Jordan and O'Grady in this volume.

AN ADAPTATIONAL FRAMEWORK FOR DEVELOPMENTAL PEDIATRICS

Adaptation is generally considered to be an ongoing or long-term process of interaction between an organism and its environment during which the organism's chances of survival are enhanced. The range of adaptive possibilities is determined not only by genetic or structural aspects of the organism but by the nature of the cultural and biophysical challenges it encounters. The adaptive capacities of an individual reflect that person's ability to "adjust to changes in the environment, to cope with internal and external stress, and generally to maintain an equilibrium in all internal physiological and psychological systems [Moore, Van Arsdale, Glittenberg, & Aldrich, 1980, p. 22]." It should be clear that the seven developmental processes listed in figure 2.1 are meant to represent the sources of adaptive flexibility across the life span. It should be clear also that the health status of an individual is one basic aspect of adaptation, as are interpersonal or vocational success. While it is widely recognized that coping with disease can divert so much of a child's (or adult's) resources that other adaptive tasks (social, academic, vocational, etc.) may suffer, it is less often noted that the process of recovery or rehabilitation as well as "good health" may be facilitated by the prior acquisition of interpersonal and intrapsychic competencies.

An adaptational model is not concerned with static characterizations of people as either "good or poor copers"; nor does it focus on time-limited outcomes per se (a cold, a fever, or an unfriendly exchange between a hospitalized child and his nurse). The reason for emphasizing temporally extended processes (*patterns* of person-environment transaction) is that these are more likely to be predictive of long-range (mal)adaptation and are less likely to serve as fuel for self-fulfilling prophecies. Further, caregivers and clinicians cannot effectively intervene in altering discrete outcomes (though behavioral interventions *appear* to do just that); but they should be capable of assessing and modifying an individual's expectancies, standards of conduct, response repertoires, and other relatively enduring features that set the stage for adaptive success or failure. The developmentalist furthermore realizes that goals, plans, incentives, and behavioral capabilities evolve and change in accordance with the demands of the culture and subculture, so that *adjustment* becomes a tentative and relativistic notion rather than a fixed product or an absolute judgment. Insofar as children with acute or chronic medical conditions are concerned, the adaptational framework is useful to the extent that it highlights neither the illness (as an unpredictable or uncontrollable stressor) nor the child's skill repertoire (factors *b* and *c*) as targets for clinical intervention; rather, the model broadens the clinician's base of understanding to include general developmental prerequisites (self-knowledge, self-regulatory skills, etc.), environmental demands, specific reaction tendencies, external supports, local standards of success, and of course age.

Because the present view of adaptation focuses upon individuals rather than populations, the operative time scale favors the analysis of individual *episodes of coping,* which can be defined as "problem-solving efforts made by an individual when the demands he faces are highly relevant to his welfare (that is, a situation of considerable jeopardy or promise), and when these demands tax his adaptive resources [Lazarus, Averill, & Opton, 1974, pp. 250–251]." What I have called "competence" (in figure 2.1) is simply the extended pattern of successful coping efforts. In that children's health and illness are the focus of this volume and of this chapter, let us consider competence to be, more specifically, the *pattern of successful coping that (cumulatively) enhances health and reduces health risk.* In my opinion, identifying this pattern of "health-related competencies" ought to be the central concern of developmental pediatrics. From a clinical standpoint, the set of physiological, instrumental, and cognitive competencies that constitutes coping (or prohealth person-environment transactions) would serve as the training targets, with the normative and acute "crises," developmental levels, external supports, and so on serving as relevant mediators to be either modified or taken into account. Remember that illness is itself viewed either as a predictor variable (in descriptive research) or as a mediator (in clinical work). The goal of coping to enhance health or reduce health risk is an ongoing one, and does not become salient only when a child (or adult) contracts an infectious disease or is otherwise incapacitated by an illness. The health status of a child depends upon his or her coping with a host of different challenges—with childhood illnesses representing only a portion of them.

But what are some of the so-called normative tasks, crises, or stresses of development that could conceivably tax the adaptive resources of the individual? Obviously, the challenges vary with the age and surroundings of the individual. During infancy, while the tasks of survival usually do not exceed the infant's reflexive "hard-wiring," there are extended periods of discomfort that require both the emission of signals to call mother forth and the display of behaviors that keep mother near (Levine, 1980; Murphy, 1974). According to White and his collaborators in the Harvard Preschool Project (White, Watts, Barnett, Kaban, Marmor, & Shapiro, 1973), by the time a child is ready for kindergarten she should have learned to deal with such challenges as gaining adult attention in "socially acceptable ways," using adults as resources, knowing when to lead, follow, or compete with peers, as well as displaying mastery of numerous other intellectual and linguistic tasks that set the stage for entry into the school experience. In school, the child is required to master the skills of academic survival (most important, reading) and of gaining peer acceptance. Failure in either area appears to carry risk of later adaptive difficulties (cf. Putallaz & Gottman, 1982). Adolescents must cope with the impact of biological changes, a new "body image," the ever-increasing complexity of the school curriculum, and the temptations of a "preadult" world (sexuality, drugs, greater mobility), among other challenges. If, as Hamburg (1980) has suggested, "the social environment of junior high school is inherently stressful," this would be a prime location for the mustering of clinical psychological methods directed toward the assessment and modification of health-related competencies and incompetencies.

The child who, in addition to the "expectable" crises, must live with cancer, diabetes, multiple sclerosis, or some other serious physical malady has tended to take on the psychological coloration of the illness, at least insofar as the pediatric literature is concerned. While it is both reasonable and productive to examine the impact of illness on such variables as self-esteem, social skills, and other aspects of adjustment, the thrust of the present chapter is to acknowledge the value of the complementary viewpoint—namely, that self-knowledge, social competence, self-regulatory abilities, and the other "adaptive resources" of the developing child can partially determine the course of an illness, just as they partially determine other adaptive outcomes across the life span.

However, before taking a closer look at the emergent constituents of adaptive success, there are several other aspects of the competence equation (figure 2.1) that require comment.

An adaptational view of health and illness places far greater emphasis on the continuing transaction between the person and the social context than does the traditional "germ theory" approach. Without minimizing the potential value of medical-surgical intervention in childhood illness, critics of traditional practice have noted the cost-ineffectiveness of many hospital-based treatments, the stigmatizing effects of special attention (even well-meaning) to children's handicaps, the lack of connectedness between medical treatment and "the rest of the child's life," and the failure of the professional services model to mobilize the efforts of natural caregivers and socializing agents or to assess the nature of the interaction between the child's treatment environment and his or her natural one (cf. Salzinger, Antrobus, & Glick, 1980). The value of consistent and effective support systems (factor *e*) and the negative effects of stressful and inconsistent relationships between children and significant social figures need to be considered essential ingredients in long-term adaptive success or failure. Maintenance of health, prevention of illness, and recovery from disease are all potentially mediated by the actions of parents, siblings, peers, teachers, neighbors, workmates, close friends, and other members of the child's *ecosystem*.

An ecological (or environmental) perspective, because it is relativistic and concerned with specific interrelationships between components of the person-environment system, also draws our attention to what I have termed *local competence criteria* (factor *d*). To a regrettably large extent, statements of what constitutes normal, acceptable, or competent performance in various life tasks have derived from untested clinical judgments. Pediatricians (and other medical professionals), clinical psychologists, and developmentalists have often been guilty of overgeneralizing from their unique data bases to domains far afield. Without knowing how active and alert a child "normally" is, a pediatrician cannot accurately evaluate the side effects of a medication she may prescribe. Without knowing how important the maintenance of eye contact is (and will be) in a child's social environment, a clinical psychologist cannot expect a behavioral program intended to increase eye contact frequency to make a significant difference in a child's current or later adjustment. And the developmentalists who have, in the words of Zigler and Muenchow (1980), "expended a great deal of energy searching for a magic critical period at which point, if intervention took place, the child would be made perfect forever after [p. 241]" cannot be relied upon to offer universal guidelines to children's caretakers or to professional interventionists. Not even medical diagnoses are context-independent. As Elliot Mishler (1981) has noted,

> broad notions of health as "harmony" or "adjustment" cannot be specified without reference to sociocultural contexts. . . . [e]ven within a more limited definition of disease as "deviations from the norm of measurable biological (somatic) variables," the biomedical model is insufficient by itself to the critical task of defining normality and deviations therefrom [pp. 5–6].

Whatever specific skills are needed for a child and adolescent to maintain physical health, they will need to be clearly specified, examined in context, and longitudinally related to indices of growth and well-being, and not presumed to be of universal relevance to children of both sexes, of all races, across varied socioeconomic strata, and for all time. Physically ill or mentally handicapped children will probably have a different set of tasks to accomplish as compared with physically healthy children in order to maximize their chances of survival, including overcoming society's tendency to lower its expectations or standards of achievement for them. However, the sick or disabled child's health competence should not be equated with society's pathology-centered definition of it.

Finally, the determinants I have termed "learned habits and motives" (factor *c*) refer to acquired, idiosyncratic styles of behavior and emotional responding which Staats (1975) has defined as being "constellations of complex skills which are evoked by many situations but also have the quality of providing the basis for additional learning [p. 63]." These specifiable foundations of growth and change may be seen as equivalent to what has traditionally been labeled "personality." Staats (1971) has discussed child development in terms of the cumulative acquisition and hierarchical organization of basic personality-like repertoires, and has used the analogy of a race to illustrate the significance of early-occurring events. If the child keeps up with the unfolding challenges and is "advanced in the acquisition of skilled repertoires" he will reap the immediate rewards (social approval) and will also create a situation conducive to further learning (and further "winning"). Chronically ill children have usually been viewed as the inevitable victims of a "downward spiral," where any early setback is taken to presage a pattern of diminishing social and vocational success. An adaptational view, on the other hand, conceptualizes illness (even life-threatening conditions like childhood cancer) as a *potential* threat to health-related competence. Whether sick children can cope or compensate (displaying what Murphy and Moriarty, 1976, call a "vulnerable but resilient" pattern) depends upon the strength and direction of their learned habits and motives along with the other components of the adaptation equation.

The framework just presented places the stress of illness alongside other life-span crises. While it would be foolish to deny that childhood disease fixes special burdens upon its victims and their families, it would be equally foolish to build our clinical models solely around the negative impacts that have garnered the bulk of attention from child psychiatrists, psychologists, and behaviorally oriented interventionists. Consider, for example, the process of coping with a life-threatening condition such as cancer. As the medical community has evolved ways to reduce the fatality rate associated with such diseases as lymphocytic leukemia, the task for pediatric clinicians has shifted from death counseling to one of assisting the stricken child, his family, and the community to maximize long-range adjustment and recovery—that is, to help the child live as normal a life as possible under the specter of an uncertain future.

In *The Damocles Syndrome* (1981), Koocher and O'Malley have provided some intriguing data on the process of survivorship in childhood cancer that are not difficult to reconcile with the adaptational viewpoint. For example, with the improved prognosis for childhood cancer has come a recognition of the need to study such "problems of living" (i.e., demands or stresses) as school and home adjustment, treatment-related changes in physical appearance, dealing with "anticipatory grief" reactions, and the like. Making use of a computerized registry of childhood cancer survivors at the Sidney Farber Cancer Institute in Boston, Koocher and O'Malley were able to identify a well-adjusted group and a group of adjustment-problem survivors. Despite the fact that the adjustment categorization was based on clinical impressions, a number of "correlates" of adjustment were found that discriminated among the 117 cancer survivors. Patients with types of cancer that occur in infancy or early childhood (neuroblastoma and Wilm's tumor) and tend not to reoccur appeared to be at reduced psychological risk. Illness that cannot be completely understood by the young child, which does not require permanent psychological readjustment, and which does not tax the resources of family support systems is apparently less debilitating than relapse-prone forms of cancer such as occur in older children (e.g., Hodgkin's disease). Adjustment problems were also associated with lower socioeconomic status of the child's family and the tendency of the family support system to express concerns about the child's future well-being. Finally, intensive interviews with adult survivors rated as having successfully coped with cancer revealed (in purely post hoc and suggestive terms) the value of social support networks and of being able, cognitively, to "make sense of" the cancer experience, placing it in proper perspective in the overall context of one's life while making liberal use of denial-suppression. Although the retrospective nature of the Koocher and O'Malley findings severely limits their utility as clinical or developmental signposts, they nonetheless underscore the value of a contextual and multidimensional perspective on the outcomes of chronic childhood illness, and a focus upon what Koocher and O'Malley call "the natural history of surviving." The material to be presented in the remainder of this chapter deals with basic aspects of child development that may serve as the fundamental mediators of survivorship. Knowledge of these developmental processes would seem to be as essential to child health professionals as an understanding of normative "stages" of growth and a facility with the specific techniques of behavioral analysis and change.

ILLNESS AND THE SELF SYSTEM

While it is not unusual to find discussions of the *emergent self* (or ego) in pediatric and developmental textbooks, it is rare for writers to couch their discourse in other than Freudian psychosexual stage-theory terms or to examine the reciprocal effects of illness and social-cognitive development across the life span. Yet is it not reasonable to assume, consistent with contemporary cognitive psychology, that individuals must employ active information-processing skills (which develop over time) that permit them to organize and interpret ambiguous stimuli, including the signs and symptoms of illness? Although the importance of patients' representations of illness as a determinant of health-related action has been emphasized (Leventhal, Meyer, & Nerenz, 1980), the point is less often made that schemas of or attributions about illness are usually indexed in terms of the experiences, emotions, and memories of the actor. A relatively stable self-referent system logically precedes the development of a self-regulatory system that theoretically constructs judgments of physical vulnerability, the seriousness of threats to well-being, and personal coping effectiveness (cf. Leventhal et al., 1980). Therefore, a critical domain of psychology in pediatrics should be the study of self-knowledge (developmental process 3, figure 2.1) and its relation to the processing of illness and disease information. The fact that little empirical work has thus far been conducted relating self-knowledge and illness does not mean that clinicians have no groundwork upon which to base their interventions, for, as I have noted, the normative and developmental approaches are perhaps the only adequate foundations upon which to build models of pediatric clinical practice.

Infancy. It has traditionally been assumed that an infant's reactions to both distal and interoceptive stimulation are relatively diffuse and undifferentiated (e.g., Werner, 1948), leaving little room for the postulation of anything so well formed as a "self-concept." However, there is no reason to presume that *individuality* is an inappropriate term to apply to infants. Organized around such parameters as activity level, sensory reactivity, neuromuscular maturity, response to strangers, and frustration tolerance, the precursors of "personhood" (or individuality) are not difficult to discern and can even be seen as useful predictors of later adjustment (e.g., Murphy & Moriarty, 1976). Assuming that the infant's "style" of engaging the environment brings about relatively consistent outcomes, there may eventually emerge a primitive "self as knower," built upon the accumulated action-outcome sequences (Lewis & Brooks-Gunn, 1979). Based upon children's responsiveness to their reflections in a mirror, developmentalists have traced the course of *self-recognition,* as an aspect of personal identity, from a rudimentary self-world differentiation to a consistent featural recognition at about 18 to 20 months of age, to the correct verbal labeling of self at about 24 months. When the child is able to transfer the skill of applying categorical labels from self to others, the beginnings of genuine social awareness can be discerned (Harter, 1982b).

It has seemed intuitively correct to conclude that physical illness or disease occurring during the period between birth and two years would invariably retard the processes of self and social awareness. However, data such as is provided in the Koocher and O'Malley (1981) studies seem to suggest no such downward spiraling. If illness occurs prior to the development of stable standards of conduct and appearance (and if the illness is successfully treated), the sick child appears to be minimally impeded in his or her sociocognitive development. I would postulate, based upon the adaptational scheme presented above, that the significant determinants of adjustmental "high risks" for sick infants would likely be familial in origin. For example, overprotective parents who knowingly limit the sick infant's range of experiences could unwittingly prevent the kind of contingency learning which Lewis and Brooks-Gunn (1979) have suggested is a prerequisite to self-knowledge and feelings of self-efficacy (cf. also Jordan and O'Grady's discussion of the "vulnerable child syndrome" in Chapter Three of this volume).

Childhood. With the emergence of language (and the capacity to elaborate verbally upon real and imagined experiences) and a more effective repertoire of instrumental skills (taking the child into a wider variety of situations), the youngster's self-labeling possibilities increase geometrically. Unfortunately, even children with impairments that restrict physical mobility are confronted with numerous opportunities for *erroneous* (inaccurate) *self-labeling* (Staats, 1971). In addition to the limits imposed by cognitive immaturity, young children would appear to be "at risk" for developing mistaken notions about themselves as a function of inconsistencies in adult-mediated and peer-mediated feedback. In fact, given the absolutistic, concrete, either-or nature of young children's thought processes, their self-centeredness, the selectivity of their memories, the unscientific manner by which they set about collecting data, and the changeableness of their environments, one is led to wonder not why some children are pathological, but why most children are not "autistic" in their construction of self.

The sparse empirical data on the emergence of self knowledge during the so-called preoperational period (roughly between two and seven years of age) suggest that identity formation is normally subject to the influence of many social variables, is something less than stable, and tends to be organized around such tangible attributes as gender, race, activity, and size (Harter, 1982b; Keller, Ford, & Meacham, 1978). In short, it is still a process in flux. Taken together with the fact that most children are *not autistic* in their dealings with themselves and the world during early childhood, we can only conclude that accuracy of self-understanding is not as critical an issue as clinical intuition would have us believe. The preoperational child with a chronic illness may indeed confront separation from parents, unusual dependency, sensory deprivation, or isolation, pain, deformity, threat of death, and a restriction of peer and school-related experiences (Steinhauer, Mushin, & Rae-Grant, 1977), but the impact of these events on self-concept may be transient, delayed, or reversible as a consequence of caretaker intervention (e.g., social support).

An interesting illustration of the mismatch between the clinical and developmental perspectives on childhood adjustment is embodied in the current debate over the meaning of *self-image disparity.* A discordance between a person's *ideal* self-image and his or her *real* (or accurate) self-perception has been considered by nondirective (Rogerian) as well as by psychodynamic theorists to be a sign of serious maladjustment. Children with incapacitating, body-altering, or restrictive symptoms of disease would be expected by traditional theory to be at risk for various forms of psychopathology, and in direct proportion to the magnitude of the discrepancy between their real and ideal self-images. However, developmentalists have offered an alternative conceptualization, wherein the real-ideal disparity is taken as a sign of a maturing cognitive system, and is expected to increase with age (Katz & Zigler, 1967; Katz, Zigler, & Zalk, 1975; Leahy & Huard, 1976; Zigler, Balla, & Watson, 1972). The evidence has generally supported the cognitive-developmental perspective, and has thus provided some empirical foundation for believing that out of the child's inevitable struggles to come to terms with the scope and limits of his or her skills and aptitudes there can arise a serviceable self-concept. Not only do scars heal, they may provide the material for genuine growth and autonomy. Keeping in mind the fact that self-images do not emerge in an interpersonal vacuum, we can again assume that a strong social support network (particularly within the family) can act as a facilitator of self-confidence and self-esteem in especially vulnerable children. While the presence of a sick child can undermine family stability (e.g., Mutter & Schleifer, 1966), a history of successful coping, a good knowledge base, and parents who focus on the tasks of surviving (in addition to the reduction of discomfort) may also provide the necessary ingredients for adaptive success.

Adolescence. Guardo and Bohan's (1971) four dimensions of self—humanity, sexuality, individuality, and continuity—are never more fully under one's scrutiny than during the many periods we have traditionally collapsed into the "era" known as adolescence. Perhaps health deserves to be considered a fifth dimension. Within the context of our multifactor, interactionist model of adaptation, the adolescent period represents a unique confluence of negative stresses and positive challenges engaging all the potential adaptive resources of the individual and setting the stage for significant health outcomes. Consider the following summary of the health status of adolescents (based on a 1974 HEW survey):

> There is a steep upsurge in bodily concerns about health. At ages 12 to 15 years, roughly 14% of both males and females have from three to five medical symptoms rated by them as definitely requiring a doctor ... ulcers, skin disorders, and neuromuscular joint disorders are far more common than previously believed ... hypertension was found to be higher than expected. ... Systolic blood pressure levels showed a mean of 105.9 mm of Hg at 6 years and increased to 134.1 mm of Hg at 17 years. ... Similarly, there is a generally consistent increase of diastolic pressure with age but less rapid than the systolic rise [Hamburg, 1980, p. 123].

Obviously the home, school, and peer group, which are important sources of support, can be breeding grounds for stress that precipitates illness. Recent evidence (Greenberger, Steinberg, & Vaux, 1981) also implicates the workplace as a potential strain on the adaptive resources of adolescents.

But once again, a simple, one-directional causal model wherein stress produces illness (or illness invariably lowers the potential for adaptive success) does not do justice to the many unfolding processes and interacting elements. As far as the adolescent self-concept is concerned, it is important to remember that teenagers, who are generally capable of using formal operational thought to deal with a host of "normative" challenges to self-understanding, should be able to cope with or overcome threats to physical well-being *given adequate social supports and a well-developed sense of personal efficacy.* Self-destructive health attitudes and practices (with long-term implications) are, however, a very real possibility in adolescents with a history of instrumental failures or unreliable social networks, or in response to sudden traumatic changes such as are occasioned by the death of a close friend or parent.

Self-focused attention, heightened by the physical and endocrine changes of adolescence, is undoubtedly a pivotal mediator of health competence during this period of life. Hardiness may therefore be a function of the individual's self-evaluative habits to the degree that (1) stress precipitates self-appraisal and (2) mobilization of defensive or coping skills depends upon the nature of that appraisal (cf. Lazarus, 1974).

Consider, for example, the health consequences of job stress in adolescence. Greenberger, Steinberg, and Vaux (1981) have argued that since adolescents typically experience normative crises over autonomy, identity, intimacy, and achievement, any job situation which "permits little autonomy, allows little initiative, provides no sense of purpose, affords little opportunity for social contact or a sense of belonging, and offers few incentives for competent performance would be especially stressful for adolescents [p. 693]." Utilizing a sample of over 500 working and nonworking 10th and 11th graders, these authors demonstrated that, although somatic symptoms do *not* appear to be the result of job stress, measures of school absence, marijuana smoking, and alcohol use (behavioral manifestations of health-related "incompetence") do appear to be related to stressful job conditions. And, in line with the present discussion, certain work stressors were found to be gender-specific (or differentially impactful as a function of learned habits and motives as they bear on self-evaluation). Specifically, boys appeared more vulnerable to autocratic modes of supervision, while teenage girls were more sensitive to the impersonal nature of the work organization. In addition, boys who work actually reported fewer physical symptoms than boys who never worked. Greenberger, Steinberg, and Vaux speculated that the self-appraisals of boys and girls under stress differed as a result of their differential socialization. Put in simplistic terms, boys suffer most when not treated like "men," and girls suffer most when not allowed to be sociable (feminine?). The ability to function in a demanding work atmosphere may likewise bolster the sense of well-being in young boys by supporting their masculine self-image, accounting for their lowered level of symptomatic complaints in comparison to their nonworking peers. Although speculative, these interpretations are consistent with the view that enduring self-evaluative habits as well as perceived competence and commitment are critical to adolescent (and adult) adjustment, and may bear a relationship to various parameters of physical and psychological well-being.

ILLNESS AND INTERPERSONAL COMPETENCE

Self-knowledge in all of its varied forms (some of which were discussed above) cannot meaningfully exist apart from accumulated life experiences of an interpersonal nature. Indeed, it has been suggested (Antonovsky, 1979) that the most basic source of adaptive resilience lies in the individual's *sense of coherence,* which has been defined as "a global orientation that expresses the extent to which one has a pervasive, enduring though dynamic feeling of confidence that one's internal and external environments are predictable and that there is a high probability that things will work out as well as can reasonably be expected [p. 123]." For Antonovsky the value of social support systems inheres in their ability to enhance the person's sense of coherence. However, it seems equally if not more plausible to view the characteristic perception of coherence as existing in a reciprocal and continuous relationship with actual social exchange. Illness and other potential life stresses may be ameliorated through successful social interaction not only because of the direct assistance others can give, but through the transmission of information and the vicarious extinction (or neutralization) of fear, as well as through the enhanced sense of purpose, of belonging, of being understood, and of having one's position confirmed (Kobasa, Maddi, & Kahn, 1982). If the survival of illness and other threats to well-being in part requires that an individual be consistently able to engage others, then a developmental perspective on interpersonal competence should be of significant utility to practitioners of child health psychology and pediatric medicine.

The literature on early (infant) development clearly suggests that the organism is "goal-directed" with respect to other people (usually the mother). The infant appears to seek proximity to a caretaker (attachment), shows fear or withdrawal to unfamiliar others (stranger anxiety), and, under certain conditions, will move away from caretakers to explore the world, within safe limits (separation-individuation). However, the infant does not act planfully, efficiently, or with great flexibility in his or her dealings with others—and hence it is debatable whether to consider the infant's selective and adaptive social behavior "skilled" (Connolly & Bruner, 1974; Turner, 1980). Further, most of the so-called skilled behaviors with which clinicians have been concerned are those with predictive implications across time and settings (cf. McFall & Dodge, 1982). It isn't clear that infants' patterns of attachment or stranger anxiety (except in extreme forms) have much influence on coping or adjustment in childhood or later life. In addition, many investigators of child behavior would assert that a "skill" is emitted rather than elicited (Fischer, 1980) and includes the ability to make use of specific performance feedback to modify future activities and to enhance a sense of "mastery" (Connolly & Bruner, 1974; Harter, 1978). Therefore, we might more profitably look to early childhood to discover the patterns of skilled and unskilled interpersonal performance that significantly influence health status. Before presenting my necessarily brief and selective account of the social skills literature, I must offer the following caveat. The empirical research dealing with children's social skills has been concerned predominantly with *training* (or therapeutic intervention). No consensus has yet been achieved on how to either *define* or *measure* the components of children's interpersonal effectiveness (Cartledge & Milburn, 1980; Gresham, 1981).

Bearing in mind the relativistic and interactional nature of the adaptational model and the fact that social skills theorists (such as McFall & Dodge, 1982) have acknowledged the value judgments inherent in labeling a performance "skillful," it is nonetheless possible to seek to identify broad categories of social behavior with adjustive implications for children. Or, as Putallaz and Gottman (1982) suggested, "The identification of those factors that are social in nature and satisfy a psychological risk criterion would seem an eminently reasonable starting point for conceptualizing social competence." Of course, our concern in the present context is with identifying dimensions of social behavior that place a child at physical as well as at psychological risk.

If we accept the position that social supports moderate the effects of stress (Cobb, 1976), it is but a short step to the conclusion that children who are *sociable* at home, at play, and at school would be at reduced health risk relative to their asocial peers. Studies of sociability or friendship suggest that such a skill may be comprised of the following subcomponents: overall positiveness, the ability to resolve conflicts or disagreements, awareness of group norms or social rules, the ability to communicate clearly and accurately, the ability to find and maintain a common bond with another person, and possibly (the evidence is weakest for this component) the presence of positive self-perception (Putallaz & Gottman, 1982). While studies have linked deficits in friendship formation (or peer unpopularity) with a number of maladaptive later-life *behavioral outcomes* (such as dropping out of school, bad conduct discharges from military service, and a high incidence of diagnosed neuroses and psychoses) as well as with *adult health outcomes* (such as the presence of tumors), there are not many studies available that link specific skill components or friendship patterns with childhood health status. However, some suggestive evidence exists.

Pennebaker, Hendler, Durrett, and Richards (1981) examined social factors mediating absenteeism due to illness in the first year of nursery school. These investigators assumed that "positive social encounters" among children and their peers and parents would serve as a buffer against the adverse effects of entering school for the first time. Parent and teacher ratings of sociability were used to predict absenteeism due to illness for 204 children, using family socioeconomic status, child's sex, birth order and early health history as covariates. Sociability was rated along the dimensions of anger-aggression, shyness, and prosocial activities. The investigators found that, as predicted, if parents perceived their child to be overly aggressive, shy, or deficient in the ability to get along (cooperate) with other children, then the child was more likely to be absent from school due to illness. While this study has a number of limitations (e.g., the seriousness or even the reality of the children's illness could not be determined merely on the basis of the parent's report to the school; the parent and teacher ratings of social skills did not agree; and all of the variables employed accounted for only 19 percent of the variance, with the sociability dimensions adding only 3 percent to the total), it is nonetheless a valuable beginning. If multiple measures of social skill were employed (including direct observations of children as well as peer nomination) and a verifiable index of health status used (e.g., emergency room visits, dental examinations, number of accidents), the nature of the putative "social skills–health status relationship" could be more clearly assessed. Also desirable, from the perspective of an adaptational model, would be the inclusion of indices of environmental stress (rather than presuming a uniform degree of pressure on children's adaptive resources).

As the nature of the child's interpersonal relationships changes, so too can we expect that maintenance of health will require modifications in patterns of social exchange. The arguments thus far presented suggest that cooperation and "fitting in" represent the young child's most useful behavioral tactics vis-à-vis the acquisition of stress-reducing social supports. But in adolescence the goals of preventing illness or protecting one's health may be best served by asserting one's relative independence from group or social pressure. In many instances, peer sociality and strong group identification are factors that facilitate drug experimentation, cigarette smoking, alcohol consumption, joyriding, and teenage pregnancy—patterns which, if they do not lead to fatal accidents or suicide, can establish the foundation for life-threatening adult lifestyles (Coates, Perry, Killen, & Slinkard, 1981).

Kohn's (1977) two-factor model of social-emotional functioning, Leary's (1957) interpersonal circumplex, Schutz's (1958) model of fundamental interpersonal relations, Benjamin's (1974) structural analysis of social behavior, and Wiggins's (1980) factor analytic studies of interpersonal trait descriptors are but some of the data sources that tend to converge upon a view of social exchange built around two independent bipolar dimensions, dominance (control, participation) versus submission (passivity, withdrawal) and friendliness (warmth, cooperation) versus hostility (defiance, coldness). It would appear, then, that successful health maintenance across the age span requires that a person adopt the age-appropriate and setting-specific attitude along the two-dimensional social space that maximizes helpful input from significant others.

Health outcomes will also require that the person manage his or her cognitive, behavioral, and emotional life and utilize his or her accumulated knowledge to generate and select alternative courses of action under conditions of conflict or uncertainty. These processes will be considered in the next two sections of this chapter.

HEALTH, ILLNESS, AND SELF-REGULATION

Among the salient reasons for the heightened involvement of psychology in general medicine and pediatrics is the emergence of lifestyle as a fundamental precursor to morbidity and mortality in contemporary industrialized societies. Lifestyle refers broadly to the "idiosyncratic and characteristic approach that a person takes toward living in his physical and social world . . . [including] the ways in which he plans, organizes, and anticipates his actions [Steffen & Karoly, 1980, pp. 16–17]." We should not lose sight of the fact that the responsibility for stimulating and protecting the health and well-being of children cannot be held solely by physicians, parents, teachers, and legislators. Socialization and education are not synonomous with external structuring and control; when outside the compass of adult monitoring, the child must chart his or her own course. Thus the self-directed or habitual pursuit of "healthy lifestyles" is an extremely important adaptive resource, deserving of special study and consideration.

In the health literature, self-regulation is often conceptualized as including the cognitive and affective components of *coping* with the stresses of illness, treatment, and posttreatment recovery (cf. Leventhal & Johnson, in press). It has also been considered particularly important in the process of *compliance* or adherence to complex medication regimens (Melamed, 1980). However, since the adaptational perspective highlights the continuity of the person-setting relationship, we should consider self-regulation of health to be relevant even when children (or adults) are not confronting a medical emergency or an obvious threat to their well-being. Health (or health lifestyle) self-regulation is perhaps best conceived of as *the ongoing process by which individuals gather, evaluate, and act upon data relevant to their physical health and formulate long-term and provisional health "objectives."*

From the point of view of a model of human action based upon feedback detection and organized self-correction (e.g., Powers, 1973), self-regulation is a fundamental characteristic of a "living system," provided the system is capable of (a) specifying a reference state or *goal,* (b) detecting goal-related information (especially discrepancies between the referent and current input), and (c) producing strategic output into the environment that contributes to the maintenance of the reference level. The apparently smooth functioning of the human control system requires higher-order problem solving because the person is often required to manage several (sometimes contradictory) reference conditions at once. It should be clear that self-regulation is a complex process that draws upon the other adaptive resources (such as self-knowledge, world knowledge, and intellectual capacities) and uses them in the service of pursuing healthful or unhealthful goals. If, for example, we examine Cohen and Lazarus's (1979) general tasks of "coping" we will discover that three of the five seem to reflect the above definition of self-regulation: to reduce harmful environmental conditions, to tolerate or adjust to negative events and realities, and to maintain emotional equilibrium. The remaining two tasks—maintaining a positive self-image and continuing satisfying relationships with others—clearly require the involvement of the previously discussed adaptive capacities (self-knowledge and social skills). A number of investigators have also pointed out that "deviant" self-regulation can occur under at least two conditions. First, individuals may be unable to gather, evaluate, or act upon health-relevant data because of inadequate learning or a process breakdown. For example, children may not know what symptoms to watch out for, or, if they do, may not have learned how to treat themselves. This failure of self-regulation has been termed the *absence of regulation,* to distinguish it from a second form of self-regulatory dysfunction wherein individuals are pursuing a health goal based upon irrelevant cues or an inappropriate evaluative standard. This latter process has been called *misregulation* (Carver & Scheier, 1982). Misregulation may occur when individuals gather information about "symptoms" unrelated to their disease (Leventhal, Meyer, & Nerenz, 1980); when they act upon short-term goals, such as anxiety-reduction, by emitting regulatory behaviors, like alcohol consumption, cigarette smoking, or overeating, which have long-term debilitating effects on health (Rodin, 1982); or when they ingest medicines for immediate symptom relief that prevent them from being focally aware of ongoing bodily signals (feedback) indicative of a systemic disease (Schwartz, 1979).

Knowledge of the processes of self-regulation should be applicable, then, to the study of acute and chronic disease as well as healthy functioning. The purpose of this section is to consider the workings of self-regulation in health and illness mainly from the perspectives of individual differences and developmental psychology. For a broader treatment of the subject, including methods of assessment and clinical intervention, the reader is referred to Karoly and Kanfer (1982).

Components and underpinnings. While the multiple-aspect process of self-regulation is built upon a number of subprocesses, such as self-awareness, attentional skills, verbal skills, instrumental competencies, and the like (cf. Karoly, 1981), the pivotal ingredients are those that reflect its motivational capacities. The conceptual and skill hierarchies and negative feedback loops that comprise a self-regulating system operate in the service of guiding the person toward the achievement of goals. Motivation, in this system, derives not from sources of powerful inner stimulation (arousal) nor from external incentives, but rather from the processes by which the individual matches input to reference levels and cancels the effects of disturbances (error). This activity is not necessarily a conservative or simply a drive-reducing one, since the individual sets standards at many different levels and is capable of introducing variability into his or her actions for the purpose of reducing error (Glasser, 1981; Powers, 1973). Thus the key to understanding successful versus deviant self-regulation of health (or any other goal) is to appreciate the processes of standard setting and feedback evaluation. How do they develop? Why do they differ? What is their effect on health and illness?

Harter (1982a), one of the few developmental psychologists to consider the childhood origins of self-regulation, has suggested that:

> Developmentally, the *order* in which the critical component processes of self-regulation are initially *acquired* is just the *reverse* of the order in which they are postulated to operate in adulthood, namely self-monitoring, self-evaluation, and self-reinforcement. That is, I am arguing that children first learn to imitate verbal approval and apply it to their own behavior before they are capable of self-evaluation, and that the process of self-evaluation must be acquired before they can fully appreciate those situations in which they should monitor their behavior [p. 173].

Assuming the validity of Harter's sequential hypothesis, the implications for health management should be obvious. First, the self-regulation of health-illness parameters is not a meaningful aspect of infant functioning. The health status of infants depends upon parental self-regulation of diet, of exposure to toxic substances and environments, of pre- and postnatal visits to the pediatrician for checkups and immunizations, and of parents' attitudes toward their infants which maximize affectionate contact and minimize the potential for accidents. Eventually, however, preschool children will come to imitate the positive and the destructive health habits of parents and other socializing agents in order to obtain reward or avoid punishment (cf. Bandura & Walters, 1963), while school-age youngsters are likely to also be influenced by comparison with peer activity (Ruble, Boggiano, Feldman, & Loebl, 1980). To the extent that accidents, which account for fully 45 percent of total childhood mortality, are the result of impulsive and careless acts, the social model who displays careful, deliberative performance in potentially dangerous situations (in a car, swimming, in the presence of medications, etc.) can facilitate child safety.

However, the "internalization" of prohealth attitudes and actions (the establishment of rudimentary *health standards*) requires more than mere exposure to virtuous models and powerful contingencies. The child must be able to understand and spontaneously generate the *rules for correct (rewardable) behavior* (i.e., specify the reference state). The child who has seemingly acquired the prohealth habit of brushing her teeth after every meal may *misregulate* by making a fuss in a restaurant because she cannot do the ostensibly rewardable act. The important lesson for caretakers and clinicians to learn is that, just because a child will very often do the "right thing" and say the "right words," flexible and realistic self-direction may not yet be possible.

Harter (1982a, b) has postulated that differences in the level of rule incorporation (standard setting) may vary as a function of whether socializing agents emphasize (through modeling and direct teaching) the *incentive* function of rewards ("You brushed your teeth, now you can watch some TV"), the *affective* function ("Doesn't it make you feel good to have clean teeth!"), or the *informational* function ("I'm glad you brushed your teeth because I want you to have strong, healthy teeth all your life, and brushing helps you to achieve that goal"). While all these functions are important, an underemphasis on the informational aspects is likely to retard the development of generalizable self-evaluative standards for health-related or other forms of conduct. The child who behaves solely in order to please others or in order to feel good is less likely to develop consistent, cross-situational health habits than the child who is capable of acting in order to preserve a view of himself as a "healthy individual." In addition to knowing the abstract principle(s) behind health-oriented activities, the developing child must also acquire the ability to anticipate long-range outcomes and to use covert speech in a self-guiding fashion (Karoly, 1981; Staats, 1971; Zivin, 1979).

Very little empirical data are available to support or disconfirm a developmental model of health self-regulation. Indeed, development is a neglected aspect of cybernetic theorizing generally. However, there is a growing body of literature on children and adolescents as rule formers and rule users (Mischel & Mischel, 1976; Weston & Turiel, 1980) that lends credence to the above line of reasoning. Similarly, children who are "accident-prone" or who are chronically unwilling to comply with parental or physician requests for health habit modification (enuretics, obese children, children with diabetes who fail to self-administer insulin or eat properly), and children who show the early signs of coronary-prone (Type A) personality, would all seem to be excellent candidates for interventions designed to enhance self-regulatory skills (cf. Magrab, 1978 Matthews & Angulo, 1980; Melamed, 1980).

PERCEPTUAL ORGANIZATION, PROBLEM SOLVING, AND CHILDREN'S HEALTH COMPETENCE

Those who refer to adaptive resources or coping skills as aspects of *intelligence* would surely expect IQ to mediate children's efforts at overcoming stress or physical trauma and at establishing a pattern of health maintenance-enhancement. Unfortunately, despite its efficacy at predicting social, academic, and vocational competencies, IQ sheds very little light upon the actual process or dynamics of adaptation. In this final section, devoted to an explication of developmental process 2 of figure 2.1, I shall address several constructs that may be more serviceable than the global concept of intelligence as components in an adaptational model of health.

Health schemata. Everything said up until now has been based on·the assumption that children and adolescents are eventually capable of unitizing, organizing, and storing aspects of their experience. Whether they are attempting to know themselves and their environments and develop a sense of mastery (process 3), attempting social inclusion or autonomy (process 5), or attempting to specify a desired health condition and minimize discrepancies from it (process 4), children are presumed to represent cognitively the regularities and invariants of their world in order to facilitate their growth and development.

Schemas (or schemata) are, in the words of Anderson (1980), "large, complex units of knowledge that organize much of what we know about general categories of objects, classes of events, and types of people [p. 129]." In the last half-dozen years cognitive psychologists have become greatly enamored of the concept of schema which, according to Rumelhart (1980), is traceable to Kant (for whom it referred to rules through which people are able to understand their sense perceptions). Vaguely equivalent terms are "script," "plan," "prototype," "format," "theme," and "cognitive map" (Landau & Goldfried, 1981). Despite the criticism that the schema notion is artificial, passive, narrow, unresearchable, and trendy (Neisser, 1980), the possibility exists that when considered with minimal complexity as a process of fitting new data to an existing pattern, it may hold a great deal of promise for understanding day-to-day symptom management (cf. also Fiske & Linville, 1980).

For example, if we recognize the fact that each of us is literally flooded by various internal sensations over the course of our daily activities, the need for a mode of "data reduction" or selective decoding should be obvious. Many of the internal stimuli are vague or ambiguous and carry little information, while many stimuli that "demand" attention may be irrelevant to the actor's purposes. Whether diffuse or focal sensations are competing for recognition, the individual remains limited in what he or she can process. Thus the cognitive apparatus, employing the same kinds of selection mechanisms as are used to perceive external signals, incorporates hypotheses, filters, or (in current parlance) schemata to guide the processing of internal bodily messages. As Pennebaker and Skelton (1981) point out:

> The information that is gleaned from the selective search is used to confirm the hypotheses and/or to create new ones. The data and hypotheses are complementary in producing integrated perception [p. 214].

Pennebaker and his colleagues have conducted a number of intriguing experiments detailing the conditions under which selective monitoring and attentional focus can influence perceptions of bodily states (symptoms), often independent of actual physiological patterns (cf. Pennebaker, Burnam, Schaeffer, & Harper, 1977; Pennebaker & Lightner, 1980; Pennebaker & Skelton, 1981).

If we make a few "leaps of faith" and assume that health schemata operate outside laboratory settings, that they operate for children (mutatis mutandis) as well as for adults, and that it is possible to identify the antecedents of adaptive and maladaptive modes of sensory processing, then the schemata notion should prove extremely important to pediatric researchers and clinicians in the years ahead.

The clinical and research questions are virtually limitless. If symptom perception is at least partly hypothesis- or schema-guided, a developmental progression in schema clarity and organization should be obtained. As is noted by Jordan and O'Grady (in Chapter Three of this volume), preoperational children do not employ realistic causal reasoning in dealing with the world of external events. Therefore, their hypotheses about internal sensations, such as pain or fatigue, may be inconsistent and their reactions to illness and treatment unpredictable. How readily do young children accept and utilize adult-structured health-illness schemata? Are they differentially susceptible to placebo effects as a function of the fluidity of their health schemata? Does having a chronic illness, such as arthritis or diabetes, tend to stabilize young children's schematic processing? Do youngsters who decode and monitor bodily signals along "negative" dimensions, such as discomfort, pain, or weakness, tend to persist in such selectivity (thereby setting the stage for adult hypochondriasis)?

Problem solving. For the most part, discussions of children's health behavior and their modes of coping with illness have focused on tactical operations. Derived hypothetically or from naturalistic observation (or both), lists of cognitive, emotive, and instrumental coping mechanisms have appeared quite frequently over the years. Some focus on direct action—seeking relevant information, applying self-hypnosis or self-relaxation, taking medicines, requesting reassurance, becoming immersed in a hobby, etc. Some describe intrapsychic maneuvers—denial, selective attention to positive outcomes, rehearsal of alternatives, acceptance, etc. However, like pills or injections, these attempts at reducing distress are discrete and ahistorical. There has been scant discussion to how children know (metacognitively) why and when to do what, in which order, and for how long. Nor do we know much about the interaction of metacognition with tasks, settings, and personal styles. However, these are the dynamic aspects of adaptive intelligence that doubtless contribute in large measure to the successful pursuit of health-related (and other) goals. While there is evidence to suggest that coping competencies are transmitted through adult modeling and direct teaching, and that certain adult teaching styles facilitate learning in their offspring (e.g., Mondell & Tyler, 1981), the *process* of problem solving and logical reasoning is one that unfolds gradually, interactively, and differentially across time and diverse settings.

The pediatrician, clinical child psychologist, pediatric nurse, parent, and any other interested caregiver would be advised therefore to examine not just the *products* of children's thinking about their health, but the sequential processes as outlined by information-processing advocates. Although complex and conceptualized in diverse ways, problem solving is usually taken to involve the child's sensitivity to task features and requirements, the process of accessing and selecting a potential strategy (specific or general, social or impersonal), the implementation of the chosen strategy, and the evaluation and (if necessary) modification of the strategy (or the problem definition) based upon observation of the strategic effects (D'Zurilla & Goldfried, 1971; Krasnor & Rubin, 1981).

While the relationship between identifiable problem-solving styles and various aspects of social and academic adjustment has been investigated widely (cf., e.g., Spivack, Platt, & Shure, 1976), and while training programs have been devised to teach specific health-oriented skills, there has been little interest in delineating empirically the natural history of the linkage between health outcomes and the problem-solving propensities of children and adolescents (mediated, of course, by personality, motives, support systems, local criteria, and the like). Such an undertaking is sorely needed.

SOME CONCLUDING REMARKS

Neither pediatrics nor clinical psychology has systematically drawn upon the data base of developmental psychology or upon the logic of an interactionist conception of life-span adaptation. The dominant biologically based model of disease has encouraged clinicians and researchers alike to focus on discontinuities and disruptions, rather than upon the essential connectedness of life tasks.

The purpose of the present chapter was to outline, in broad strokes, the configuration of an alternative perspective which, as Rudolf Virchow noted over a century ago, might provide a foundation for medical intervention via the knowledge of "the normal course of the phenomena of life and of the conditions under which this course is possible."

In the U.S. surgeon general's report on health promotion and disease prevention (U.S. Department of Health, Education, and Welfare, 1979), a number of national goals were set, including the reduction of infant mortality by at least 35 percent, the reduction of deaths among children 1 to 14 years of age by at least 20 percent, and among adolescents 15 to 24 years of age by the same percentage by the year 1990. The essential preventability and controlability of many health risks was presumed, and the optimistic tone of HEW's mandate seemed predicated on the availability of a technology for altering environments and for socializing health lifestyles. The findings, trends, explanations, and suggestions contained in this chapter were offered as tentative guidelines for determining *where, when,* and *to what* aspects of children's thought and behavior such technologies might best be applied.

REFERENCES

Anderson, J. R. *Cognitive psychology and its implications.* San Francisco: Freeman, 1980.

Antonovsky, A. *Health, stress, and coping.* San Francisco: Jossey-Bass, 1979.

Bandura, A., & Walters, R. H. *Social learning and personality development.* New York: Holt, Rinehart & Winston, 1963.

Benjamin, L. S. Structural analysis of social behavior. *Psychological Review,* 1974, **81,** 392–425.

Brown, G. W. Developmental and behavioral pediatrics: A realistic challenge? *Journal of Developmental and Behavioral Pediatrics,* 1980, **1,** 3–10.

Cartledge, G., & Milburn, J. F. (Eds.), *Teaching social skills to children: Innovative approaches.* New York: Pergamon Press, 1980.

Carver, C. S., & Scheier, M. F. An information-processing perspective on self-management. In P. Karoly & F. H. Kanfer (Eds.), *Self-management and behavior change: From theory to practice.* New York: Pergamon Press, 1982.

Coates, T. J., Perry, C., Killen, J., & Slinkard, L. A. Primary prevention of cardiovascular disease in children and adolescents. In C. K. Prokop & L. A. Bradley (Eds.), *Medical psychology: Contributions to behavioral medicine.* New York: Academic Press, 1981.

Cobb, S. Social support as a moderator of life stress. *Psychosomatic Medicine,* 1976, **38,** 300–314.

Cohen, F., & Lazarus, R. S. Coping with the stresses of illness. In G. C. Stone, F. Cohen, & N. E. Adler (Eds.), *Health psychology.* San Francisco: Jossey-Bass, 1979.

Connolly, K., & Bruner, J. Competence: Its nature and nurture. In K. Connolly & J. Bruner (Eds.), *The growth of competence.* London: Academic Press, 1974.

Denzin, N. K. *Childhood socialization.* San Francisco: Jossey-Bass, 1977.

Depue, R. A., Monroe, S. M., & Shackman, S. L. The psychobiology of human disease: Implications for conceptualizing the depressive disorders. In R. A. Depue (Ed.), *The psychobiology of depressive disorders: Implications for the effects of stress.* New York: Academic Press, 1979.

D'Zurilla, T. J., & Goldfried, M. R. Problem-solving and behavior modification. *Journal of Abnormal Psychology,* 1971, **78,** 107–128.

Engel, G. L. *Psychological development in health and disease.* Philadelphia: W. B. Saunders, 1962.

Engel, G. W. The need for a new medical model: A challenge for biomedicine. *Science,* 1977, **196,** 130–136.

Fischer, K. W. A theory of cognitive development: The control and construction of hierarchies and skills. *Psychological Review,* 1980, **87,** 477–531.

Fiske, S. T., & Linville, P. W. What does the schema concept buy us? *Personality and Social Psychology Bulletin,* 1980, **6,** 543–557.

Glasser, W. *Stations of the mind.* New York: Harper & Row, 1981.

Greenberger, E., Steinberg, L. D., & Vaux, A. Adolescents who work: Health and behavioral consequences of job stress. *Developmental Psychology,* 1981, **17,** 691–703.

Gresham, F. M. Validity of social skills measures for assessing social competence in low status children: A multivariate investigation. *Developmental Psychology,* 1981, **17,** 390–398.

Guardo, C. J., & Bohan, J. B. Development of a sense of self-identity in children. *Child Development,* 1971, **42**, 1909–1921.

Hamburg, B. A. Early adolescence as a life stress. In S. Levine & H. Ursin (Eds.), *Coping and health.* New York: Plenum Press, 1980.

Harter, S. Effectance motivation reconsidered: Toward a developmental model. *Human Development,* 1978, **1**, 34–64.

Harter, S. A developmental perspective on some parameters of self-regulation in children. In P. Karoly & F. H. Kanfer (Eds.), *Self-management and behavior change: From theory to practice.* New York: Pergamon Press, 1982. (a)

Harter, S. Developmental perspectives on the self-system. In M. Hetherington (Ed.), *Carmichael's manual of child psychology.* New York: Wiley, 1982. (b)

Howie, V. M. Developmental sequelae of chronic otitis media: A review. *Journal of Developmental and Behavioral Pediatrics,* 1980, **1**, 34–38.

Karoly, P. Self-management problems in children. In E. J. Mash & L. G. Terdal (Eds.), *Behavioral assessment of childhood disorders.* New York: Guilford, 1981.

Karoly, P., & Kanfer, F. H. (Eds.), *Self-management and behavior change: From theory to practice.* New York: Pergamon Press, 1982.

Katz, P. A., & Zigler, E. Self-image disparity: A developmental approach. *Journal of Personality and Social Psychology,* 1967, **5**, 186–195.

Katz, P. A., Zigler E., & Zalk, S. R. Children's self-image disparity: The effects of age, maladjustment, and action-thought orientation. *Developmental Psychology,* 1975, **11**, 546–550.

Keller, A., Ford, L.H., & Meacham, J. Dimensions of self-concept in preschool children. *Developmental Psychology,* 1978, **14**, 483–489.

Kenny, T. J., & Clemmens, R. L. *Behavioral pediatrics and child development: A clinical handbook* (2nd ed.). Baltimore: Williams & Wilkins, 1980.

Kobasa, S. C., Maddi, S. R., & Kahn, S. Hardiness and health: A prospective study. *Journal of Personality and Social Psychology,* 1982, **42**, 168–177.

Kohn, M. *Social competence, symptoms, and underachievement in childhood: A longitudinal perspective.* Washington: V. H. Winston & Sons, 1977.

Koocher, G. P., & O'Malley, J. E. *The Damocles syndrome: Psychosocial consequences of surviving childhood cancer.* New York: McGraw-Hill, 1981.

Krasnor, L. R., & Rubin, K. H. The assessment of social problem-solving skills in young children. In T. V. Merluzzi, C. R. Glass, & M. Genest (Eds.), *Cognitive assessment.* New York: Guilford, 1981.

Landau, R. J., & Goldfried, M. R. The assessment of schemata: A unifying framework for cognitive, behavioral, and traditional assessment. In P. C. Kendall & S. D. Hollon (Eds.), *Assessment strategies for cognitive-behavioral interventions.* New York: Academic Press, 1981.

Lazarus, R. S. Psychological stress and coping in adaptation and illness. *International Journal of Psychiatry in Medicine,* 1974, **5**, 321–333.

Lazarus, R. S., Averill, J. R., & Opton, E. M. The psychology of coping: Issues of research and assessment. In G. V. Coelho, D. A. Hamburg, & J. E. Adams (Eds.), *Coping and adaptation.* New York: Basic Books, 1974.

Leahy, R. L., & Huard, C. Role-taking and self-image disparity in children. *Developmental Psychology,* 1976, **12**, 504–508.

Leary, T. *Interpersonal diagnosis of personality.* New York: Ronald Press, 1957.

Leventhal, H., & Johnson, J. E. Laboratory and field experimentation: Development of a theory of self-regulation. In R. Leonard & P. Woolridge (Eds.), *Behavioral science and nursing theory.* St. Louis: C. V. Mosby, in press.

Leventhal, H., Meyer, D., & Nerenz, D. The common sense representation of illness danger. In S. Rachman (Ed.), *Contributions to medical psychology,* Vol. 2. Oxford: Pergamon Press, 1980.

Levine, S. A coping model of mother-infant relationships. In S. Levine & H. Ursin (Eds.), *Coping and health.* New York: Plenum Press, 1980.

Lewis, M., & Brooks-Gunn, J. *Social cognition and the acquisition of self.* New York: Plenum Press, 1979.

Magrab, P. R. (Ed.), *Psychological management of pediatric problems,* Vol. 1. Baltimore: University Park Press, 1978.

Matthews, K. A., & Angulo, J. Measurement of the type A behavior pattern in children: Assessment of children's competitiveness, impatience-anger, and aggression. *Child Development,* 1980, **51,** 466–475.

McFall, R. M., & Dodge, K. A. Self-management and interpersonal skills learning. In P. Karoly & F. H. Kanfer (Eds.), *Self-management and behavior change: From theory to practice.* New York: Pergamon Press, 1982.

Melamed, B. G. Behavioral psychology in pediatrics. In S. Rachman (Ed.), *Contributions to medical psychology,* Vol. 2. Oxford: Pergamon Press, 1980.

Melamed, B. G., & Siegel, L. J. *Behavioral medicine: Practical applications in health care.* New York: Springer, 1980.

Mischel, W., & Mischel, H. N. A cognitive social-learning approach to morality and self-regulation. In T. Lickona (Ed.), *Moral development and behavior.* New York: Holt, Rinehart & Winston, 1976.

Mishler, E. G. Viewpoint: Critical perspectives on the biomedical model. In E. G. Mishler, L. R. Amara Singham, S. T. Hauser, R. Liem, S. D. Osherson, & N. E. Wexler, *Social contexts of health, illness, and patient care.* Cambridge: Cambridge University Press, 1981.

Mondell, S., & Tyler, F. B. Parental competence and styles of problem-solving/play behavior with children. *Developmental Psychology,* 1981, **17,** 73–78.

Moore, L. G., Van Arsdale, P. W., Glittenberg, J. E., & Aldrich, R. A. *The biocultural basis of illness.* St. Louis: C. V. Mosby, 1980.

Murphy, L. B. Coping, vulnerability, and resilience in childhood. In G. V. Coelho, D. A. Hamburg, & J. E. Adams (Eds.), *Coping and adaptation.* New York: Basic Books, 1974.

Murphy, L. B., & Moriarty, A. E. *Vulnerablity, coping, and growth: From infancy to adolescence.* New Haven: Yale University Press, 1976.

Mutter, A. Z., & Schleifer, M. J. The role of psychological and social factors in the onset of somatic illness in children. *Psychosomatic Medicine,* 1966, **28,** 333–343.

Neisser, U. On "social knowing." *Personality and Social Psychology,* 1980, **6,** 601–605.

Pennebaker, J. W., Burnam, M. A., Schaeffer, M. A., & Harper, D. C. Lack of control as a determinant of perceived physical symptoms. *Journal of Personality and Social Psychology,* 1977, **35,** 167–174.

Pennebaker, J. W., Hendler, C. S., Durrett, M. E., & Richards, P. Social factors influencing absenteeism due to illness in nursery school children. *Child Development,* 1981, **52,** 692–700.

Pennebaker, J. W., & Lightner, J. M. Competition of internal and external information in an exercise setting. *Journal of Personality and Social Psychology,* 1980, **39,** 165–174.

Pennebaker, J. W., & Skelton, J. A. Selective monitoring of physical sensations. *Journal of Personality and Social Psychology,* 1981, **41,** 213–223.

Powers, W. T. *Behavior: The control of perception.* Chicago: Aldine, 1973.

Putallaz, M., & Gottman, J. M. Conceptualizing social competence in children. In P. Karoly & J. J. Steffen (Eds.), *Improving children's competence.* Lexington, Mass.: Lexington Books, 1982.

Richmond, J. B. Child development: A basic science for pediatrics. *Pediatrics,* 1967, **39,** 649–658.

Rodin, J. Biopsychosocial aspects of self-management. In P. Karoly & F. H. Kanfer (Eds.), *Self-management and behavior change: From theory to practice.* New York: Pergamon Press, 1982.

Ruble, D. N., Boggiano, A. K., Feldman, N. S., & Loebl, J. H. Developmental analysis of the role of social comparison in self-evaluation. *Developmental Psychology,* 1980, **16,** 105–115.

Rumelhart, D. E. Schemata: The building blocks of cognition. In R. J. Spiro, B. C. Bruce, & W. F. Brewer (Eds.), *Theoretical issues in reading comprehension.* Hillsdale, N.J.: Erlbaum, 1980.

Salzinger, S., Antrobus, J., & Glick, J. (Eds.), *The ecosystem of the "sick" child.* New York: Academic Press, 1980.

Santostefano, S. *A biodevelopmental approach to clinical child psychology: Cognitive controls and cognitive control therapy.* New York: Wiley, 1978.

Schutz, W. C. *The interpersonal underworld.* Palo Alto, Calif.: Science and Behavior Books, 1958.

Schwartz, G. The brain as a health care system. In G. C. Stone, F. Cohen, & N. E. Adler (Eds.), *Health psychology.* San Francisco: Jossey-Bass, 1979.

Spivack, G., Platt, J. J., & Shure, M. B. *The problem-solving approach to adjustment.* San Francisco: Jossey-Bass, 1976.

Staats, A. W. *Child learning, intelligence, and personality: Principles of a behavioral interaction approach.* New York: Harper & Row, 1971.

Staats, A. W. *Social behaviorism.* Homewood, Ill.: Dorsey Press, 1975.

Steffen, J. J., & Karoly, P. Toward a psychology of therapeutic maintenance. In P. Karoly & J. J. Steffen (Eds.), *Improving the long-term effects of psychotherapy: Models of durable outcome.* New York: Gardner Press, 1980.

Steinhauer, P. D., Mushin, D. N., & Rae-Grant, Q. Psychological aspects of chronic illness. In P. D. Steinhauer & Q. Rae-Grant (Eds.), *Psychological problems of the child and his family.* Toronto: Macmillan, 1977.

Task Force on Pediatric Education. *The future of pediatric education.* Denver: Hirschfeld, 1978.

Turner, J. *Made for life: Coping, competence, and cognition:* London: Methuen, 1980.

U.S. Department of Health, Education, and Welfare. *Healthy people: The surgeon general's report on health promotion and disease prevention.* DHEW Publication no. 79-55071. Washington: Government Printing Office, 1979.

Virchow, R. Concerning standpoints in scientific medicine. *Archiv für Pathologische Anatomie und Physiologie und für Klinische Medizin,* 1847, **1**, 3–7.

Weiner, H. *Psychobiology and human disease.* New York: Elsevier, 1977.

Werner, H. *Comparative psychology of mental development.* Chicago: Follett, 1948.

Weston, D. R., & Turiel, E. Act-rule relations: Children's concepts of social rules. *Developmental Psychology,* 1980, **16**, 417–424.

White, B. L., Watts, J. C., Barnett, I. C., Kaban, B. T., Marmor, J. R., & Shapiro, B. B. *Experience and environment: Major influences on the development of the young child.* Englewood Cliffs, N.J.: Prentice-Hall, 1973.

Wiggins, J. S. Circumplex models of interpersonal behavior. In L. Wheeler (Ed.), *Review of personality and social psychology,* Vol. 1. Beverly Hills: Sage, 1980.

Williams, B. J., Foreyt, J. P., & Goodrick, G. K. *Pediatric behavioral medicine.* New York: Praeger, 1981.

Wohlwill, J. F. *The study of behavioral development.* New York: Academic Press, 1973.

Wright, L. Health care psychology: Prospects for the well-being of children. *American Psychologist,* 1979, **34**, 1001–1006.

Zigler, E., Balla, D., & Watson, N. Developmental and experiential determinants of self-image disparity in institutionalized and noninstitutionalized retarded and normal children. *Journal of Personality and Social Psychology,* 1972, **23**, 81–87.

Zigler, E., & Muenchow, S. H. Principles and social policy implications of a whole-child psychology. In S. Salzinger, J. Antrobus, & J. Glick (Eds.), *The ecosystem of the "sick" child.* New York: Academic Press, 1980.

Zivin, G. (Ed.) *The development of self-regulation through private speech.* New York: Wiley, 1979.

3

Children's Health Beliefs and Concepts: Implications for Child Health Care

Mary Kay Jordan
and
Donald J. O'Grady

It is only within the past century that comprehensive child health care has been established as a national priority. During this time one of the greatest challenges to children's health has been infectious disease; however, recent developments in immunization and antibiotic therapy have all but eradicated many of these previously fatal diseases. At present pediatric health professionals are faced with a dramatically different set of problems. The current leading cause of death among children is accidents, killing 16,000 and permanently injuring 40–50,000 each year (*Health U. S.,* 1978; Mofenson & Greensher, 1978). Chronic physical illness strikes approximately one in ten children by the age of 15 (Pless, 1978). Accidents and chronic illness are unique as health care problems because behavior, rather than medical technology, is often the major factor contributing to their prevention, treatment, and outcome. This shift in emphasis toward behavior as the key to health has strengthened the role of the psychologist as a health care professional.

Psychological research has been focused primarily on two factors related to health behavior, namely, health beliefs and health knowledge. Social psychologists have suggested that voluntary health behaviors are determined by an individual's (in this case, either parents' or children's) beliefs about the likelihood of illness, its severity, and the benefits of prevention or treatment (Becker, 1974a). Developmental psychologists have examined systematic changes in children's health and illness concepts within the context of general cognitive maturation. Contributions from both these traditions have been critical for understanding and modifying health behaviors. The present chapter is concerned with the implications of health beliefs and knowledge for the practice of child health psychology.

PREDICTING HEALTH BEHAVIORS
FROM HEALTH BELIEFS

The notion that an individual's behavior can be predicted from his or her beliefs is not new. In the 1930s Kurt Lewin suggested that behavior was determined by subjective perceptions and the expected value of particular actions. Later Hochbaum applied Lewin's approach to health behavior. He suggested that health behaviors were a function of the perception of illness as a threat (i.e., an area of negative valence that was to be avoided) and the expected value of preventive health action for reducing that threat. In a study of participation in a tuberculosis screening program, Hochbaum (1956) found that three health beliefs were expressed by adults who voluntarily submitted to chest x-rays. First, these individuals believed that they were personally vulnerable to tuberculosis. They also believed that tuberculosis could be diagnosed asymptomatically by chest x-ray. Finally, participants believed in the benefits of early diagnosis, that is, that the prognosis for recovery was better if the disease was detected early. The formal statement of the relationship between health beliefs and behavior was called the Health Belief Model (Becker, Haefner, Kasl, Kirscht, Maiman, & Rosenstock, 1977; Maiman & Becker, 1974; Rosenstock, 1974b; Rosenstock & Kirscht, 1979; Stone, 1979). According to this model, an individual's health beliefs determined his or her "readiness to act." Certain demographic characteristics (e.g., higher socioeconomic status and education) were also correlated with the use of health services because positive health beliefs were more common among individuals of higher education and income. Participation in health behaviors was most likely among individuals who possessed the optimal combination of health beliefs and demographic characteristics; nevertheless, given the proper constellation of beliefs, preventive health behavior occurred regardless of socioeconomic status (Rosenstock, 1974a). Over the years investigators have amassed substantial evidence implicating the role of health beliefs in the use of preventive, diagnostic, and treatment services by adults (cf. Becker, 1974a; Becker, Haefner et al., 1977; Kasl & Cobb, 1966; Rosenstock, 1966).

As one might expect, the predictive power of certain health beliefs varies according to the specific outcome measure used (i.e., type of health action being predicted). Preventive and illness behaviors, for example, constitute distinct behavioral dimensions that are associated with different constellations of health beliefs (Becker, Nathanson, Drachman, & Kirscht, 1977). For this reason it is important to distinguish among various types of health behaviors. One of the more popular taxonomies includes three categories: preventive health behaviors (activities undertaken by asymptomatic persons for the purpose of preventing or detecting disease), illness behavior (activities engaged in by symptomatic individuals for the purpose of defining and treating illness), and sick-role behavior (actions undertaken by individuals with diagnosed illness for the purpose of getting well; Kasl & Cobb, 1966). For the present discussion, the range of behaviors typically included in each of these categories will be expanded somewhat to include other clinically relevant child health behaviors such as accidents and risk taking.

Preventive Health Behavior

Most investigations of preventive health behavior have been retrospective studies of adult participation in public health screening programs or medical examinations. These studies have suggested consistently that the likelihood of engaging in preventive health behavior was determined by health beliefs—specifically, the perceptions of personal susceptibility to illness and of the benefits of preventive action (Rosenstock, 1974a).

In one of the few prospective studies of preventive health behavior, Haefner and Kirscht (1970) attempted to modify the health beliefs of adults and to determine subsequent changes in health behavior. Subjects responded to questions about their past health-related actions and their health beliefs (e.g., perceptions of illness susceptibility, illness severity, and the benefits of action) and then were exposed to threatening films about heart disease, cancer, and tuberculosis. Individuals who viewed the films reported immediate increases in their perceptions of susceptibility and of the benefits of preventive action. These changes were sustained over an unannounced eight-month follow-up period. Individuals exposed to the films also engaged in a recommended health behavior (routine checkup) significantly more often than did individuals in a control group that had not seen the films.

The role of health beliefs for explaining and predicting health behaviors in adults has gained much empirical support. By comparison, there is a conspicuous lack of information about the influence of children's health beliefs on their preventive health behaviors. One of the few investigations of children's health behaviors was concerned with the relationship between mothers' health beliefs and their use of preventive medical services for their children. Becker, Nathanson, Drachman, and Kirscht (1977) conducted a prospective study of 250 primarily black mothers of low socioeconomic status. Three dimensions of mothers' health beliefs were assessed in an initial interview: degree of preventive orientation (i.e., belief that illness could be prevented), attitudes toward medical care (i.e., degree of agreement with a medical diagnosis made during the index visit), and perceptions of their children's general health and susceptibility to illness. For three and a half years after collecting the attitudinal data, Becker and his coworkers recorded the children's preventive, acute illness, and accident-related clinic visits. Although the correlations between beliefs and behavior were rather modest, well-child care was more frequent among mothers who expressed a preventive orientation, mothers who tended to agree with diagnoses, and mothers who perceived their children as healthy and unsusceptible to illness. The latter finding apparently differed from studies of adults that indicated more preventive actions among individuals who perceived themselves as vulnerable to illness. It is not clear whether this discrepancy reflected a significant developmental difference or simply a difference in the measurement of vulnerability. In most studies of adults' preventive behavior, subjects have been asked to rate their susceptibility to very serious illnesses (e.g., cancer and heart disease), whereas Becker and his colleagues defined susceptibility in terms of mothers' ratings of their children's health (from excellent to poor) and their perceptions of whether their children "get sick easily." Given the frequency of minor illnesses among children, it is probable that this index of susceptibility differed from that of the previous example. Moreover, mothers' reports of excellent general health in their children may have reflected the success of past preventive actions. Nevertheless, the 1977 study by Becker and his colleagues demonstrated the utility of assessing mothers' health beliefs for predicting their use of preventive clinic services for their children.

Using a somewhat different approach, Pratt (1973) studied the relationship between child-rearing methods and children's personal health practices such as toothbrushing and exercising. She hypothesized that these practices would be more frequent among children whose parents encouraged self-reliance and esteem (e.g., by granting autonomy, using reason and explanation, rewarding desired behavior) than among children whose parents maximized their own control (e.g., by using punishment). In interviews with 510 families, Pratt asked 9- to 13-year-old children to report their health practices and their parents' child-rearing methods. The results supported the original hypothesis and also indicated a stronger relationship between children's health practices and child-rearing characteristics than between children's and parents' health practices or between children's practices and socioeconomic status. Thus the influence of child-rearing methods on children's health habits appeared to extend beyond that of socioeconomic advantage or the imitation of parental behaviors. Pratt concluded that sound health behavior was an expression of competency and active coping that could be developed only through autonomy.

To date, the study of children's preventive health behaviors has been limited to activities that may prevent the occurrence of disease (well-child care, personal health practices, etc.). However, there are a host of other behaviors that are necessary for the preservation and promotion of health. These include the performance of healthful behaviors, such as eating a balanced diet or wearing a seat belt, as well as the avoidance of dangerous activities. Because children maintain primary responsibility for these behaviors, it is likely that their own health beliefs assume a more prominent role than do well-child visits, which are determined primarily by parents' health beliefs. The role of health beliefs in these behaviors has been virtually ignored in previous research but is particularly relevant for pediatric psychologists.

Children's tendency to have accidents has probably received more study than any other self-initiated health behavior. Accidents are the predominant cause of mortality and morbidity among children (Wright, Schaefer, & Solomons, 1979). For this reason, accident prevention is considered the key to pediatric health care efforts. Certain physical and emotional stresses are known to be related to the occurrence of accidents in children. These include hunger, fatigue, recent substitution in the caretaker, and the illness or death of a family member (Mofenson & Greensher, 1978). Beyond these factors, investigators have attempted to find personal characteristics that may be associated with repeated accidents. Approximately 30 percent of all young accident victims have had one or more previous accidents. This alarming rate has led many investigators to reject the notion that accidents are due to stress or mere chance. Instead, they have suggested the concept of the "accident-prone" child. In general, this child has a high activity level, neuromuscular immaturity, and difficulty anticipating, assessing, and adapting to the consequences of behavior (Wright et al., 1979). Although the belief correlates of accident repeating have not yet been demonstrated empirically, there are known clusters of health beliefs, behaviors, and personal characteristics that readily place some individuals at risk for accidents. For example, adolescent boys (for whom the accident rate is quite high) are more likely than other age-sex groups to take excessive risks, to deny pain, and to fail to seek medical care (*Health U. S.*, 1978; Mechanic, 1964).

Illness Behavior

It is well known that the use of medical services is not correlated perfectly with either the presence or severity of illness (Pless, 1978). Rather, utilization is a behavioral response to the perception of symptoms (Rosenstock, 1974a). Individual variations in the interpretation of and response to symptoms are regarded as learned behavior (Fabrega, 1973; Mechanic, 1962). Mechanic (1962) proposed the concept of "illness behavior" to describe "the ways in which given symptoms may be differentially perceived, evaluated, and acted (or not acted) upon by different kinds of persons [p. 189]." Similarities in the willingness to report pain and the inclination to seek medical advice have been found among individuals of common ethnic, religious, and socioeconomic backgrounds (cf., Mechanic, 1962). For example, low socioeconomic status has been associated with a disbelief in the efficacy of medical treatment. This negative orientation has resulted in discontinuity of care, untreated episodes of illness (Kirscht, 1974), and greater severity of illness when treated (Roghmann & Pless, 1975).

The influence of health beliefs on illness behavior has been very difficult to determine. In part this difficulty reflects the fact that the Health Belief Model was designed to account for preventive behavior. The overwhelming problem, however, is a methodological one. "Illness behavior" is an extremely variable concept, including everything from emergency room visits to an individual's willingness to admit pain. As one might expect, the relationship between health beliefs and illness behaviors depends on the outcome measures employed. For the use of medical services, the most important health belief is the perception of increased symptom severity. This is true for adults responding to their own symptoms as well as for parents responding to their childrens' symptoms (Kirscht, 1974; Rosenstock & Kirscht, 1979). The relationship between this belief and illness behavior (at least for adults) may be curvilinear, however, because anxiety is correlated with delay in seeking treatment (Kasl & Cobb, 1966).

Mechanic (1964) explored the relationships among demographic characteristics, mothers' health beliefs, stress, and the use of pediatric medical services. Mothers' education was positively correlated with the belief that illness could be prevented and with specific health behaviors such as taking the child's temperature. Mothers with a relatively high inclination to use medical services for themselves expressed a similar tendency to use services for their children, although given the same circumstances of illness mothers were more likely to actually use services for their children than for themselves. Mothers under stress reported more illness symptoms both for themselves and for their children and tended to use pediatric services more frequently than did mothers not experiencing stress. Unfortunately, there were no data in Mechanic's study to indicate whether children of mothers under stress experienced more illness or whether these mothers simply reported more illness. Others have suggested that maternal stress does not increase the incidence of illness; rather, it raises mothers' tendency to perceive and report it (Roghmann & Haggerty, 1973, 1975; Rosenstock & Kirscht, 1979). Roghmann and Haggerty (1973, 1975) reported that the probability of initiating medical contacts was greater on stressful days independent of the occurrence of illness. In particular, stress was associated with the use of accessible sources of care (e.g., phone calls, emergency room visits).

Parents' beliefs about their children's vulnerability to illness have also been suggested as a predictive factor for illness behavior (Becker, Nathanson, et al., 1977; Green & Solnit, 1964; Levy, 1980). Green and Solnit (1964) described a "vulnerable child syndrome" in children with histories of early life-threatening illness or accident whose parents subsequently considered them extraordinarily vulnerable and destined to die before maturity. Levy (1980) reported that among the nearly 800 inner city children in her sample, those designated particularly vulnerable by their parents used more medical services than their nonvulnerable peers. Moreover, for cases in which parents' perceptions of vulnerability could not be substantiated by impartial inspection of medical records, the pattern of utilization included less comprehensive consultation with primary care facilities and more reported dissatisfaction with care. This tendency toward dissatisfaction was also noted by Becker, Nathanson, et al. (1977). In a prospective study of health beliefs among mothers of low socioeconomic status, they found less satisfaction with care and less agreement with diagnoses among mothers who used services for care of acute illnesses rather than for prevention. Mothers who used more illness services also reported that they "worry a lot" about their children's health and that their children "get sick easily." Unfortunately, in spite of the prospective nature of their study, it could not be ascertained from the data whether mothers' health beliefs were the antecedent or the consequence of behavior.

It is not surprising that mothers' health beliefs have been correlated with use of pediatric medical services because they most often decide when and how to obtain medical care. For illness behaviors such as the reporting of pain or symptoms, however, the child's own health beliefs probably assume a more influential role. Mechanic (1964) asked fourth and eighth grade students about their willingness to report pain, their willingness to report illness symptoms, and their fear of being hurt. (Note the similarity between the latter variable and what some investigators have called "perceived vulnerability.") The most impressive findings of the study were the relationships between the children's responses and their age and sex. A greater proportion of boys than girls in both age groups reported that they had "no fear of getting hurt" and did not "pay attention to pain." Risk taking and pain denial were higher among eighth grade than fourth grade students among children of both sexes. The willingness to report symptoms of illness was not related to age or sex except among older boys. Nearly half of the eighth grade boys indicated that they would not admit illness. The clear implication of these findings was that boys had learned to deny pain and illness and to appear invulnerable. Kasl and Cobb (1966) reached the same conclusion from evidence that boys experienced more illness but used fewer services than girls. Perceptions of invulnerability to illness have also been reported more frequently among inner city than non–inner city children (Gochman, 1972). Apparently these relationships among social characteristics, health beliefs, and illness behaviors change little during adolescence because in adulthood the individuals most likely to delay in seeking diagnoses are men of low socioeconomic status (Rosenstock, 1974a).

Sick-role Behavior

The recognition and diagnosis of illness often necessitates adjustments in lifestyle. An acute illness may demand relatively few changes in the daily routine (e.g., taking medication according to a prescribed schedule, modifying school and play activities, and visiting the pediatrician). A chronic illness, on the other hand, may involve significant emotional adjustment in addition to medical treatment. Compliance with treatment regimens (both acute and chronic) and adjustment to chronic illness are the most challenging problems associated with the sick role and are likely to come to the attention of pediatric psychologists.

Compliance. As generally defined, compliance refers to the extent to which a patient adheres to a prescribed therapeutic regimen. The regimen may include such diverse behaviors as taking medication, modifying diet, and keeping appointments for follow-up care. Some authors have also considered cognitive elements of compliance, such as learning the name of the medication and the dosage schedule (Becker, Drachman, & Kirscht, 1974). Overall, cognitive and behavioral elements of compliance are positively correlated, although behavioral measures such as administering medication and keeping appointments are not necessarily related to one another (Becker et al., 1974) or stable over time (Kasl, 1974). For this reason it is important to distinguish among the elements of compliance both conceptually and empirically (Becker et al., 1974; Becker, Maiman, Kirscht, Haefner, & Drachman, 1977). Compliant behaviors such as keeping appointments and pursuing referrals have been studied in pediatric populations and are reviewed elsewhere (cf. Becker, Drachman, & Kirscht, 1972; Becker et al., 1974; Fy, 1978; Kasl, 1974; Mattar & Yaffe, 1974; Rosenstock & Kirscht, 1979). In general, these behaviors appear rather easily facilitated by appropriate structural interventions to ensure care by the same physician at each visit, convenient appointment times with specifically named providers, and external reminders of appointment times (e.g., postcards or phone calls).   ·

The compliant behavior of greatest import to physicians and psychologists is that of taking medication. Drug noncompliance constitutes a significant health risk, precludes determination of a drug's effectiveness, and, in the case of antibiotic therapy, may increase the disease organism's resistance to treatment. In addition to its direct effect on quality of care and outcome, noncompliance may undermine the physician-patient relationship and satisfaction with care (Becker & Maiman, 1975). Among the many techniques used to assess drug compliance are direct measurement of the drug or its metabolites in blood or urine, pill counts, and subjective reports. Estimates of compliance have varied widely depending on the definition (i.e., partial versus total) and measurement of compliance, the duration and complexity of treatment, and a host of psychosocial influences. Pediatric compliance has been estimated between 20 and 80 percent, with a modal estimate around 50 percent (Haggerty & Roghmann, 1972; Litt & Cuskey, 1980; Mattar & Yaffe, 1974). Parents' most frequent reason for terminating drug administration is that the child "feels better" (Becker, 1974b; Litt & Cuskey, 1980). As a result, compliance is often less than 50 percent in asymptomatic children (Mattar & Yaffe, 1974). Compliance is generally lower among children than adults (Mattar & Yaffe, 1974) and is especially poor among adolescents (Litt & Cuskey, 1980).

Physicians have had a notoriously difficult time predicting pediatric compliance (Charney, Bynum, Eldridge, Frank, MacWhinney, McNabb, Scheiner, Sumpter, & Iker, 1967; Ey, 1978). Unlike preventive and illness behaviors, compliance has not been related in any consistent way to demographic characteristics of the child or parents (Becker, 1974b; Charney et al., 1967; Kasl, 1974; Marston, 1970; Mattar & Yaffe, 1974). Neither the particular illness, the physician's rating of severity at onset, nor the type of medication has been predictive of compliance (Charney et al., 1967), although compliance was often lower in the case of long-term or complex regimens (Litt & Cuskey, 1980; Mattar & Yaffe, 1974). Compliance with recommendations for acute illness decreased over time (Charney et al., 1967), and in general, compliance with short-term regimens was greater than with long-term regimens (Ey, 1978). Some relatively simple interventions, such as giving verbal and written instructions, labeling drugs precisely, and giving patients a calibrated measure, have been effective in increasing medication compliance (Mattar & Yaffe, 1974). Beyond these structural features, psychosocial characteristics involving the physician-patient relationship, family functioning, and mothers' health beliefs offer the greatest promise for the facilitation of compliance.

A modified version of the Health Belief Model has been applied successfully to the explanation and prediction of pediatric compliance (Becker, 1974b; Becker et al., 1972, 1974). Several health beliefs have been related to compliant behavior. First, compliant mothers believed that their ill children were vulnerable to the progressive effects of illness or were susceptible to the recurrence of illness (Becker et al., 1972, 1974; Becker, Haefner et al., 1977; Becker, Maiman et al., 1977). In the case of chronic illness, compliance was generally best among mothers who recognized that their ill children were more vulnerable than others and would require medication for their lifetime (Radius, Becker, Rosenstock, Drachman, Schuberth, & Teets, 1978). Second, although there was no evidence that compliance was related objectively to illness severity or to physicians' assessment of seriousness, there was a strong relationship between compliance and mothers' belief in the seriousness of illness (Becker, 1974b; Becker, Maiman et al., 1977; Becker et al., 1972, 1974; Charney et al., 1967; Mattsson, 1972; Radius et al., 1978). A note of caution is necessary, however, because mothers' perceptions of extreme vulnerability or severity may produce anxiety sufficient to inhibit acceptance of recommendations (Becker, Haefner et al., 1977), decrease recall of instructions (Becker, 1974b), and induce feelings of helplessness (Leventhal, 1973). Finally, compliance was associated with mothers' belief in the benefits and efficacy of treatment, agreement with diagnosis, and satisfaction with care (Becker et al., 1972, 1974). In addition to beliefs about their children's health, mothers' perceptions that it was "easy to get through the day" has been strongly related to behavioral compliance in acute treatment regimens (Becker et al., 1972, 1974). Mothers who reported that treatment regimens were personally disruptive were also poor compliers with chronic treatment recommendations for their children (Radius et al., 1978).

Adjustment to chronic illness. An illness is considered chronic if it persists longer than three months. At any given time, 10 to 20 percent of the children under 18 years of age have a chronic physical disorder (Pless & Satterwhite, 1975). If sensory and speech impairments, mental retardation, and learning and behavior disorders are included, 30 to 40 percent of children under age 18 suffer from one or more chronic disorders (Mattsson, 1972). Chronic illness causes disability and interference with ordinary daily activities in a significant number of children (Battle, 1975). Almost one-half of all chronically ill children are judged by their parents to be unable to participate in activities in which they otherwise would have (Pless & Satterwhite, 1975). Repeated exacerbations and remissions, permanent physical disfigurement or impairment, and shortened life expectancy are among the stresses imposed by chronic illness. These children are at risk for underachievement and emotional maladjustment, although the latter appears directly related to parents' knowledge about the disease and to family functioning (Pless, Roghmann, & Haggerty, 1972; Pless & Satterwhite, 1975).

The use of cognitive and emotional functions to cope with chronic illness is more significant for psychosocial adaptation to illness than is the nature of the illness itself. Mattsson (1972) identified some of the coping mechanisms associated with adequate and poor adaptation. In general, well-adapted children tended to display little need for secondary gains from illness, used cognitive skills to understand and accept their limitations realistically, participated in compensatory intellectual and motor activities, relied on their families for support, and released emotions appropriately. In contrast, poorly adapted children tended to demonstrate one of three behavioral patterns: fearfulness, inactivity, and dependency; denial of realistic dangers and risk-taking behaviors; or loneliness and resentment (Mattsson, 1972). Suicide has been attempted by children who were extremely depressed or resentful as well as by those who perceived their physical illness as disfiguring or as an obstacle to vocational or academic achievement (Weinberg, 1970). Children who harbored resentment about illness occasionally used noncompliance, passivity, or excessive risk-taking as weapons against self or others (Mattsson, 1972).

Chronic illness requires relatively sophisticated cognitive functioning in addition to emotional coping mechanisms. For example, chronically ill children must recognize and avoid risk even in the absence of symptoms, continue to take medication even if they "feel better" (or even if they know that the medication will not help them to feel better), and comply with treatment regimes indefinitely (Kasl, 1974). Totally compliant behavior depends on a sophisticated set of beliefs and knowledge about health. As Leventhal (1973) cogently pointed out:

> There is a difference between receiving, understanding and memorizing information and having that information change one's evaluations and desires. People are told that smoking causes cancer, that consuming butter and animal fats leads to

cholesterol deposits and cardiac disease; and they hear, understand and remember. But they do not necessarily believe that cigarettes are dangerous, nor do they taste the danger in the butter [p. 572].

In order to avoid a health threat, one must possess both the knowledge to identify the dangerous agent or activity and the belief that it in fact constitutes a threat. This task is many times more difficult for children than for adults due to the limitations of the developing cognitive system. To extend Leventhal's example, adults may choose to eat butter despite their knowledge of the connection between butter, cholesterol deposits, and cardiac disease. Young children, on the other hand, may not be capable of comprehending that causal link. It is not surprising, then, that chronically ill children often forget or refuse medication when they "feel better," because for them "feeling better" necessarily implies the absence of disease or illness. For all children, the understanding of illness causality is basic to their adjustment to illness and treatment. Therefore it is essential that pediatric psychologists appreciate the developmental history of health and illness concepts.

DEVELOPMENTAL CONCEPTIONS OF HEALTH AND ILLNESS

Knowledge and beliefs about health and illness develop gradually during childhood. As they grow and experience their share of illness, children begin to postulate cause-and-effect relationships. For young children the temporal or spatial contiguity of two events is sufficient for the presumption of causality. Thus a youngster may conclude that "I got sick because I was bad" or "I caught a cold because I went outside without wearing a hat." These statements are not the result of erroneous learning or reasoning. On the contrary, they reflect the perfectly normal use of developing cognitive processes to understand causality.

Jean Piaget has provided the most comprehensive developmental framework within which to consider children's health knowledge and beliefs (Phillips, 1969; Piaget, 1959, 1969; Piaget & Inhelder, 1969; Sigel & Cocking, 1977). According to Piaget, the acquisition of knowledge depends on complementary processes with which the child integrates new elements of the environment into existing mental structures and modifies existing mental structures to conform to the new elements. These dynamic processes enable the child to interact with the environment in increasingly complex ways, thereby creating, altering, and objectifying knowledge (Sigel & Cocking, 1977). Cognitive development progresses through an invariant sequence of age-related stages, each of which is characterized by a qualitatively different mode of reasoning. Rational notions of causality constitute a sophisticated and relatively late acquisition during childhood. Before a child develops the ability to reason causally, he or she demonstrates precausal reasoning involving fantasy, belief in magic, and attribution of life to inanimate objects. A brief review of Piaget's stages will illustrate the development of health knowledge and beliefs.

In Piaget's *sensorimotor* stage (birth to two years), a child does not distinguish between the self and the external world and consequently believes that his or her own actions are the source and cause of all events. During the *preoperational* stage (two to seven years of age), the child begins to experience the world as distinct from self. He or she is not yet capable of assuming the perspective of another person and is preoccupied with immediate sensory experiences. Reasoning is concrete, irreversible, and centered on single aspects of an event to the exclusion of the whole.

Bibace and Walsh (1979) identified two substages in the preoperational child's understanding of illness causality. The first, phenomenism, is characterized by the belief that illness is caused magically by a single external sensory event that was associated with it. For example, the child may explain that the wind caused illness, or describe a heart attack as "falling on your back [p. 291]." During the second preoperational substage, contagion, illness is believed to be caused by physical proximity to (although not necessarily contact with) an external agent; thus one may catch a cold simply by walking near someone who has a cold. Children at this level tend to apply the concept of contagion uncritically (Nagy, 1951) and are not likely to understand the effect of distance between people on the likelihood of contracting illness (Kister & Patterson, 1980). They may also overextend the concept of contagion to accidents and noncontagious illnesses (Kister & Patterson, 1980).

Along with the development of logical reasoning, Piaget postulated age-related changes in the emergence of moral reasoning. Preoperational children typically comply with rules because they believe them to be unalterable. Violations of social norms are necessarily followed by immediate punishment, which may be delivered in the form of misfortune, accidents, or illness (Peters, 1978). This tendency to invoke the concept of immanent justice for illness causality decreases with age as the child learns to understand the rational causes of illness (Kister & Patterson, 1980), although there is some evidence that anxious and ill children retain a belief in immanent justice longer than do their healthy, nonanxious peers (Brodie, 1974).

During Piaget's stage of *concrete operations* (7 to 11 years), the child begins to distinguish between the internal and external worlds and may identify specific external causes of illness. The first concrete operational substage, contamination, is characterized by the child's suggestion that illness is caused by physical contact between some contaminating agent and an external body surface (e.g., one catches measles by rubbing against someone who has them). Later, during the substage of internalization, the child begins to realize that contaminants must be taken inside the body for infection to occur. For example, one may become sick by "breathing in germs that get in your blood." It is also during the stage of concrete operations that the child begins to conceive of the reversibility of physical or mental processes. Therefore, he or she begins to entertain notions that illness is curable and preventable (Bibace & Walsh, 1979).

During Piaget's final stage, *formal operations* (11 to 15 years and beyond), the child is no longer bound by sensory experience or external stimuli. Thus the formal operational child is able to reason logically and hypothetically, and to consider possibilities beyond concrete reality. He or she develops an understanding of internal body functioning and multiple causality. During the physiological substage, the child may explain illness in terms of physiological causes (e.g., blockage of heart valves may precipitate a heart attack). During the final substage, psychophysiological, the young adult recognizes that personal actions and psychological factors affect health and illness. It is during this period that the individual may hypothesize that thoughts, feelings, and stress can influence bodily function (Bibace & Walsh, 1979). Similar developmental stages have been described for children's understanding of body parts (Williams, 1979), self-awareness (Gilbert & Finell, 1978), procreation (Bernstein & Cowan, 1975), medical procedures (Steward & Regalbuto, 1975), and death (Childers & Wimmer, 1971; Koocher, 1973; White, Elsom, & Prawat, 1978). Likewise, there is a gradual emergence during childhood of various beliefs related to health. For example, before age 10 children often fail to recognize their vulnerability to illness, but by age 17 they can estimate the probability of illness realistically (Gochman, 1970, 1971, 1972; Gochman, Bagramian, & Sheiham, 1972).

Piaget proposed that cognitive stages were linked to chronological age; nevertheless, there is some evidence of cognitive regression in sick and hospitalized children (cf. Blos, 1978; Brodie, 1974; Myers-Vando, Steward, Folkins, & Hines, 1979; Parrish, 1978). It has also been suggested that health history interacts with age to influence illness concepts, producing less sophisticated concepts in younger ill children and more sophisticated concepts in older ill children (Campbell, 1975).

IMPLICATIONS FOR CHILD HEALTH CARE

Since its recognition as a national priority, significant contributions to child health care have been made by medical and public health professionals. Their efforts have produced overwhelming improvements in the care of high-risk infants, the prevention of fatal diseases, and the treatment of infectious diseases. However, current child health care needs (e.g., accident prevention, compliance) extend beyond the scope of medical technology and are appropriately within the domain of child health psychology.

In years past a strictly medical approach has defined health as the absence of disease and symptoms as the manifestation of disease. The use of medical services was thought to be a function of illness severity. Acceptance of this orientation implied that medical care was the appropriate intervention for all health needs. As an alternative to this model, consider the assumptions underlying the Health Belief Model. Health is not only the absence of disease, but is a positively valued state of physical and emotional well-being that can be promoted through changes in behavior and attitudes. The Health Belief Model also assumes that the report of illness does not necessarily imply the presence of disease. When disease is present, there are almost certainly other factors involved in the decision to take action: learned responses to pain, stress, or a sudden change in the individual's perception of the seriousness of the symptoms. Likewise, the use of medical services is a function of the collective influence of the individual's health beliefs and demographic characteristics and the availability and cost of services. A shift in emphasis from an entirely medical to a psychosocial approach has clear implications for the improvement of health care. Children's health behaviors may be promoted through modification of beliefs and knowledge of both children and their parents.

A significant portion of pediatric psychological service is devoted to the modification of children's health behaviors. Application of the Health Belief Model suggests two strategies for changing behavior, both of which are based on the modification of health beliefs (Rosenstock & Kirscht, 1974). First, health beliefs may be modified directly by the induction of fear of the negative consequences of illness. The rationale for this approach is that fear (in some sufficient but not excessive amount) will motivate the individual to engage in health behaviors. This has been demonstrated successfully in adults (Haefner & Kirscht, 1970) and children (Haefner, 1965) by using messages designed to increase perceptions of vulnerability, the seriousness of illness, and the benefits of health actions. As a qualifier to this strategy, Leventhal (1973) has suggested that fear acts only to change health *beliefs*. In order to effect a change in behavior, a specific structure or plan for action must be provided in addition to the fear messages. In using this approach, it is also important to recognize that the "optimally motivating" level of fear differs for each health belief and behavior. For example, an individual who already perceives himself or herself as susceptible to illness may be incapacitated by a high fear message that will increase the perception of vulnerability. Moreover, individuals who feel vulnerable may choose to participate in behaviors that will decrease their anxiety (e.g., toothbrushing for the prevention of tooth decay) but may not participate in activities that will increase anxiety (e.g., a dental examination). In addition, the optimal level of fear may be influenced by demographic characteristics such as age and socioeconomic status.

The second strategy for changing health beliefs is through modification of the health care delivery system. This approach is based on the assumption that discontinuous, costly, inaccessible, or inadequate care leads to parental dissatisfaction, a fatalistic attitude, and a lack of faith in the health care system. Improvement in the delivery of services may encourage health behaviors by preventing the development of these negative beliefs. Since health behaviors and health beliefs share a reciprocal influence, regular participation in health actions (e.g., routine medical examination) may reinforce adaptive health beliefs.

For the most part, the strategies suggested by the Health Belief Model affect parent-initiated health behaviors through modification of parents' health beliefs. Child health care may be improved through direct modification of children's health beliefs and self-initiated behaviors as well. Drawing on psychological research concerning accidents, compliance, adjustment to chronic illness, and so on, it is possible to identify children at risk for maladaptive health behaviors. For example, it is known that young children (particularly boys) who are extremely active and aggressive tend to become involved in accidents repeatedly (Wright et al., 1979). On a cognitive level, these children fail to recognize their vulnerability to accidents (Gochman, 1970, 1971, 1972; Gochman et al., 1972). Older boys are even more vulnerable because they also tend to deny pain and to delay in seeking medical help (*Health U. S.,* 1978; Mechanic, 1964). Another possible target population for modification of health behaviors is chronically ill adolescents. Compliance with long-term treatment regimens is notoriously poor among adolescents, but may be encouraged somewhat by granting the child autonomy and self-responsibility for medical care (Litt & Cuskey, 1980).

Prevention must be a primary focus for clinical and educational service to parents and children. Well-child care is effective for the prevention and early diagnosis of many diseases and is less traumatic and less costly than illness care. In addition, preventive behavior may be easier to modify because it is fundamentally a planned, goal-directed behavior. Illness behavior is often impulsive and may be more difficult to predict or modify. Educational efforts must begin early and continue throughout life. Although obedience and conformity may elicit some health behaviors, education of children and parents is more likely to foster the health beliefs that result in lasting and responsible health behaviors.

It is important to consider children's health knowledge and beliefs within the more general context of cognitive development. Young children's health concepts and beliefs may seem to have no basis in reality. They may even sound amusing to the adult. Nevertheless, they cannot be dismissed as wrong or as developmentally inappropriate. Statements about health constitute an important source of information for the physician or psychologist because they reflect the child's general level of cognitive and emotional functioning. The clinician or educator who realizes that learning may be limited by developmental stage can devise appropriate methods for explaining health practices and medical procedures as well as for obtaining cooperation and compliance. Awareness that the stress of illness may produce cognitive regression is also helpful in evaluating children's cognitive functioning and emotional adaptation to illness.

The need for scientific study of children's health behaviors is overwhelming. There is a paucity of information about the frequency and types of self-initiated behaviors, the role of children's health beliefs in these behaviors, the optimal limits of each belief, the ways in which health beliefs might interact to determine behavior, and the most effective strategies for changing these beliefs and behaviors. Accidents, risk taking, and noncompliance are among the most challenging problems confronting health care professionals, yet we know little about their psychological correlates.

To date there have been two distinct approaches to research on child health behaviors: what one might call a public health approach, exemplified by social psychologists and public health physicians, and the developmental approach, exemplified by cognitive-developmental psychologists. Investigators using the former approach have provided useful information about group differences in observable behaviors such as the use of medical services. Investigators in the latter group have concentrated primarily on individual differences in knowledge, health beliefs, and emotional adjustment to illness. A fruitful approach for future research may be some integration of these two traditions. This would enable us to identify risk factors (including those involving interactions between beliefs and demographic characteristics) and to test various intervention strategies experimentally in large groups of children. In addition, knowledge of individual differences in cognitive and emotional functioning would enable us to apply these research findings optimally to each child. It is imperative that we continue these efforts in order to achieve our goal of optimal child health care.

REFERENCES

Battle, C. U. Chronic physical disease. *Pediatric Clinics of North America,* 1975, **22**, 525–531.

Becker, M. H. (Ed.) *The health belief model and personal health behavior.* Thorofare, N.J.: Charles B. Slack, 1974. (a)

Becker, M. H. The health belief model and sick role behavior. In M. H. Becker (Ed.), *The health belief model and personal health behavior.* Thorofare, N.J.: Charles B. Slack, 1974. (b)

Becker, M. H., Drachman, R. H., & Kirscht, J. P. Predicting mothers' compliance with pediatric medical regimens. *Journal of Pediatrics,* 1972, **81**, 843–854.

Becker, M. H., Drachman, R. H., & Kirscht, J. P. A new approach to explaining sick-role behavior in low-income populations. *American Journal of Public Health,* 1974, **64**, 205–216.

Becker, M. H., Haefner, D. P., Kasl, S. V., Kirscht, J. P., Maiman, L. A., & Rosenstock, I. M. Selected psychosocial models and correlates of individual health-related behaviors. *Medical Care,* 1977, **15**, 27–46.

Becker, M. H., & Maiman, L. A. Sociobehavioral determinants of compliance with health and medical care recommendations. *Medical Care,* 1975, **13**, 10–24.

Becker, M. H., Maiman, L. A., Kirscht, J. P., Haefner, D. P., & Drachman, R. H. The health belief model and prediction of dietary compliance: A field experiment. *Journal of Health and Social Behavior,* 1977, **18**, 348–366.

Becker, M. H., Nathanson, C. A., Drachman, R. H., & Kirscht, J. P. Mothers' health beliefs and children's clinic visits: A prospective study. *Journal of Community Health,* 1977, **3**, 125–135.

Bernstein, A C., & Cowan, P. A. Children's concepts of how people get babies. *Child Development,* 1975, **46,** 77–91.

Bibace, R., & Walsh, M. E. Developmental stages in children's conceptions of illness. In G. C. Stone, F. Cohen, N. E. Adler, & Associates (Eds.), *Health psychology.* San Francisco: Jossey-Bass, 1979.

Blos, P. Children think about illness: Their conceptions and beliefs. In E. Gellert (Ed.), *Psychosocial aspects of pediatric care.* New York: Grune & Stratton, 1978.

Brodie, B. Views of healthy children toward illness. *American Journal of Public Health,* 1974, **64,** 1156–1159.

Campbell, J. D. Illness is a point of view: The development of children's concepts of illness. *Child Development,* 1975, **46,** 92–100.

Charney, E., Bynum, R., Eldridge, D., Frank, D., MacWhinney, J. B., McNabb, N., Scheiner, A., Sumpter, E. A., & Iker, H. How well do patients take oral penicillin? A collaborative study in private practice. *Pediatrics,* 1967, **40,** 188–195.

Childers, P., & Wimmer, M. The concept of death in early childhood. *Child Development,* 1971, **42,** 1299–1301.

Ey, J. L. Compliance with recommendations. In R. A. Hoekelman, S. Blatman, P. A. Brunnell, S. B. Friedman, & H. M. Seidel (Eds.), *Principles of pediatrics.* New York: McGraw-Hill, 1978.

Fabrega, H. Toward a model of illness behavior. *Medical Care,* 1973, **11,** 470–484.

Gilbert, D. C., & Finell, L. Young child's awareness of self. *Psychological Reports,* 1978, **43,** 911–914.

Gochman, D. S. Children's perceptions of vulnerability to illness and accidents. *U. S. Public Health Reports,* 1970, **85,** 69–73.

Gochman, D. S. Children's perceptions of vulnerability to illness and accidents: A replication, extension, and refinement. *HSMHA Health Reports,* 1971, **86,** 247–252.

Gochman, D. S. Development of health beliefs. *Psychological Reports,* 1972, **31,** 259–266.

Gochman, D. S., Bagramian, R. A., & Sheiham, A. Consistency in children's perceptions of vulnerability to health problems. *Health Services Reports,* 1972, **87,** 282–288.

Green, M., & Solnit, A. J. Reactions to the threatened loss of a child: A vulnerable child syndrome. *Pediatrics,* 1964, **34,** 58–66.

Haefner, D. P. Arousing fear in dental health education. *Journal of Public Health Dentistry,* 1965, **25,** 140–146.

Haefner, D. P., & Kirscht, J. P. Motivational and behavioral effects of modifying health beliefs. *Public Health Reports,* 1970, **85,** 478–484.

Haggerty, R. J., & Roghmann, K. J. Noncompliance and self-medication: Two neglected aspects of pediatric pharmacology. *Pediatric Clinics of North America,* 1972, **19,** 101–115.

Health United States 1978 (Public Health Service Publication no. 78-1232). Washington: U. S. Department of Health, Education, and Welfare, 1978.

Hochbaum, G. M. Why people seek diagnostic x-rays. *Public Health Reports,* 1956, **71,** 377–380.

Kasl, S. V. The health belief model and behavior related to chronic illness. In M. H. Becker (Ed.), *The health belief model and personal health behavior.* Thorofare, N.J.: Charles B. Slack, 1974.

Kasl, S. V., & Cobb, S. Health behavior, illness behavior, and sick-role behavior. I. Health and Illness Behavior. *Archives of Environmental Health,* 1966, **12,** 246–266.

Kirscht, J. P. The health belief model and illness behavior. In M. H. Becker (Ed.), *The health belief model and personal health behavior.* Thorofare, N.J.: Charles B. Slack, 1974.

Kister, M. C., & Patterson, C. J. Children's conceptions of the causes of illness: Understanding of contagion and use of immanent justice. *Child Development,* 1980, **51,** 839–846.

Koocher, G. P. Childhood, death, and cognitive development. *Developmental Psychology,* 1973, **9,** 369–375.

Leventhal, H. Changing attitudes and habits to reduce risk factors in chronic disease. *American Journal of Cardiology,* 1973, **31,** 571–581.

Levy, J. C. Vulnerable children: Parents' perspectives and the use of medical care. *Pediatrics,* 1980, **65,** 956–963.

Litt, I. F., & Cuskey, W. R. Compliance with medical regimens during adolescence. *Pediatric Clinics of North America,* 1980, **27,** 3–15.

Maiman, L. A., & Becker, M. H. The health belief model: Origins and correlates in psychological theory. In M. H. Becker (Ed.), *The health belief model and personal health behavior.* Thorofare, N.J.: Charles B. Slack, 1974.

Marston, M. V. Compliance with medical regimens. *Nursing Research,* 1970, **19,** 312–323.

Mattar, M. E., & Yaffe, S. J. Compliance of pediatric patients with therapeutic regimens. *Postgraduate Medicine,* 1974, **56,** 181–188.

Mattsson, A. Long-term physical illness in childhood: A challenge to psychosocial adaptation. *Pediatrics,* 1972, **50,** 801–811.

Mechanic, D. The concept of illness behavior. *Journal of Chronic Diseases,* 1962, **15,** 189–194.

Mechanic, D. The influence of mothers on their children's health attitudes and behavior. *Pediatrics,* 1964, **33,** 444–453.

Mofenson, H. C., & Greensher, J. Childhood accidents. In R. A. Hoekelman, S. Blatman, P. A. Brunell, S. B. Friedman, & H. M. Seidel (Eds.), *Principles of pediatrics.* New York: McGraw-Hill, 1978.

Myers-Vando, R., Steward, M. S., Folkins, C. H., & Hines, P. The effects of congenital heart disease on cognitive development, illness causality concepts, and vulnerability. *American Journal of Orthopsychiatry,* 1979, **49,** 617–625.

Nagy, M. H. Children's ideas of the origin of illness. *Health Education Journal,* 1951, **9,** 6–12.

Parrish, R. A. M. Constructs of self-image. In J. Curry & K. K. Pepe (Eds.), *Mental retardation: Nursing approaches to care.* St. Louis: C. V. Mosby, 1978.

Peters, B. M. School-aged children's beliefs about causality of illness: A review of the literature. *Maternal-Child Nursing Journal,* 1978, **7,** 143–154.

Phillips, J. L., Jr. *The origins of intellect: Piaget's theory.* San Francisco: W. H. Freeman, 1969.

Piaget, J. *Judgment and reasoning in the child.* Peterson, N.J.: Littlefield, Adams, 1959.

Piaget, J. *The child's conception of physical causality.* Totowa, N.J.: Littlefield, Adams, 1969.

Piaget, J., & Inhelder, B. *The psychology of the child.* New York: Basic Books, 1969.

Pless, I. B. Current morbidity and mortality among the young. In R. A. Hoekelman, S. Blatman, P. A. Brunell, S. B. Friedman, and H. M. Seidel (Eds.), *Principles of pediatrics.* New York: McGraw-Hill, 1978.

Pless, I. B., Roghmann, K., & Haggerty, R. J. Chronic illness, family functioning, and psychological adjustment: A model for the allocation of preventive health services. *International Journal of Epidemiology,* 1972, **1,** 271–277.

Pless, I. B., & Satterwhite, B. B. Chronic illness. In R. J. Haggerty, K. J. Roghmann, & I. B. Pless (Eds.), *Child health and the community.* New York: Wiley, 1975.

Pratt, L. Child rearing methods and children's health behavior. *Journal of Health and Social Behavior,* 1973, **14,** 61–69.

Radius, S. M., Becker, M. H., Rosenstock, I. M., Drachman, R. H., Schuberth, K. C., & Teets, K. C. Factors influencing mothers' compliance with a medication regimen for asthmatic children. *Journal of Asthma Research,* 1978, **15,** 133–149.

Roghmann, K. J., & Haggerty, R. J. Daily stress, illness, and the use of health services in young families. *Pediatric Research,* 1973, **7,** 520–526.

Roghmann, K. J., & Haggerty, R. J. The stress model for illness behavior. In R. J. Haggerty, K. J. Roghmann, & I. B. Pless (Eds.), *Child health and the community.* New York: Wiley, 1975.

Roghmann, K. J., & Pless, I. B. Acute illness. In R. J. Haggerty, K. J. Roghmann, & I. B. Pless (Eds.), *Child health and the community.* New York: Wiley, 1975.

Rosenstock, I. M. Why people use health services. *Milbank Memorial Fund Quarterly,* 1966, **44,** 94–127.

Rosenstock, I. M. The health belief model and preventive health behavior. In M. H. Becker (Ed.), *The health belief model and personal health behavior.* Thorofare, N.J.: Charles B. Slack, 1974. (a)

Rosenstock, I. M. Historical origins of the health belief model. In M. H. Becker (Ed.), *The health belief model and personal health behavior.* Thorofare, N.J.: Charles B. Slack, 1974. (b)

Rosenstock, I. M., & Kirscht, J. P. Practice implications. In M. H. Becker (Ed.), *The health belief model and personal health behavior.* Thorofare, N.J.: Charles B. Slack, 1974.

Rosenstock, I. M., & Kirscht, J. P. Why people seek health care. In G. C. Stone, F. Cohen, N. E. Adler, & Associates (Eds.), *Health psychology.* San Francisco: Jossey-Bass, 1979.

Sigel, I., & Cocking, R. R. *Cognitive development from childhood to adolescence: A constructivist perspective.* New York: Holt, Rinehart & Winston, 1977.

Steward, M., & Regalbuto, G. Do doctors know what children know? *American Journal of Orthopsychiatry,* 1975, **45**, 146–149.

Stone, G. C. Psychology and the health system. In G. C. Stone, F. Cohen, N. E. Adler, & Associates (Eds.), *Health psychology.* San Francisco: Jossey-Bass, 1979.

Weinberg, S. Suicidal interest in adolescence: A hypothesis about the role of physical illness. *Journal of Pediatrics,* 1970, **77**, 579–586.

White, E., Elsom, B., & Prawat, R. Children's conceptions of death. *Child Development,* 1978, **49**, 307–310.

Williams, P. D. Children's concepts of illness and internal body parts. *Maternal-Child Nursing Journal,* 1979, **8**, 115–123.

Wright, L., Schaefer, A. B., & Solomons, G. *Encyclopedia of pediatric psychology.* Baltimore: University Park Press, 1979.

The Epidemiology of Childhood Diseases

Marc S. Lewis
and
Suzanne Craft

One of the greatest detectives of all time was John Snow, a physician who lived in 19th-century London. In 1848 Snow faced his most difficult adversary: an epidemic of cholera that killed more than 500 people in ten days. At that time almost nothing was known about the cause of cholera and there seemed little that could be done to prevent the death of thousands within a short time. Despite the apparent hopelessness of the situation, Snow began to gather clues. He found that most deaths had occurred in a small area near Broad Street. This seemed to fit one of the popular theories of the day, which suggested that cholera was transmitted by warm air. But then a contradiction arose. Not one death had occurred among the workers in a brewery located near the center of the epidemic. Snow learned that the brewery workers differed from the local residents in one important way: residents drank water from a public pump, brewery workers drank only malt liquor or water from a private well. Even more significant was the following item that Snow found among the death reports for the epidemic: "At West End on 2nd September, the widow of a percussion cap maker, aged 59 years, diarrhea two hours, cholera epidemica sixteen hours." This woman, who had lived far from the affected area, had often sent for water from the Broad Street pump because it tasted better than water from pumps near her house. These and other clues led Snow to conclude that cholera was transmitted by water. At some risk to his reputation, he convinced the Parish Guardians to remove the handle from the guilty pump. This ended the epidemic and established a precedent that has saved many thousands of lives.

Those who, like Snow, study disease on a community level are called epidemiologists; the deductive method that they use is called epidemiology. The list of diseases prevented or cured by epidemiology is long, and includes smallpox, polio, typhoid fever, typhus, and bubonic plague.

But despite these successes, new diseases continue to evolve and some-times a significant part of the population has no immunity from them. Such a case occurred only seventy years ago, when swine flu killed twenty million people in less than two years. Even today the potential exists for an epidemic such as plague, a disease that killed one of every four Europeans in the 14th century. The aim of epidemiology is to discover the nature of such diseases and to prevent or cure them. In the following chapter we introduce some of the deductive methods that epidemiologists use.

Explorers sometimes carry diseases to the people that they find. There were about 25 million Aztecs in Mexico when Cortez arrived; less than a century later 24 million were dead from measles, smallpox, and other Western diseases (Crosby, 1972). About a hundred years later, those same diseases destroyed most of the North American Indians. For example, in just three years (1616–19) diseases carried by French, English, and Dutch traders killed nine-tenths of the Indians living on the coast of New England between Maine and Rhode Island. Consequently, when the Pilgrims arrived in 1620 the few Indians left on hand in Massachusetts were understandably reluctant to give them a warm welcome—especially since many of them had come to believe that the guns of the Pilgrims were the cause of disease (since both guns and disease killed mysteriously). In fact Squanto, the only member of the Pawtuxet Indians to survive both guns and disease, made his reputation among neighboring villages by claiming special protective powers. Two centuries later, in 1875, the king of the Fiji Islands visited New South Wales and brought home measles. The disease killed a quarter of his 160,000 subjects.

Like the king of the Fijis, children are visitors to a foreign country. At birth they possess some of their mothers' immunities, but after a time they become susceptible to a large body of diseases. This is why most childhood diseases occur in childhood. Measles can occur at any age, but children, like Aztecs, are highly susceptible because they lack immunity. It follows that the development of a vaccine against measles would change it from a childhood disease to a "disease of the unvaccinated" of all ages, and that is precisely what has happened in recent years. Similarly, smallpox (now believed extinct) was a childhood disease in the 18th century, but with the development of a vaccine in the 19th century it became a disease of all ages.

In many cases, then, the distinction between disease and childhood disease is fictitious. Often childhood diseases are simply those that attack the most vulnerable groups, and children are highly vulnerable. A corollary to this proposition is that if there were no children the pool of susceptible people would not be replenished and many diseases would become extinct.

Thus the epidemiology of childhood disease is like that of disease in general. Both use powerful techniques that are as closely allied to detective work as they are to the scientific method. The purpose of this chapter is to introduce some of those techniques within the framework of several childhood diseases. The primary focus will be on kuru, one of the most peculiar childhood diseases ever discovered.

KURU

After World War II, several aborigine tribes were discovered in the highlands of New Guinea. The people of those tribes were primarily hunters (pigs), farmers (sweet potatoes), and cannibals (relatives). These tribes also possessed something new to the outside world. In an area of roughly 2,000 square kilometers, a new disease was discovered among the Fore people. The Fore called the disease "kuru," a word which in their language meant trembling or shaking. Trembling is indeed a prominent early symptom of kuru, but the symptoms that follow are more dramatic.

> In the more advanced stage of the disorder it is impossible to stand erect and sitting becomes difficult. A stake is driven into the ground in front of the patient and he clutches precariously to this rigid support. In their huts a rope suspended from the ceiling serves the same purpose. Even this support eventually proves inadequate and the patient remains recumbent [Hornabrook, 1976, p. 66].

The cause of these symptoms can be traced to peculiar changes in brain tissue, changes that are similar to those seen in progressive degenerative diseases such as Creutzfeldt-Jacob disease and scrapie. As in those diseases, neurons are lost or degenerate, subcortical areas wither, and much of the tissue that remains grows spongy.

Kuru appears to have both an adult and a childhood form. The childhood form strikes both sexes equally and its course is rapid, with death usually occurring within four to eight months after onset. The adult form strikes women far more often than men and its course is slower than that of the childhood form, with death occurring about three years after onset.

THEORIES ABOUT KURU

The Fore believe that kuru is caused by magic. A "magician" makes a bundle of hair clippings, clothing, or other items taken from the victim, adds magic leaves, ties the bundle with vines, and buries it. As this fetish rots, the Fore believe, the victim's coordination deteriorates, and when it has completely rotted the victim dies.

The cure for kuru sorcery is a kind of environmental surgery—find the bundle and remove it from its burial place before it rots completely. However, since there is usually no bundle to be found, alternative courses of action have been developed. One school advises the victim to identify the sorcerer by casting charms with woodchuck meat, bamboo, and fire. A second school advises the victim to eat a medicinal meal of pork, ginger, and forest products. In addition, tiny arrows are shot into the victim's limbs, head, and any other areas where the kuru symptoms are strong (figure 4.1).

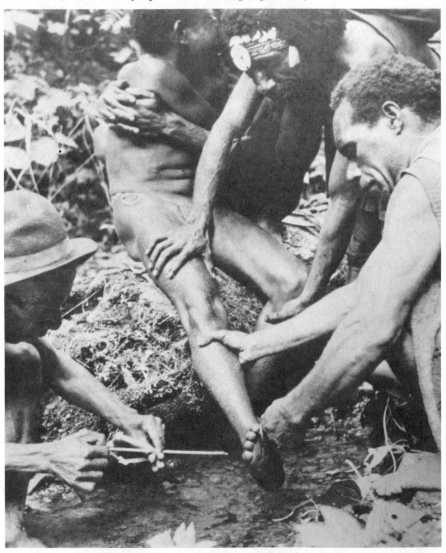

Fig. 4.1. A standard native treatment for childhood kuru. (From *Essays on Kuru* by R. W. Hornabrook. Faringdon, Oxfordshire: E. W. Classey Ltd. Copyright 1976 by E. W. Classey Ltd. Reprinted by permission.)

The magical theories and cures of the Fore strongly influenced the first Westerners on the scene, who saw kuru as a psychological disorder with death somehow caused by suggestion and by the victim's belief in magic. This theory did not survive long because it failed to explain some peculiarities of kuru. For example, the theory could not explain why kuru was rarely observed in members of nearby tribes whose belief in magic rivaled that of the Fore.

Another early Western theory postulated kuru as a genetic disease. This theory had some explanatory power, but a suspiciously complicated pattern of inheritance had to be invoked to explain the differences between the childhood and adult forms of the disease. Basically, kuru was attributed to a Mendelian trait carried by an autosomal allele (Ku) that was recessive in males but dominant in females. This hypothesized trait explained the rarity of kuru in adult males given the further postulate that male hetcrozygotes (Ku ku) were resistant to the disease. The childhood form of kuru would then be free to occur in homozygotes (Ku Ku) of either sex.

In addition to the genetic hypothesis, a number of less complicated non-genetic hypotheses were proposed, most of which blamed kuru on toxic substances in the environment, on nutritional deficits, or on biochemical abnormalities. These hypotheses, however, suffered from a common problem: none adequately explained the sex differences in the rate of kuru among adults and the lack of sex differences in the rate among children. We will consider some theories that do explain these sex differences, but first we turn to the general concept of disease rates.

RATES

Epidemiologists distinguish three broad types of disease rates: an endemic or normal rate; an epidemic or abnormally high rate; and a pandemic or extraordinarily high rate. The swine flu that killed 20 million people in 1918 is a recent example of a pandemic. For an interesting example of an epidemic we turn to a mysterious disease called the English swets. Between 1485 and 1551 the swets appeared about every 20 to 30 years and killed thousands of people, many of them children (Geddes, 1941). The disease was characterized by minor symptoms such as fever and excessive perspiration, but the familiarity of those symptoms was deceptive; the disease had an incredibly high case fatality rate— more than 99 percent of the people who contracted the swets died within a day or two. In England the preferred treatment for the swets was bed rest, a remedy that was raised to a high art in Germany, where it was believed that the patient should be kept under as many blankets as was necessary to "sweat" the fever out. To this end, some patients were simply sewn into their beds until they had recovered or died. The blanket treatment of the Germans aggravated the process of dehydration in patients and added to the already extraordinary fatality rate. In 1551 the swets suddenly disappeared and was never seen again. It remains one of the most mysterious epidemics in history.

The term "epidemic" is often misapplied to diseases that are pandemic (such as the Black Plague) and occasionally also misapplied to diseases that are epizootic (an epizootic is an epidemic that occurs in animals) as well. Some epidemics are indeed almost pandemics, but other epidemics are so subtle that they almost pass unnoticed. For example, in early December 1952 a polluted fog settled over London and killed 4,000 people (MacMahon, Pugh, & Ipsen, 1960). At the time no one believed that the fog was dangerous because the rise in deaths was small compared to the total population of the city. It was only in retrospect, when deaths in December 1952 were compared to deaths in previous years, that it became clear that the fog had produced a lethal epidemic.

In order to uncover subtle epidemics such as that of the London fog, many fine-grained methods for reporting rates have been developed. A sample of them is given in table 4.1. Typically these rates compare a group of interest (e.g., new cases of disease) to some relevant group (e.g., the number of people in the population). Thus, if 500 cases of measles occurred in 1980 in a population of 50,000, the one-year incidence rate for measles would be 500/50,000, or one case per 100 people in the population.

Epidemiologists are more than disease accountants, however, and it is not rates that are important but differences in rates compared across different populations or at different times. For example, the fact that nuns experience a low rate of cervical cancer is not as important a clue to the etiology of that disease as is the fact that they experience a far lower rate than prostitutes.

Using disease rates, we can develop clues about the etiology of kuru. For example, the kuru mortality rates shown in table 4.2 yield two such clues. First, the Fore have much greater rates than either the neighboring Gimi or Keiangana-Kanite tribes. This suggests that a comparison of the cultural, physiological, and environmental differences among the three tribes might help to uncover the cause of kuru. The second clue yielded by table 4.2 is that in each tribe the mortality rate for kuru followed an unusual pattern. Mortality decreased gradually until 1944, but then suddenly began to decrease far more dramatically than it had in the past. This decrease occurred at about the same time that the New Guinea tribes were first discovered, and it suggests that the decline might be connected to that discovery. Perhaps, for example, the scientific teams sent to study the Fore corrected a nutritional deficit that was responsible for kuru. Or perhaps simply the presence of such teams caused a change in some tribal custom that was important to the etiology of the disease. The two clues yielded by table 4.2 are not by themselves enough to solve the problem of kuru, but they are a first step in that direction.

Of the rates shown in table 4.1, the most commonly used are incidence, period prevalence, and point prevalence. Incidence refers to the number of new cases that occur in a population over a selected period (often one year). Period

Table 4.1.   Some Epidemiological Measures of Disease Rates

Measure	Numerator	Denominator
Crude birth rate	Live births during a selected interval	People in the population at the midpoint of the selected interval
Crude fertility rate	Live births during a selected interval	Women aged 15–44 at the midpoint of the selected interval
Low birth weight ratio	Live births under 2,500 grams (about 5.5 pounds) during a selected interval	Live births reported during the same interval
Incidence	New cases reported during a selected interval	People at risk at the midpoint of the selected interval
Point prevalence	All cases (new and old) in population during a selected point in time	People at risk at the selected point
Period prevalence	All cases (new and old) in the population during a selected interval	People at risk at the midpoint of the selected interval
Crude death rate	Total deaths reported during a selected interval	Risk during the selected interval
Case fatality ratio	Deaths caused by a given disease during a selected interval	Cases reported during that interval
Fetal death ratio	Fetal deaths at 20 (sometimes 28) weeks or more during a selected interval	Live births during that same interval
Infant mortality rate	Deaths under one year of age during a selected interval	Live births during that same interval

prevalence is similar to incidence, but includes old cases as well as new ones. Thus, for example, if in a population of 1,000 Fore there were 52 new cases of kuru in 1969 and 33 cases of kuru left over from previous years, then the one-year incidence for kuru would be 5.2 per 100 and the one-year period prevalence would be 8.5 per 100.

Point prevalence is like period prevalence in that it is a count of both old and new cases. However, in point prevalence the period of observation is very short (e.g., one day). Thus, for example, the point prevalence of kuru on June 1, 1969 might be 6.3 per 100 and on July 1 it might be 6.6 per 100.

When the course of a disease is fairly constant over time, an interesting relationship exists between its incidence (I), point prevalence (P) and duration

Table 4.2   Kuru Mortality Rates among Women
in Selected Census Districts
(Per 1,000)

Year of Birth	South Fore	North Fore	Gimi	Keiagana-Kanite
1954–58	2	—	1	—
1949–53	10	1	2	<1
1944–48	18	4	2	<1
1939–43	28	8	—	1
1934–38	53	3	3	2
1929–33	58	11	5	2
1924–28	71	30	4	3
1919–23	62	29	9	2
1914–18	26	29	2	3

Source: McArthur (1976)

(D) (duration is usually measured from time of onset to time of recovery or death). This relationship is expressed by the equation:

$$P = I \times D. \tag{4.1}$$

To illustrate the use of this equation, let us apply it to kuru among the Fore people. We have introduced no incidence rates for kuru, but since the disease is almost invariably fatal within three years, the mortality rate provides a reasonable estimate of incidence. Thus, from table 4.2 we have an estimated incidence of 71 cases per 1,000 females among the South Fore between 1924 and 1928 and an average duration of about three years. The estimated point prevalence (i.e., number of cases in the population at a given time) is, therefore, 213 cases per 1,000 women. Thus, we estimate that in the mid-1920s about 21 percent of the South Fore women had kuru at any given time.

Given the incidence and prevalence of a disease we can, of course, use the equation to calculate its average duration. This type of calculation can produce striking results. For example, MacMahon et al. (1960) report that near the middle of this century the average yearly incidence of acute childhood leukemia was 32.4 cases per million and the point prevalence was 6.7 cases per million. The duration of the disease was, therefore, surprisingly brief—about .21 years or about 2.5 months. Further, since the time that these figures were reported, improvements in treatment methods have increased the duration of acute childhood leukemia. From equation 4.1 it can be seen that an increase in the duration of a disease produces a comparable increase in prevalence. For example, a treatment which added just 2.5 months to the life expectancy of the average acute leukemia patient would double the number of patients on hand at any given time. This illustrates an epidemiological irony: improvements in treatment increase the point prevalence of a disease that create the false impression that the disease is becoming a greater problem.

FREQUENCY CURVES:
THE INCIDENCE OF NICKNAMES

Rates of disease are not as important as changes in rates. Those changes are usually expressed as frequency curves such as the ones shown in figure 4.2. The shape of these types of curves can be a clue to the etiology of a disease. To illustrate this point, consider which curve best describes the incidence of nicknames.

The first curve suggests that the number of people who receive a nickname in a given year increases with age. According to this curve a thirty-year-old grown man is more likely to find himself called "Blinky" than a ten-year-old child. That is, of course, not what happens with nicknames, but it is what happens when a disease is caused by repeated exposure to some causal agent. For example, it is what happens with lung cancer where, as one ages, repeated exposure to tobacco raises the incidence rate. Thus if kuru followed this curve we might suspect that the disease was the result of repeated exposure to an environmental toxicant or to the accumulation of a nutritional deficit.

According to the second curve, the risk of receiving a nickname is the same at all ages. Here a nickname is something of a chance event—more a matter of running into the wrong person at a party than a matter of some internal characteristic that cries out for recognition. This curve is somewhat like the one that describes the incidence of deaths from lightning; by analogy, if the incidence of kuru resembled this curve we would want to look at chance environmental agents to which the Fore might be exposed.

The third curve is called a point source epidemic, and it often occurs when a group of susceptible people are exposed to a disease at a single point (e.g., at a single time, place, and/or age). In the case of nicknames, the curve might reflect the occurrence of nicknames in a group of people, some of whom attend the party of the last paragraph. People who are too young or too old to attend the party are unlikely to meet the nicknamer and consequently they are unlikely to receive a nickname. This creates the large age group at the center of the curve. Thus if this curve typified kuru we might conclude that the disease was caused by exposure to some agent which was accessible to certain age groups but not to others.

Often the abscissa of a point source epidemic is time rather than age. When that is the case, the curve suggests that a large group of people have been exposed to a disease at a single time and place. Consequently, the curve creates a strong presumption that the disease is contagious and that the group of cases represents people who have been exposed to a single carrier or to a contaminated object (in epidemiology, living carriers of disease are called *vectors* and nonliving carriers are called *vehicles*).

The fourth curve is called a propagated epidemic and it has two distinct stages. The first stage is like that of the point source epidemic: a large number

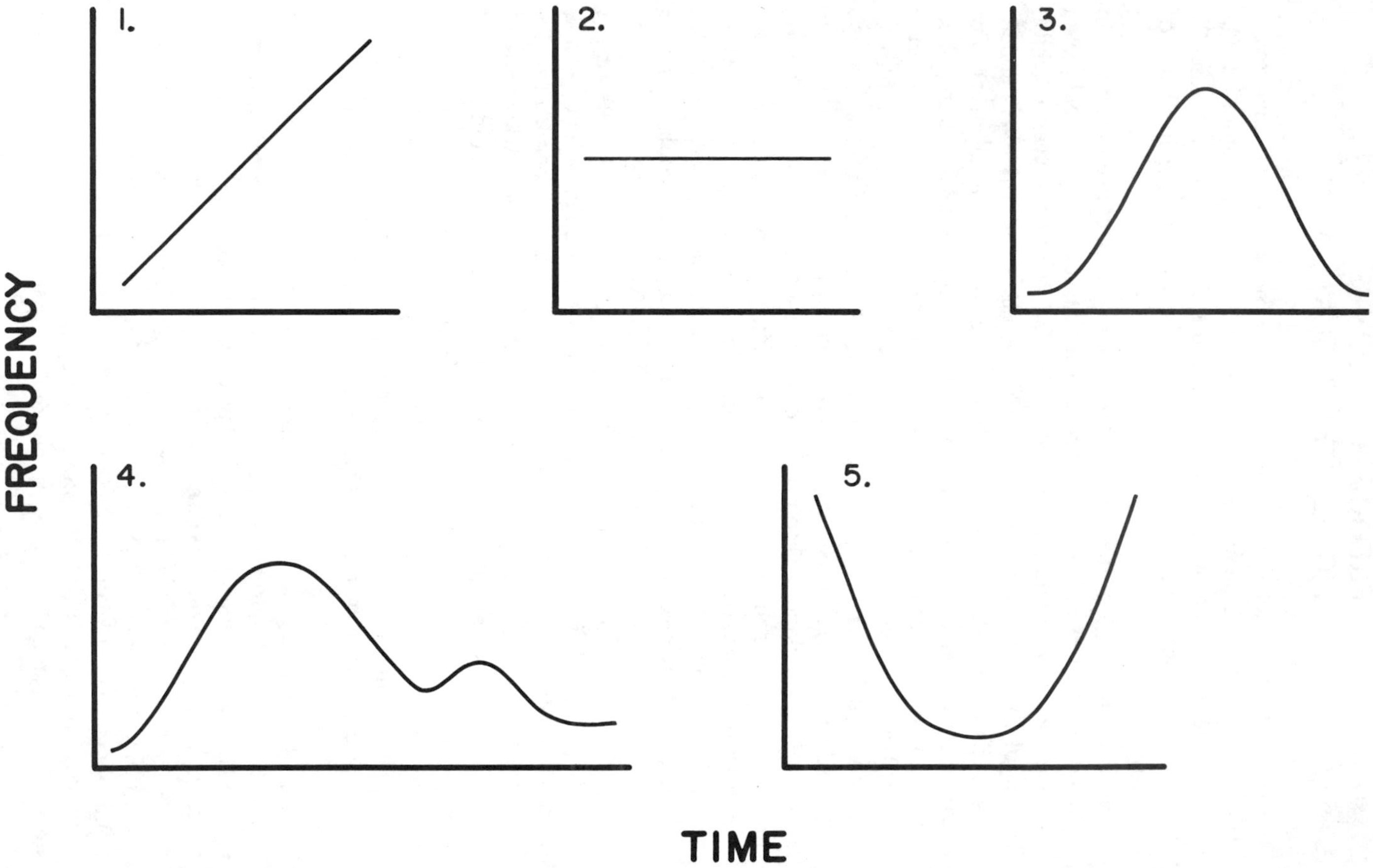
1.
2.
3.
4.
5.
FREQUENCY
TIME

Fig. 4.2. Five types of disease curves. The horizontal axes of such curves are usually some measure of time such as age or date of

of cases occurs at a single age. These cases then pass on the disease to a second group of people, creating a bimodal curve. As before, when the abscissa of this curve is time (rather than age) the curve suggests that the disease is infectious—that the large group has passed on the infection to the small one. Moreover, the distance between the two modes of the curve sometimes gives a good estimate of the disease's incubation period.

The fifth curve describes a disease that has an elevated risk period among children and adults with a period of decreased risk between the two age groups. The curve suggests that there are two types of nicknames—one type given to children, the other given to adults. This agrees with reality, in that the nicknames that children give to each other are quite different from those that lovers give to each other. When diseases are at issue rather than nicknames, this curve suggests that there could be a childhood and an adult form of a disease. In some cases this suggestion may be true—there may indeed be two forms of the disease. But often this type of curve occurs when the childhood and adult forms are actually two different diseases that mimic one another. For example, leukemia has a childhood and adult form that together produce a pattern somewhat like the one seen in this curve. Therefore, many epidemiologists suspect that the two types of leukemia are distinct diseases. The same is true of childhood and adult forms of other diseases such as schizophrenia.

The incidence curve that most closely describes kuru is that of a propagated epidemic (i.e., the fourth curve in figure 4.2). Earlier we noted that when time is the abscissa of this curve, the disease may be infectious. In the present case, however, the abscissa of the curve is age rather than time and a different interpretation is called for. One hypothesis is that Fore mothers are in close contact with children of certain ages and the two groups pass the disease back and forth. This is the strongest etiological hypothesis that we have yet considered because it fits what is known about the sex differences in the incidence of that disease. That is, the hypothesis predicts that the disease will be prominent in adult women and in children of both sexes but rare in adult men. Although this hypothesis is promising, it is not without problems. For example, one problem is that the curve for kuru has changed over the years; the average age at onset for childhood kuru has risen, while the average age at onset of adult kuru has remained constant. In addition, incidence rates for both the child and adult forms of kuru have diminished considerably in recent years. It is difficult to explain these changes in terms of transmission of the disease from mother to child. But regardless of whether the curve fits the hypothesis of transmission from mother to child, we should note that it does help rule out the genetic hypothesis, since it is difficult to attribute a rapid change in the age of onset and incidence rates to genetic features.

A MIDPOINT HYPOTHESIS

The epidemiological information that we have gathered so far has produced evidence that would be difficult to obtain by experiment. Instead, using a deductive process we have gathered and examined clues and retained only those theories that survive the examination. One surviving and plausible explanation is that kuru is caused by exposure to an environmental agent. If that agent were available to adult women and to children of both sexes, but unavailable to adult men, then the fourth curve of figure 4.2 would result. This situation again demonstrates how frequency curves can lead to clues about etiology. Here the curve leads us to a specific question: what agent in the environment is highly accessible to women and children, but inaccessible to men? There are probably only a few features in the environment of the Fore that meet these criteria, and any that do meet it become important etiological possibilities.

Consider the following possible explanation. As the Fore cultivate more land they destroy forest. The birds of the forest lose their sources of food and are forced to feed upon the seeds planted in the fields. The birds carry a kuru virus which is transmitted when mosquitoes bite the birds who enter the fields and subsequently bite the workers of those fields. If women are the primary field workers, they will develop kuru more often than men; and if those women bring their children with them to the fields, then the childhood form of the disease will occur in both sexes and the adult form will occur primarily in women. Finally, a change of ideas about how old a child should be before its mother can work in the fields will mean that only the older children will be exposed to the kuru virus and the age of onset will increase for children but not necessarily for mothers. This would account for some of the changes that have occurred in the kuru curve since 1944.

The foregoing chain of events may seem tenuous, but there are many precedents for it. Consider, for example, the way in which plague came to Borneo just a few decades ago. In an attempt to control flies and mosquitoes, the World Health Organization spread DDT over large areas of that country. The DDT was effective, but the poisoned flies were eaten by gecko lizards who sickened and became easy prey for local cats. The cats died from the DDT-laden reptiles and the absence of cats, in turn, allowed rats to flourish. The rats carried plague, which was transmitted to the local populace via rat fleas. (A digression: rats not only carry plague, but die from it as well. However, rats are more resistant to plague than men are and they live longer after they have contracted it. This allows them to build a reserve of plague bacteria in their blood, which then becomes available to fleas. Men, however, die before a reserve can be built. This is why fleas can carry plague from rat to man but not from man to man. Any living creature that succumbs to the same disease that it gives to man is known as a biological vector. The rat is a biological vector and the rat flea is another, because it too dies of the plague that it carries. This is not the case for all diseases. For example, the mosquito that carries yellow fever does not itself contract that disease. Any living creature that carries a disease without contracting it is called a mechanical vector.) It was not until the World Health Organization parachuted groups of cats into the stricken areas that the disease was finally controlled.

MATHEMATICAL MODELS

If a disease is transmitted from case to case, some interesting observations can be made. For one thing, we can predict the size of an epidemic, that is, the number of cases that are likely to occur over the course of the epidemic. Suppose that in a given population there are S people who are not immune to a disease (i.e., there are S susceptibles), that these people are mixing at rate C, and that some number, R, of them are removed from the susceptible population (through cure, emigration, death, or recovery). In such a case, an epidemic cannot occur unless the following relationship is true of the population:

$$\frac{R}{C} < S \qquad\qquad (4.2)$$

The mixing and removal rates, C and R, are technical terms that are defined in detail by Bailey (1975). For the moment, however, we can think of the mixing rate as the probability of meeting someone who can transmit the disease and the removal rate as the probability that a case is removed from the population within a given time. It makes sense that when cases are removed from the population faster than they can pass the disease on to other susceptibles, an epidemic will not start. This is the theory behind large immunization programs. Vaccination removes susceptibles from the population so that S decreases and makes an epidemic less likely. Note that in such a case unvaccinated persons are *also* less likely to become diseased, since they are less likely to be exposed to a person who can transmit the disease. Thus, the unvaccinated person benefits from what is called *herd immunity*.

Equation 4.2 is called the threshold density for an epidemic. The concept of threshold density has produced an interesting observation called the Kermack-McKendrick Threshold Theorem. Again, let S be the theoretical number of susceptibles needed to initiate an epidemic, and let the actual number of susceptibles in the population be P. The theorem states that at the end of the epidemic the appropriate number of susceptibles left in the population will be $2S - P$. For example, if 1,000 susceptibles are needed for an epidemic of measles to start (as computed by R/C in equation 4.2), and there are 1,200 susceptibles in a given population, then at the end of the epidemic there will be about $2,000 - 1,200 = 800$ susceptibles remaining. Or, to put it still another way, about 400 cases of measles will occur during the epidemic.

The foregoing is no more than a brief introduction to the kinds of observations that can be made using mathematical models of epidemics. More detailed models described by Bailey (1975) give insight into other properties of diseases. For example, it can be shown that a population of about 250,000 is a critical point for measles. When the population is that size, the disease becomes endemic—there are enough people available to support that disease in the population for an indeterminate time, without an epidemic.

MILL'S CANONS

The first step is an epidemiological exploration is often the recognition of an oddity—an unusual set of circumstances or coincidences that catches the eye of an alert observer. These initial clues can play a critical role in discovering the etiology of a disease. Take, for example, the case of a mother who brought her severely retarded twin sons in for a routine physical examination. One of the observations that the woman made while describing her sons' condition to the consulting physician was that she had noticed an unusually pungent odor to their urine. The doctor, his interest piqued by this casual remark, ordered an extensive urinalysis. The tests revealed a substantial excess of phenylalanine, one of the essential amino acids. This clue led to further tests of similarly afflicted children, and the ultimate identification of phenylketonuria—a treatable syndrome resulting from a genetically determined inability to metabolize phenylalanine (Følling, 1971).

It is not too often that a single clue reveals a direct path of causation. More frequently, the pattern of a disease is embedded within a web of variables. The job of the epidemiologist is to determine which variables play pivotal roles in the disease and to clarify the nature of those roles. To accomplish this goal the epidemiologist uses a number of methods based on creative deductive reasoning. Many of the most widely used methods were first elaborated by John Stuart Mill and hence are known as Mill's canons. We present four of those canons next.

Method of similarities. If two groups of people in different circumstances have the same incidence of a disease, it is possible that these circumstances share a common quality that plays a part in causing the disease. The aim of the epidemiologist who uses this method is to identify the common factor.

This line of reasoning was crucial in unraveling the cause of a puzzling and lethal disease known as erythroblastosis fetalis (Zimmerman, 1973). Most of those afflicted with this disease die before birth or in the first few weeks of life. The few infants who survive suffer severe mental and physical impairment. Doctors came to recognize the disease's presence by the newborn's swollen, misshapen appearance and increasingly jaundiced color. Although it was correctly inferred from the jaundice that the condition resulted from a blood disorder, the cause of the disorder and the means by which it was transmitted were unknown. Prior to 1930 there seemed to be no clear pattern to the disease. Afflicted infants were found in all social classes and all regions of the country. Finally investigators recognized a common thread connecting the seemingly unrelated cases.

One such investigator was Dr. Ruth Darrow, whose dedicated efforts were rooted in personal tragedy: at the age of 40 she gave birth to her first son and watched helplessly as he succumbed to erythroblastosis. She channeled her grief into a search for some understanding of the nature and cause of the disease. For two years she pored over reports covering hundreds of cases, among them the autopsy report on her son's body. It was through the collaborative efforts of Dr. Darrow and other researchers that clinical and epidemiological features of the disease began to emerge. One important feature that appeared was that most of the parents of affected babies had previously had stillborn babies or children who had died from severe newborn jaundice. This simple observation immediately ruled out existing theories, which had hypothesized that the disease was caused by exposure to some pathogenic agent or to dietary insufficiency during pregnancy. The new line of inquiry ultimately led to the identification of the Rh antibody–antigen reaction responsible for the disease and the development of the Rh vaccine, which has made erythroblastosis fetalis a defeated disease.

Applying the method of similarities to kuru yields some interesting observations. If we divide the women living in the Fore villages into those who are native-born and those who immigrated to the Fore as adults, we find the same incidence of kuru in the two groups. Similarly, if we divide native-born Fore women into those who remain with the Fore and those who emigrate to foreign villages, we find approximately the same rate of kuru. These observations are subject to the method of similarities. In the first case we have two groups who have different circumstances (i.e., different childhood experiences) but who have the same incidence of a disease. In the second case we again have two groups who have different circumstances (i.e., different adult experiences) but who have the same incidence of the disease.

Another observation derived from the method of similarities is that when microepidemics of kuru occur within the Fore population, they usually involve neighboring villages. That is, villages that are immediately adjacent to each other show similar increases in the rate of kuru.

Method of differences. If two groups of people differ on certain dimensions and one group gets a particular disease more often than the other, it is possible that the etiology of the disease may be related to the differences between the two groups.

The potential power of this method is illustrated by the following example. During the three-year period from 1966 to 1969, several gynecologists in Boston noted that eight young girls had been diagnosed as suffering from vaginal cancer, more cases in that age group than had been reported for the entire century. Comparing the eight patients yielded no obvious explanation. Puzzled, the doctors decided to compare the girls to another group who showed no indications of cancer. This second group was closely matched with the first on a number of variables, including birth date, birth weight, and mother's age. After the matching, detailed interviews with the members of both groups and their parents were conducted. Analysis of the information obtained from these interviews revealed one major difference between the two groups. All the mothers of the affected girls had been treated with the synthetic hormone stilbestrol in order to prevent miscarriage during pregnancy. As a result of this discovery, the sale of stilbestrol was banned and public announcements were made to alert other individuals at risk.

The method of differences also provided important clues that led to the discovery of the cause of pellagra. Pellagra is an Italian word meaning "rough skin," a condition that characterizes the disease's early stages. Later symptoms include painful running sores, foul odor, vomiting, diarrhea, and gradual neurological and mental detoriation. In the early 1900s, 100,000 people, most of them children, died from pellagra each year in the southern United States. It was thought at the time that pellagra was an infectious disease. Joseph Goldberger, then surgeon general of the United States, visited a South Carolina hospital hoping to identify the means by which the disease was transmitted. Instead, he found such peculiar differences in the incidence of pellagra across age groups that he was forced to completely abandon the idea that the disease was infectious. Very few children below the age of 6 or above the age of 12 developed pellagra, while practically all the children between the ages of 6 and 9 were affected. Similarly, he noted that none of the nurses, even those in daily contact with the sick children, became sick.

After close scrutiny, Goldberger determined that one of the major differences between the groups was their diet. The nurses did not live at the hospital and ate most of their meals at home. The children ate the institution fare, a diet relying heavily on starch and exceptionally deficient in animal proteins. Children below the age of 6, however, received a dietary supplement of milk and children above the age of 12 were able to supplement their daily intake by foraging for food on their own.

On the basis of these observations, Goldberger hypothesized that pellagra was caused either by severe protein deficiency or by a deficiency in some undiscovered substance that was contained in animal protein. The medical community strongly rejected both hypotheses, with most doctors clinging to the then current theory of infectious transmission (and a few supporting a competing theory that pellagra was caused by eating spoiled corn). To prove that pellagra was not infectious, Goldberger conducted a dramatic experiment. He, his wife, and several volunteers consumed feces, urine, and nasal discharges taken from pellagra patients. Goldberger also inoculated himself with blood taken from those patients. None of these efforts produced pellagra in the volunteers. But while this demonstration captured the attention of the medical community, most physicians remained convinced that pellagra was infectious. Therefore, to further substantiate his nutritional hypothesis, Goldberger conducted an experiment in which he created pellagra in a group of convicts by feeding them a protein-deficient diet. He also demonstrated that pellagra disappeared in affected children who were fed sufficient amounts of animal protein.

In later years the cause of pellagra was pinpointed further and found to be caused by a dietary deficiency of what was first called vitamin G (for Goldberger) and later renamed niacin. This later discovery illustrates an interesting point, for in the final analysis Goldberger's animal protein theory was incorrect, but his remedy for pellagra was effective. This is a common outcome when deductive epidemiological methods of analysis are used, and it is one of the strengths of the epidemiological approach.

For another illustrative example, we need only turn to John Snow (1855), the 19th-century British physician who attributed cholera to contaminated water and thereby found a way to prevent that disease almost 30 years before its bacterial cause was known. One major strength of epidemiology is, therefore, that it does not focus solely on a disease, but rather on the entire web of causation that leads to the disease. Even today it is easier to prevent cholera by sanitation than it is to treat individual cases, and it is easier to kill mosquitoes than it is to treat yellow fever. The promise of epidemiology lies in its ability to prevent or cure disease in many ways, even when the cause of the disease is unknown.

We have strayed a bit from the method of differences, so let us return to that topic and to kuru. Applying that method to the riddle of kuru yields several observations. One observation is that the Fore have a much higher rate of kuru than a neighboring tribe, the Awa. A comparison of the two groups reveals several differences, the most obvious of which are cultural. For example, among the Fore there exists a deeply ingrained antagonism between the sexes. From the age of seven Fore males live in houses separate from the females, and customarily go into periodic seclusion to rid themselves of the polluting effects of female contact. Relations between the sexes are characterized by two beliefs. First, the male is considered superior and dominant in all social interactions. Second, it is believed that the male must continually protect himself from evil female influences. Sexual intercourse is thought to be so dangerous that it can only be practiced by married men who possess the magic necessary to protect themselves. More than anything, Fore men fear contact with menstrual blood (Megget, 1964):

They believe that contact with it or a menstruating woman will, in the absence of counter-magic, sicken a man and cause persistent vomiting, turn his blood black, corrupt his vital juices so that his skin darkens and wrinkles as his flesh wastes, permanently dull his wits, and eventually lead to a slow decline and death [p. 207].

On the other hand, relationships between men and women in the neighboring Awa tribe (where kuru is rare), while far from egalitarian, are much less antagonistic. Husband and wife live together, each assuming some of the tasks necessary to run a household. It is thought that the difference in the nature of male-female relationships in the two tribes may be rooted in the way tribes encourage men to select their mates. Both tribes encourage men to select as wives their mother's brother's daughter or a girl who belongs in the same kinship category. However, among the Awa this choice is based on true genetic kinship, while the Fore adhere to a much looser definition of kinship. Because the Fore are frequently at war with neighboring tribes, they welcome the addition of any newcomers to strengthen their forces, elevating these "adoptees" to the status of true relatives. It is possible that the characteristic antagonism between the sexes among the Fore may be attributed to the fact that many of the females in the tribe were originally members of conquered enemy tribes.

The foregoing differences in customs and beliefs among the two tribes provide a source of hypotheses about the nature of kuru. To choose just one of many possibilities, the sexual segregation practices by the Fore may account for sex differences in the incidence of kuru in adults. There are also, however, other tribal customs that raise additional hypotheses. For example, the Fore live in small villages that function as the focus of social activity. Weddings and funerals often bring together friends and relatives of neighboring villages. Fore funerary rites were of particular interest to the Western anthropologists who first encountered the tribe. This interest was piqued by the peculiar way in which the Fore paid tribute to the deceased—namely, by eating them. This tradition, which first appeared in 1915 and showed a rapid gain in popularity, followed certain prescribed patterns. The primary participants in cannibal feasts were female relatives, and the body parts that they consumed were determined by their relationship to the deceased. For example, sisters were entitled to the brains of their brothers, while brothers' wives laid claim to the buttocks, intestines, and vulvas of their sisters-in-law. Distant relatives were usually relegated body parts considered less valuable, such as legs and hands.

Method of concomitant variation. If the frequency or strength of a characteristic or event in a population varies with the frequency of a disease, it is possible that the characteristic is related to the etiology of the disease.

In 1961 three German gynecologists independently noted the appearance of large numbers of babies with severe deformities that followed the characteristic pattern of an extremely rare syndrome. This syndrome was known as phocomelia (from the Greek *phokos*, "seal," and *melia*, "limbs") because of the flipper-like appearance of the legs and arms. Additionally, these babies often had heart and intestinal tract dysfunction. About half of the afflicted infants died; those who survived were physically deformed but had normal intelligence. The number of cases reported soon reached epidemic proportions. It was estimated that in one year 6,000 to 8,000 cases occurred in West Germany alone. Large numbers of cases were also reported in Australia, Canada, South America, Africa, and Japan. The disorder was finally traced to the use of the sedative thalidomide by the infant's mother during the early stages of pregnancy. The pharmaceutical company that produced the drug protested this conclusion, refusing at first to withdraw it from the market, but the evidence soon proved overwhelming. Specifically, investigators found that the first cases of the epidemic had been reported approximately nine months after the drug was first sold in Germany in 1956. In addition, in each country the sales volume of the drug closely paralleled the frequency of the syndrome with a time lag of about nine months. Finally, the epidemic ended in each country approximately nine months after thalidomide was taken off the market. Experiments with animals confirmed the conclusions first indicated by the method of concomitant variation.

If we return once again to the New Guinea highlands, we find that several climatic factors seem to vary with the incidence of kuru. For example, it has been noted that the onset of kuru is most likely to occur in the dry months of the year. It has also been observed that the mortality rate for kuru is correlated with the amount of rainfall that occurred one and a half to two and a half years previous. It is doubtful that rain is a direct cause of kuru, but the method of concomitant variation might indicate that the disease is caused by factors that are indirectly related to rainfall, for example plant and insect growth.

Other aspects of Fore life also raise hypotheses based on concomitant variation. For example, kuru first appeared in the early part of the 20th century at about that same time that the sweet potato became an important part of the Fore diet. It is possible that something about sweet potatoes is responsible for kuru (there are similar theories that link potatoes to other childhood diseases, for example anencephaly), but the major problem with this hypothesis is that men eat as many sweet potatoes as women but get kuru far less often. It is also possible that the growing taste for sweet potatoes had secondary repercussions that resulted in kuru. We consider that possibility next.

As the Fore began to cultivate the sweet potato in great numbers, they destroyed the forest around their village. This forest was the natural habitat of the feral pig, a main source of protein in the Fore diet. Wild pigs grew scarce and Fore men began to claim first right to the pork that was available. Fore women were left to forage for themselves and their children as best they could. It is thought that the custom of cannibalism may have developed in part as a means of supplementing the protein intake of the Fore women and children.

The prevalence of cannibalism among the Fore has steadily diminished in the last 25 years and in recent times is practiced only very rarely by older members of the tribe who find it hard to relinquish their taste for human flesh. This decline is due to the increasing influence of the Australian administration, which has made concerted efforts to discourage the practice. The concomitant variation of the decline of cannibalism with the decline of kuru raises the possibility of a relationship. However, the Australian administration made many other changes at the same time that it began to discourage cannibalism, and any one of them could also be responsible for the decline in kuru. For example, the government introduced improvements in the general standard of living, such as better sanitation and housing and more efficient farming methods, which in turn led to bigger crops and the domestication of the feral pig.

Method of analogy. If a disease has certain features that are similar to those of another disease whose cause is already known, it is possible that the two diseases may have the same or highly similar etiologies.

This method was instrumental in constructing the clinical picture of poliomyelitis (Paul, 1971). This disease, which immediately conjures images of a child condemned to a life of leg braces and wheelchairs, reached epidemic proportions in the late 1800s and early 1900s. During epidemics in the 1930s and 1940s it was estimated that poliomyelitis was responsible for varying degrees of paralysis in more than 10,000 children annually in the United States alone. Because the disease most often strikes children from two to four years old, early investigators believed it to be related to the process of teething. However, Duchenne de Boulogne, a French orthopedist, reported an observation in 1853 that had great impact on later research. He pointed out that acute paralysis in these children was followed by the same sort of muscular degeneration and electromuscular irritability seen in patients who had suffered traumatic spinal cord injuries. He concluded from this analogy that the spinal cord might also be the affected site in paralytic poliomyelitis. Many of de Boulogne's contemporaries rejected his conclusions because examination of the spinal cords of children for whom the disease proved fatal revealed no observable lesions. It was not until ten years later that the theory received confirmation, when Corbil detected microscopic spinal cord lesions that were invisible to the naked eye.

The symptoms of kuru have been analogized to several diseases of known etiology. Kuru was first compared to Parkinson's disease because of the involuntary athetoid and choreiform jerks and tremors characteristic of both diseases. However, later investigators noted several symptomatic discrepancies. The gait of the kuru victim is different from that of the Parkinson victim. The pill-rolling movements so characteristic of Parkinson's are absent in kuru, as are the voice tone changes suggestive of extrapyramidal disorder.

Surprisingly, a disease whose clinical picture most closely parallels that of kuru is one found in sheep. Scrapie is reported to have an incubation period of three years or more. The disease begins with occasional fits of trembling, followed by increasing incoordination and emaciation. As the disease progresses, the sheep develop a staggering gait, which deteriorates into paralysis. Death follows shortly. Scrapie is transmitted in several ways, but the principal methods are by physical contact and through the mouth. The agent that is transmitted seems to be similar to a virus in some ways. However, the agent remains potent after being exposed to a temperature of 99.5 C for eight hours and after exposure to a number of chemical substances, any of which should obliterate the infectivity of any virus.

KURU: THE CLUES

The list of diseases that have yielded to the epidemiological approach is long and in the mid-1970s kuru was added to it. The evidence that we have dispersed throughout this chapter represents most of what was known about kuru and about the Fore people at the time that the etiology of the disease was confirmed. This information is sufficient to allow the mystery to be solved, and to that end we will gather the most important clues together in this section. However, these clues are presented without the environmental, cultural, and physiological facts about the New Guinea Highlands that are also dispersed throughout the chapter. We leave the reader to make his own list of those that seem important to the problem.

The clues:

1. Kuru is a degenerative disease that resembles scrapie.
2. There might be two forms of kuru—a childhood form and an adult form.
3. The disease is markedly limited to the Fore people.
4. Among adults, kuru occurs almost entirely in women.
5. Among children, kuru occurs equally often in both sexes.
6. Kuru runs in families.
7. Women who immigrate to the Fore tribe contract kuru about as often as women who are born into the tribe.
8. Women who emigrate from the Fore contract kuru about as often as those who remain in the tribe.
9. When microepidemics of kuru occur within the Fore village they also occur in neighboring villages where the disease is normally rare.
10. Kuru rates vary with the amount of rainfall that occurred one and a half to two and a half years previously.
11. The mortality curve for kuru resembles that of a propagated epidemic.
12. In recent years the average age of onset for childhood kuru has risen. The average age of onset for adult kuru has remained the same.
13. The incidence of kuru (measured indirectly by mortality rates) has declined dramatically since 1950.

Not all of these clues are equally important, and some even appear contra-dictory. In particular, clues 3, 6, 7, and 8 form a tangle of contradictions that appear to be unexplainable by any single theory. You are advised that there is a solution that satisfies all of the clues, but that the solution may not be easy and that some of the information needed has been presented subtly. For those who have no need of subtlety, we have described the etiology of kuru on the following pages.

KURU: THE CAUSE

The psychogenic theory. This is the weakest of the theories that were proposed, with only one item of support. It is possible that belief in magic has declined since the coming of modern times and that that decline would be concomitant with the decline in the incidence of kuru. However, whether in fact belief in magic has actually declined is an unproven hypothesis, and against it we have at least two counterclues. First, tribes that are neighbors to the Fore have a strong belief in magic but a low incidence of kuru. Second, adult men have at least as strong a belief in magic as adult women but the men contract kuru far less often than the women do. Thus the psychogenic theory fails because it explains too little and what it does explain is not convincing.

The genetic theory. The genetic theory explains the fact that kuru runs in families, it explains the sex differences in adult kuru, and it explains why women who emigrate from the Fore develop kuru as often as those who remain. It does not, however, explain why women who immigrate to the Fore develop kuru as often as those who are born in the tribe, nor does it explain why kuru occurs in the adopted members of a family as often as it occurs in the blood members. We might amend the theory in an attempt to repair these problems, but the genetic theory was already unwieldy with its need for recessive genes having unusual properties. Thus this theory remains viable only if we abandon Occam's razor.

The environmental theory. There may be unknown environmental agents that are responsible for kuru but we have uncovered very little evidence to either support or deny that hypothesis. It is easy to generate environmental hypotheses that would explain the sex differences in the incidence of kuru, the resemblance of kuru to a propagated epidemic, the link between kuru and rainfall, or, for that matter, the link between kuru and scrapie. It is difficult, however, to think of a single environmental theory that would simultaneously account for all of these clues. In addition, there are results that do not support the environmental hypothesis. These counterclues include the fact that kuru runs in families and the fact that neighboring tribes with apparently similar environments to those of the Fore have a low incidence of kuru. We might invoke microenvironments to explain these problems, but that route, once taken, can never be abandoned, for we can always oppose negative evidence by shrinking our microenvironments until they are the size of a single person. In addition, the environmental hypothesis is antithetical to the genetic hypothesis, in that the strengths of one are the weaknesses of the other. In essence, the two hypotheses cancel each other.

The genetic-environmental theory. This approach attempts to save both the genetic and environmental theories by combining them. In that way one part of the theory watches out for the other. This is a good try and it fits many of the clues. In a sense, however, the strength of this theory is also its weakness, since it fits almost any other set of clues well. That is why we find one version or another of this theory for almost every disease whose cause is unknown. In the present case, however, we are not even afforded that solace, since even the genetic-environmental theory cannot explain why immigrants to the Fore tribe contract kuru as often as those born into the tribe (who presumably have a hereditary predisposition to kuru).

The nutritional deficit theory. Basically this is a weaker version of the environmental theory. It has very little explanatory power.

The infection theory. Kuru is cousin to scrapie, which is an infectious disease, so we can turn to scrapie for hypotheses. Scrapie is caused by what has been called a "slow virus." Here the word "slow" refers to the fact that the virus may lie dormant in the body for many years before it becomes active. Scrapie, for example, usually takes at least two to three years to become active.

Although there is very little question that slow viruses are slow, there is some question as to whether they are viruses. They behave much like viruses but they remain potent after exposure to conditions that would destroy the infectivity of any virus and they seem to be composed of a material that is found in no other type of virus.

The cause of scrapie is not known, but it does appear to be contagious by contact. This suggests that kuru might also be contagious by contact, since the two diseases are so similar. As it happens, however, this cannot be true, because we can be certain that Fore men have some contact with Fore women, and therefore both sexes should be equally susceptible to kuru. Scrapie, however, can also be transmitted orally, a fact that leads us to look at the Fore diet. Here we find one item of note. Fore women and children are cannibals; Fore men are not. This fits what we know about the sex differences in the incidence of kuru, it explains why there appears to be both an adult and a childhood form of the disease, and it explains why the curve for kuru resembles that of a propagated epidemic.

The fact that kuru runs in families was originally seen as evidence for the genetic hypothesis, but that hypothesis failed when we learned that the incidence of kuru was as great among adopted members of those families as it was among blood members. The weakness of the genetic hypotheses is, however, the strength of the cannibalism hypothesis, because both adopted and blood relatives participate in the funeral meal. This interpretation also fits what we know about immigrants to the Fore, who probably contract kuru when they take part in their adopted tribe's funeral customs.

The cannibalism hypothesis does not at first appear to explain why women who emigrate from the Fore develop kuru as often as those who remain. However, it is now known that there are two reasons for the emigration data, both related to cannibalism. First, like scrapie, kuru is a slow virus and the time between exposure to the disease and the first onset of symptoms can be lengthy—as long as twenty years or more. Therefore, it often happens that a woman will contract kuru before leaving the Fore but will not display symptoms until long after she has joined her new tribe. This delay can make it appear that Fore emigrants contracted kuru while living in their adopted tribes. The second explanation for kuru among Fore emigrants also explains another difficult clue—the existence of microepidemics of kuru among neighboring tribes of the Fore. As we noted earlier, women who emigrate often return home for funerals, where they participate in cannibalism. Some carry kuru home with them. Later, when these women first show symptoms of kuru, it appears that the disease originated in the adopted tribe rather than in the visit to the home tribe.

In recent years the incidence of cannibalism has declined dramatically, and the average age of onset for childhood kuru has increased. Both events were caused by the Australian administration's attempts to eliminate cannibalism. These attempts have been successful. Thus, there are fewer cases of both adult and childhood kuru, and the cases of childhood kuru that are now seen were probably in incubation for many years. Finally, the fact that the incidence of kuru varies with rainfall of previous years is again indirectly related to cannibalism. A dry season reduces the available wildlife and therefore has the double effect of increasing the death rate among the Fore and encouraging the survivors to supplement their diets by cannibalism.

The link between kuru and cannibalism was suspected very early in the course of research, although for a long time it was no more than one of a dozen or so competing theories. Two decades after the discovery of the Fore, Gajdusek, Gibbs, and Alpers (1966, 1967) demonstrated that when brain tissue from kuru victims was injected into chimpanzees, they died of the disease in about two years. This experiment was part of a careful research program that led to the final understanding of the disease in the mid-1970s, and it earned Gajdusek a share of the Nobel prize for medicine in 1976.

REFERENCES

For interested readers, we have included a representative list of books and articles that illustrate various epidemiological ways of thought. This list is representative, but of course not exhaustive. Starred items are references presented in this chapter.

*Bailey, N. *The mathematical theory of infectious diseases and its applications.* New York: Hafnner Press, 1975.

Blumberg, B. S. Differences in the frequency of disease in different populations. *Annual Review of Medicine,* 1964, **15**, 387-404.

*Crosby, A. W. *The Columbian exchange.* Westport, Conn.: Greenwood Press, 1972.

Craelius, W. Comparative epidemiology of multiple sclerosis and dental caries. *Journal of Epidemiology and Community Health,* 1978, **32**, 155-165. (An application of the method of analogy that is somewhat different from the one that we have described.)

Feinstein, A. Clinical epidemiology. *Annals of Internal Medicine,* 1968, **69**, 1037-1061.

Feinstein, A. Methodologic problems and standards and case-control research. *Journal of Chronic Diseases,* 1979, **32**, 35-44.

*Følling, A. The original detection of phenylketonuria. In H. Bickel, F P Hudson, & L. I. Woolf (Eds.), *Phenylketonuria.* Stuttgart: Georg Thieme Verlag, 1971.

Frost, W. H. The age selection of mortality from tuberculosis in successive decades. *American Journal of Hygiene,* 1930, **30**, 91-96.

*Gajdusek, D. C., Gibbs, C. J., & Alpers, M. Experimental transmission of a kuru-like syndrome to chimpanzees. *Nature,* 1966, **209**, 794-795.

*Gajdusek, D. C., Gibbs, C. J., & Alpers, M. Transmission and passage of experimental "kuru" to chimpanzees. *Science,* 1967, **155**, 212-213.

*Geddes, S. *Plague on us.* New York: Commonwealth Fund, 1941.

Gordon, J. E. The epidemiology of accidents. *American Journal of Public Health,* 1949, **39**, 504-515.

Greenwald, P., Rose, J. S., & Daitch, P. B. Acquaintance networks among leukemia and lymphoma patients. *American Journal of Epidemiology,* 1979, **110**, 162-177. (An unusual approach to determining infectiousness.)

Hippocrates upon Air, Water, and Situations, Upon Epidemical diseases, and upon prognosticks in acute cases especially. London: J. Watts, 1734.

*Hornabrook, R. W. Kuru: The disease. In R. W. Hornabrook (Ed.), *Essays on kuru.* Farington, Berks.: E. W. Classey, 1976.

Horwitz, O. Disease, cure and death: Epidemiologic and clinical parameters for chronic diseases illustrated by a model—tuberculosis. *American Journal of Epidemiology,* 1973, **97**, 148-159.

Lillienfeld, A. M. The distribution of disease in the population. *Journal of Chronic Diseases,* 1960, **11**, 471-483.

Lillienfeld, A. M. Epidemiology of infectious and non-infectious disease: Some comparisons. *American Journal of Epidemiology,* 1973, **97**, 135-147.

Lillienfeld, A. M., & Lillienfeld, D. What else is new? *American Journal of Epidemiology,* 1977, **105**, 169-179.

Lillienfeld, A. M., & Lillienfeld, D. A century of case control studies: Progress? *Journal of Chronic Diseases,* 1979, **32**, 5-13.

*MacMahon, B., Pugh, T., & Ipsen, J. *Epidemiologic methods.* Boston: Little, Brown, 1960.

*McArthur, N. Cross-currents. In R. W. Hornabrook (Ed.), *Essays on kuru.* Farington, Berks.: E. W. Classey, 1976.

*Megget, M. J. Male-female relationships in the highlands of Australian New Guinea. *American Anthropologist,* 1964, 204-224.

Niles, G. M. *Pellagra.* Philadelphia: W. B. Saunders, 1912.

*Paul, J. R. *A History of poliomyelitis.* New Haven: Yale University Press, 1971.

Platt, J. R. Strong inference. *Science,* 1964, **146,** 347–352. (Not exactly epidemiology, but related and worth reading.)

*Snow, J. *On the mode of communication of cholera.* (2nd ed.) London: John Churchill, 1855. Reproduced in *Snow on Cholera.* New York: Commonwealth Fund, 1936.

Zinsser, H. *Rats, lice and history.* New York: Bantam, 1934. (A lyrical approach.)

*Zimmerman, D. R. *The intimate history of disease and its conquest.* New York: Macmillan, 1973.

GLOSSARY: SOME EPIDEMIOLOGICAL TERMS

Biological vector: A living organism that carries a disease and succumbs to it as well.

Endemic rate: The usual frequency with which a disease is found in a population. The number of cases is unimportant; an endemic rate may be very high or very low.

Epidemic: A disease frequency that is greater than usual. An epidemic need not involve large numbers of cases; it is only necessary that the number of cases be greater than usual.

Epidemiology: The study of diseases in groups of people in order to find methods of prevention or cure.

Enzootic: An epidemic among animals.

Incidence: The number of new cases of a disease that occur within a selected observation period (often one year). Incidence is usually expressed as the number of new cases divided by the number of people at risk for the disease during the observation period.

Kermack-McKendrick Threshold Theorem: A method for predicting the size of an epidemic.

Mechanical vector: A living organism that carries a disease but does not succumb to it.

Method of analogy: States that if a disease whose etiology is unknown has symptoms that are similar to those of a disease whose etiology is known, the antecedents of the known disease may be similar to those of the unknown one.

Method of concomitant variation: States that if the frequency of a disease rises and falls in concordance with some feature of the environment, then the disease may be caused by that feature.

Method of similarities: States that if people in different circumstances have the same frequency of disease, then those circumstances may have a common factor that is responsible for the disease.

Method of differences: States that if the incidence of disease is greater for one group of people than for another, the etiology of the disease may be related to differences between the two groups.

Pandemic: A disease that affects a major part of the population.

Period prevalence: The total number of cases in a population during a given observation period. This total includes new cases that occur during the observation period and old cases that began before the observation period.

Point prevalence: The number of cases of a disease in the population at a given moment.

Point source epidemic: An epidemic caused by the simultaneous exposure of a group of people to a disease agent.

Propagated epidemic: An epidemic caused by a disease that propagates itself as one generation of cases infects the next.

Threshold density: The number of susceptible people necessary for an epidemic to take place.

5

Methodological Issues in Behavioral Pediatrics Research*

Edward R. Christophersen

The field of pediatrics has its credentialing procedures, its national and local organizations, its journals, and all of its subspecialty areas. Singly and jointly, these various divisions have gone about the task of solving the most pressing clinical and research questions of the day, drawing heavily from other fields of medicine where appropriate and applicable.

The entry of behavioral pediatrics as a new area within pediatrics has followed the path laid out by its many predecessors. In the beginning, individual pediatric practitioners, out of personal interest, elected to alter their practices in order to accommodate this new facet (cf. Brazelton, 1975) and to offer services related to behavioral, emotional, and school-based problems that they encountered. Pediatricians have often been presented with problems they were not trained to handle (Green, 1980). However, before an area of interest becomes a formal part of pediatric training, several vaguely defined criteria must generally be met. The burden of proof for both the necessity of the new area and the effectiveness and cost-effectiveness of its procedures rests with existing practitioners. Generally, in areas like endocrinology and nephrology commonly accepted definitions for establishing the presence of disease in the patient (e.g., abnormal CBC values, abnormal serum or urine assays, and abnormal or remarkable radiographic findings) are initially used to establish which treatment is indicated. These same definitions are later used in clincial trials to demonstrate, as outcome measures, the subsequent absence of, or control of, the disease. Only then are studies employing experimental designs conducted to demonstrate beyond a reasonable doubt that the treatment paradigm under investigation was in fact responsible for the improvement in the patient's presenting symptoms.

*Preparation of this manuscript was partially supported by a grant from NICHD (HD 03144) to the Bureau of Child Research, University of Kansas. The editorial assistance of Barbara Cochrane and Jack W. Finney is gratefully acknowledged.

For example, in a patient who presents with the symptoms of polyuria (excessive urine production), polydipsia (excessive thirst), weakness, and dry skin, appropriate blood tests can be run for hyperglycemia (elevated blood sugar) and glycosuria (sugar in the urine). These tests are used to assist the physician in making the original diagnosis of diabetes mellitus. After the original diagnosis is made, the blood sugar and urine sugar levels are then used to determine how well controlled the patient's diabetes is. Now, as new procedures are developed for better management of the juvenile diabetic (e.g., the use of feedback to the patient on periodic HbA_{1c} levels, or two insulin injections per day instead of one), they can be evaluated by assessing what the effect is on the blood sugar and urine sugar levels.

Later much more sophisticated experimental procedures, such as parametric analyses and double blind studies, are usually conducted to define more clearly the specific parameters that can be used to account for the patient's improved functioning. As has been pointed out for a long time (e.g., Bernard, 1865/ 1957; Risley, 1970), measurement procedures become the basis for much of this later, more sophisticated research.

Behavioral pediatrics, like many other areas of behavioral medicine, is responsible for dealing with a wide range of problems that mandate a wide range of investigative procedures. These range from the laboratory analysis of biofeedback procedures, which depend upon well-established instrumentation for documentation, to the use of office consultation with parents for establishing instructional control over a behaviorally noncompliant child. Because of this wide range of procedures, investigators have limited their research interests to a relatively narrow area. This has resulted in "gaps" in the scientific base for behavioral pediatrics, gaps that are often filled with common-sense medical or behavioral advice that may or may not be effective. What is needed is the integration of more pediatric practitioners into the research practices of this area. Research methodology historically has not been emphasized in pediatric training.

What follows is a discussion of some methodological issues that may stimulate the design of research investigations for behavioral pediatric interventions. When adequately designed studies are available to demonstrate a specific point, these studies will be described in some detail to illustrate the research methodology within the context of pediatrics.

EXPERIMENTAL DESIGN

The reason for insisting on the use of an adequate experimental design is that the researcher and the clinician need to distinguish between what is thought to be true and what is known to be true. As research progresses in sophistication from simple case studies with a single patient to complex double blind crossover designs that include random assignment to alternative treatment groups, investigators experience a corresponding increase in confidence that the results are clearly related to the independent variables that were manipulated. For example, when a well-intentioned clinician treats a known disease and obtains a favorable outcome, the tendency is to conclude that it was his treatment that was responsible for the improvement. Bernard (1865/1957) calls this "the clinician's fallacy."

> A physician, who tries a remedy and cures his patients, is inclined to believe that the cure is due to his treatment. . . . But the first thing to ask them is whether they have tried doing nothing, i.e., not treating other patients; for how can they otherwise know whether the remedy or nature cured them [p. 194]?

Although the experimental method has grown enormously in its complexity over the years, particularly through the development of statistics and, later, computer analyses, the same basic question must be addressed: how do you know that it was your treatment that changed the patient's condition? Case studies, however well described, will never be able to answer this question satisfactorily. Nor will collections of case studies. Two basic types of experimental designs are available that adequately address the issue of causality. The first and probably most widely recognized is the group design. The second is the single subject or time series analysis design. Each will be briefly explained here.

Group Designs

All of the elaborate designs that fall under this basic category have a single feature in common—at least two groups that are treated differently in at least one respect are compared with each other. If the two groups are identical in all but one way, and one group does significantly better than the other, then the experimenter has garnered some support for the hypothesis that one treatment is "better" than the other. Rarely is a single experiment sufficient to establish, beyond reasonable doubt, that the better treatment is also the treatment of choice, for many other factors must be considered before such a sweeping generalization can be justified. While many investigators accept this point only with chagrin, it remains true. With the explosion in the number of articles published in the medical behavioral sciences, it is all too easy to overlook the fact that, unless the study was performed correctly (that is, unless numerous scientific criteria are met), the article contributes little, if anything, to medical science.

In the traditional experimental control group design, one group usually is subjected to the procedures under investigation while the other group remains untouched, i.e., a no-treatment control group. A second possibility involves alternative treatment groups, where two or more groups are subjected to different treatments and the outcomes are compared.

There are several conditions that require group designs: first, when studying the occurrence and prevalence of disease in medicine, i.e., epidemiological studies; second, when actuarial data are needed (e.g., the percentage of patients that can be expected to react favorably to a drug or the number and variety of side effects that are associated with a particular drug); third, when comparing treatments where serial or order effects are known or suspected to occur; fourth, when the intent is to draw generalizations to a much larger population; and fifth, when comparing two or more treatment strategies for the same disease entity or problem area.

Conversely, group designs have the disadvantage that they do not allow the prediction of the response or side effects of an individual patient to a treatment protocol; they deal with averages, which can be misleading at times. Also, in the pilot stages of development of entirely new interventions it may be difficult to justify subjecting an entire group of subjects to an untried procedure since very little is known about it. For a detailed discussion of group experimental designs, the reader is referred to Campbell and Stanley (1963).

Single Subject Design

In these intervention designs, subjects are usually used as their own control. That is, a measure or a set of measures is taken, usually several over time (repeated measures), and then some change is introduced and the measure or set of measures is repeated. By comparing the pretreatment, or baseline, performance of subjects with their later performance after intervention, the researcher is able to evaluate the effect of the intervention. The researcher may return to the baseline condition (a reversal design) for a more powerful demonstration of cause and effect (cf. Bernard, 1865/1957). For situations where a reversal design is not practical or desirable, three different multiple baseline designs are available: across subjects, situations, or responses (cf. Baer, Wolf, & Risley, 1968). A multiple baseline design includes data on three or more components (subjects, situations, or responses). The independent variable (e.g., treatment) is introduced in the first component, but not in the other two. At a later point in time, the independent variable is introduced for the second component, and, still later, for the third. In this way the second and third components serve as a control for the first, and the third component serves as a control for the second. If the patient's behavior *only* changes when the researcher manipulates the independent variable, then a cause-effect relationship has been demonstrated by replication.

Some conditions which require the use of a single subject design include: (1) when only a single subject is available for research about a particular condition or disease, e.g., a single patient in a burn trauma center, because it is simply not possible to wait until enough patients are available to form two groups; (2) when a new disease or behavior problem or an entirely new treatment protocol is being developed, in which case the researcher inevitably begins with one subject and studies that subject in painstaking detail prior to introducing the procedure to yet another subject. Only after the investigator has carefully detailed what results and side effects can be anticipated can the procedures be attempted with a large group of subjects. For a detailed discussion of single subject designs, the reader is referred to Hersen and Barlow (1976).

In actual practice, single subject designs typically precede the use of group designs. For example, early investigations of the effects of biofeedback procedures for the control of anal sphincter pressure involved only one or a few subjects (Engel, Nikoomanesh, & Schuster, 1974; Kohlenberg, 1973) using single subject experimental designs. When the effectiveness of the procedures was evident in a number of single cases, larger-scale investigations were conducted to demonstrate further the generality of the procedures (Cerulli, Nikoomanesh, & Schuster, 1979).

Each set of experimental designs plays an important role in the development of behavioral medicine. The advantage of first investigating a number of single cases intensively is the ability to assess for subtle, or not so subtle, effects associated with the treatment procedures that would not be obvious within a group design. The later group designs, when random assignment is incorporated into the subject selection, are necessary to determine generality to a larger sample. Selection issues for research subjects is an important component of any design.

SELECTION OF SUBJECTS

When researchers and clinicians provide written reports of investigative studies, often too little detail is provided regarding how the patients in those studies were selected. Ideally, if a pediatric group is reporting on a topic like enuresis, then either every enuretic in the practice will be studied or a sample of enuretics will be selected randomly from the total number of enuretics who meet the entry criteria for the study. The entry criteria can be misleading, depending upon the site in which the study takes place. If the study is conducted by selecting enuretics from the local public school system, then there is a high probability that it is a representative sample, since, by law, every child must attend school. However, such a study would omit any children enrolled in a nonpublic school, and may influence the generalizability of the results to this population due to some selection factor.

If all of the enuretics seen through a pediatric clinic are eligible, then some description should be provided of the demographic characteristics of the patient population served. Some university-based pediatric clinics serve almost exclusively low-income families, whereas some private practice groups, by virtue of their office location and fee schedule, serve middle- or upper-middle-income families. Obviously, enuretics seen in a university-hospital-based psychiatry department that serves indigent families or families on public assistance could hardly be called a representative sample of the sort of "average" enuretics that a pediatrician in a different setting could be expected to encounter.

Since most investigators are quite limited in their selection of sites at which their research can be conducted, the description of the site where the study was done becomes mandatory. Whether a single case, a group of cases, or a "representative sample" of cases is being presented, the investigator needs to identify clearly how the cases were selected. A similar responsibility must be borne by the reader or reviewer who is seeking "incidence" estimates for an individual disease or problem. For example, in Wright, Schaeffer, and Solomons's (1979) discussion of the incidence of "encopresis," they distinguish between the incidence reported from psychiatric clinics, institutionalized children, hospital-based pediatric groups, and the general population.

The more restrictive the selection is for a population under study, the less generalization can be made to other populations. However, if the population is clearly defined, as in the case of Azrin, Sneed, and Foxx's (1973) study of enuresis treatment with institutionalized retardates, then the likelihood is increased that other professionals dealing with identical or very similar populations will find that the procedures could be implemented with their populations. The real issue here is that investigators need to describe clearly how the subjects were selected, i.e., by what criteria and from what population, for inclusion in a particular study.

STUDY SETTING

Frequently studies are described in the literature without real concern for the setting in which they were conducted. For example, many studies have been conducted on the use of "time out" as a disciplinary procedure for young children (e.g., Bernal, 1969; Forehand, Flanagan, & Adams, 1979; Patterson, 1974). All of these studies were conducted by behavioral psychologists through psychology treatment programs of one type or another. The question of whether these procedures would be as effective when implemented, for example, by pediatricians in a general pediatric practice, is left unanswered (cf. Drabman & Jarvie, 1977). Similarly, in Olness's (1975) description of the use of hypnosis in the management of childhood enuresis, the procedures were implemented by a pediatrician (well trained in the therapeutic use of hypnosis) in a general pediatric practice. The question of whether similar hypnosis procedures would be as effective when implemented by behavioral psychologists in a psychological clinic remains unanswered.

Ideally, since many problems are usually detected by the patient's primary care physician (either pediatrician or family practitioner), procedures for management of the specific problems should be piloted by these practitioners in the setting in which they normally practice. To the extent that these procedures are adequately addressed by the investigator, the practitioner can probably be confident that the treatment recommended will generalize to a practice setting.

The case of Azrin and Foxx's (1974) *Toilet Training in Less than a Day* provides an illustrative example. The pilot work and the research on the "dry pants training" procedure described by Azrin and Foxx was implemented by professionals well trained in the dry pants procedures. Yet the book was marketed for use by parents in the privacy of their own homes. As several subsequent studies have shown (Matson & Ollendick, 1977), the dry pants training procedures when implemented by parents were not nearly as effective as they were reported to be by Azrin and Foxx. In fact, the parents who both read the book and had some professional supervision had the best outcomes.

As with the other issues raised in this chapter, the point here is that, when the original work was conducted in a setting different from the one in which it is being introduced, the clinician or researcher needs to be cognizant of the change in setting and, perhaps, take appropriate precautionary measures that may not have been alluded to in the original work.

MEDICAL COMPLIANCE

The issue of medical compliance has been called one of the best documented but least understood phenomena in medicine (Becker & Maiman, 1975). When a study is conducted in a clinical research unit with inpatients, or with inpatients supervised by well-trained and well-motivated medical and nursing staffs, some caution must be exercised in attempts to generalize the results to general outpatient practices. While much of the basic work on control of such disease entities as diabetes and asthma is usually done in well-staffed hospital settings, the general implementation of the findings with outpatients is usually done under less than ideal circumstances with less than optimal results. In fact, the problem of medical compliance has been an unknown influence that has undoubtedly biased drug studies as well as medical-behavioral or behavioral treatment programs.

Ideally, investigators will include some reliable measure of patient compliance when they report the results of their intervention efforts. The most prevalent measure, patient report or physician estimate, is usually no better than chance and cannot be depended upon (Gordis, 1979). Unfortunately, much of the literature in behavioral pediatrics depends upon parents for either the collection of "data" or for reports of cures or outcome. For example, the work done by Olness (1975) with enuretics and Levine and Bakow (1976) and Wright (1973) with encopretics depended entirely on parent report as did Foxx and Azrin (1973a) for their outcome data on toilet training.

More objective measures of compliance include pill counts (Sackett, 1979), actual observation of parent implementation of procedures (Patterson, 1974; Barnard, Christophersen, & Wolf, 1976), and urine, serum, or saliva biochemical assays (McKenney, 1979). To date, one of the most sophisticated measures of compliance is the long-term assay, best represented by the Hemoglobin A_{1c} to measure the control of diabetics. Since this measure actually assesses the patient's state during the three-month period prior to the assay, there is virtually nothing that the patient can do, other than comply with his treatment regimen, to affect appreciably the HbA_{1c} measure.

Unfortunately, objective measures such as pill counts and biochemical assays still have their drawbacks. With pill counts, a patient who is aware that the pill count is to be done can destroy some of the pills so as to appear more compliant. Conversely, if the patient starts the medication regimen one day late but thereafter complies perfectly, he will be considered partially noncompliant when, in fact, the regimen was followed very carefully. With most of the biochemical assays, e.g., blood sugar levels or urine sugar levels, compliance in the 24-hour period immediately preceding the assay will usually result in an assay with normal or near-normal values, which may be misleading.

For a complete review of the factors affecting compliance with pediatric patients, the reader is referred to Rapoff and Christophersen (in press).

OBSERVATION-MEASUREMENT PROCEDURES

Whatever the form of measurement used, from biochemical assays to observation of the rate of occurrence of behavior problems, interobserver reliability checks are not a luxury—they are absolutely essential. In the behavioral literature, the general rule of thumb is that, on a random basis, at least 20 percent of the observations should have independent reliability checks, preferably with the checks evenly distributed over subjects and over experimental conditions.

The purpose of interobserver reliability checks is to reduce the likelihood that any of the experimenter's biases might have inadvertently influenced the data collection. For example, if hired observers are being paid to conduct observations of the effects of a particular medication on the hyperactivity levels of preschoolers, the observers may unknowingly allow their definitions or their procedures to change just enough to demonstrate an improvement over baseline when the child is started on medication. The commonly accepted control procedure in such cases is the double blind crossover design. With this design, neither the patient nor the physician knows whether any individual coded packet contains a placebo or one of the drugs under investigation. At a preselected point in time, the patient is changed from one set of packets to another, with the patient and physician still "blind" as to the contents of the packet. In this way neither the physician nor the patient can alter their observations in any systematic way, since they have no knowledge of what treatment is in effect. Although the double blind crossover design is a very sophisticated procedure, its use does not obviate the need for interobserver reliability checks. Nor is it always possible to keep the parent or physician blind to the treatment condition, since commercially prepared placebo drugs are frequently a slightly different color, to avoid the inadvertent substitution of a placebo for the real drug.

Also, with behavioral procedures the professional observer can usually tell during observation periods whether a given patient is in the baseline or no-treatment phase or in the treatment phase. For example, the difference between parent-child interactions before and after the implementation of a behavior management protocol for hyperactivity is usually quite easy to see. Thus the observer can frequently tell from the context of the observations what experimental condition is in effect.

Of course, no study can be done perfectly, without flaws or shortcomings, but every effort must be made to control for any unplanned entry of experimenter or observer bias.

GENERALITY OF TREATMENT EFFECTS

"A behavioral change may be said to have generality if it proves durable over time, if it appears in a wide variety of possible environments, or if it spreads to a wide variety of related behaviors [Baer et al., 1968, p. 94]." Thus if an intervention procedure produces both immediate and long-term improvement, then that procedure is said to have generality. Clearly, the majority of research studies only report the immediate effects of the procedures under investigation. Occasionally an author will provide anecdotal reports from family members that a behavior change was maintained for an extended period of time. Rarely do authors provide long-term follow-up data (i.e., for a period of *years*) using the same data acquisition procedures that were used in the initial intervention, including interobserver reliability checks. As an example, one area of pediatric research has dealt with getting parents to use safety restraint seats every time they transport their infants or children in an automobile. Most of the literature published to date has only reported on the short-term effects of procedures—usually no more than four to six weeks after intervention. Yet to be fully protected, children must be transported in safety restraint seats throughout their entire childhood. Christophersen and Gyulay (in press) reported on a procedure for getting parents to comply with the health care provider's instructions on the use of car seats and furnished data immediately after intervention, three months later, six months later, and one full year later. Although this type of follow-up data is difficult to obtain and delays publication of research findings, it provides the best assurance that a procedure will stand the test of time.

Similarly, much of the published literature is concerned with treatment procedures that are implemented in a hospital or laboratory setting. However, unless the results generalize to the natural environment, many of these reported procedures will have extremely limited utility. Many practitioners are all too familiar with the lack of generalization of compliance with chronic disease regimens from the inpatient setting to the natural home. Numerous articles have recently appeared that address this issue. For example, a juvenile-onset, insulin-dependent diabetic is admitted to an endocrinology service for the purpose of regulating his insulin requirements. Under these near-ideal circumstances, where meals are planned and prepared under the direction of a registered dietitian and served by a registered or licensed practical nurse, and where insulin injections and urine testing are supervised by the nursing staff, all but the most recalcitrant juvenile diabetics can be well regulated. All too often, however, not long after discharge from the hospital the results of the inpatient hospitalization are not found to generalize to the home.

Obviously, in the situations just described one alternative that needs to be considered is that short-term and long-term results, or hospital versus home results, may represent two different but related problems. The task of providing parents with the impetus for initial change may have to be approached with entirely different procedures than those necessary for long-term maintenance. Likewise, the hospitalized juvenile diabetic probably is under a totally different set of circumstances than the same diabetic in his own home. The delineation of the parameters of generalization is an important but often neglected task in behavioral pediatrics.

SIGNIFICANCE

The issue of whether a finding is significant can be addressed in two distinctly different ways. From the statistical standpoint, the question of significance means whether the observed change was due to a chance variation or to the intervention efforts of the investigator. Elaborate mathematical computations are currently available for estimating the statistical significance of the change. Usually researchers, with the help of statisticians, are able to arrive at a figure that expresses significance, such as the .01 level, which means that on only one time out of 100 will a change of a given magnitude occur due to chance variation: thus, although the possibility exists that the change was due to chance, it is not very likely.

A totally different but equally important question is whether the change was socially significant (cf. Baer et al., 1968). That is, assuming that during the baseline or preintervention period the patient's behavior was unacceptable, because of (1) the type of behavior (e.g., head banging or other self-injurious behavior), (2) the situation in which the behavior occurs (e.g., toilet training), or (3) the rate at which the behavior occurs (e.g., certain self-care behaviors), then the researchers would not consider the change to be significant unless the posttreatment behavior was within normal limits.

Thus three distinct possibilities emerge. One is that the investigator can produce a statistically significant change that is also socially significant (e.g., teaching a child enough self-help skills that the child can now take care of himself). The second is a change that is not statistically significant but is socially significant (e.g., in toilet training a child, reducing bowel accidents from one per day to none would not be statistically significant but would certainly please the parents). The third is a change that is statistically significant but not socially significant (e.g., reducing self-injurious head banging from 200 times per day to only 20 times per day is still unacceptable to most parents).

Ideally, most of the treatment programs described in the behavioral pediatrics literature should be both socially significant and, within appropriate experimental designs, statistically significant. In actuality, many do not meet these two criteria.

ADEQUATE DESCRIPTION OF TREATMENT

Baer et al. (1968) categorized the technological description of treatment or intervention procedures (i.e., the independent variable) as an important dimension for behavioral research. By "technological description" they meant simply that the techniques were completely and adequately described. Foxx and Azrin's (1973b) book *Toilet Training the Retarded* provides an eloquent illustration of a technological description. They provided step-by-step directions for implementing procedures to train self-initiated toileting, included definitions of most terms that might not be generally understood, and provided flow charts detailing exactly what to do and when. While research papers published in journals cannot be expected to detail procedures as clearly as a book, more concern for inclusion of detailed descriptions would benefit many articles.

The medical literature frequently has an advantage in that there is a long history of using clearly described, highly reliable procedures. For example, when a researcher describes a decrease in the white blood cell count after administration of a commercially available drug, most researchers reading or hearing this description would be able to administer the same drug under the same conditions and note the corresponding changes in the white blood cell count. However, a behavioral scientist may describe the use of a "time out" procedure for discipline, but there is no commonly accepted standard of how to use "time out." The easiest way to rectify this problem is to provide detailed descriptions of the procedure (or reference an earlier published description) and conduct and report the results of interobserver reliability checks on the actual use of a procedure like "time out." While such a requirement may initially appear to be too expensive or too time-consuming, the overall savings in terms of the ability of researchers to communicate accurately what they did and what happened will probably more than offset the initial added expense. Although there has been a tendency for some behavioral scientists to try to simplify protocols by dropping previously required reliability checks, few medical laboratories would consent to drop their use of "quality control checks." The concern for technological rigor exemplified by medical technologists might very profitably be carried over into the behavioral sciences.

CONCLUDING REMARKS

The field of behavioral medicine is unique in that there really isn't a "typically trained reader." Rather there are some readers with a strong medical background (which may be research oriented or clinically oriented) or a strong social science background (either research or clinical). Also, much of the literature reviewed in discussions regarding behavioral medicine was originally conducted and written to appeal to a specialized audience, e.g., pediatricians, pediatric nurses, psychiatrists, psychologists, social workers, or medical educators. Therefore the potential for misunderstanding is great. Oftentimes psychologists have little background knowledge of anatomy, physiology, or the components of a thorough medical examination. Similarly, the pediatric health care provider may have at best an outdated view of what social scientists do, predicated on exposure to traditional psychiatric approaches that were in vogue during his or her years of medical and residency training.

Although some of the work in behavioral pediatrics is done as a collaborative effort by a multidisciplinary team, most professionals individually review and write about the literature in their area of interest—not with teams. Thus the potential for misunderstanding or lack of comprehension is great. To further complicate the situation, journals like *Pediatrics* are written and edited for pediatricians, and, as such, will not allow lengthy descriptions of standard medical procedures that would be necessary for many social scientists to be able to comprehend specifically what was done. Even standard abbreviations such as UTI, URI, and IVP will be beyond the average, traditionally trained social scientist.

One answer to this dilemma is for various pediatric departments that are interested in behavioral pediatrics to welcome "outsiders" to their ambulatory seminars. Since there is little objection to the basic premise that, at least administratively, behavioral pediatrics belongs in pediatric departments under the general auspices of pediatricians (cf. Green, 1980), the social scientist who is interested in behavioral pediatrics will have to establish alliances that will foster and nurture true collaborative or interdisciplinary efforts.

A related issue has to do with the training of the professional who implemented the treatment procedures described in a particular article. When Davidson (1958) discusses the need for "cleaning out the colon" of a child seen for fecal incontinence or constipation, the average social scientist might not know what this means, much less have the personnel available to carry out the appropriate procedures. Likewise, when a behavioral psychologist describes the use of contingent praise, the pediatrician may have only the most elementary understanding of what is involved. Frequently, both disciplines tend to gloss over procedural details, assuming that the reader is familiar with the procedures.

Rather than presenting a major obstacle, these problems of collaborative research and clinical endeavors point to the real strength of any behavioral medicine program—the perennial concern for cross-fertilization among the various disciplines involved. It is exactly this effort that appears to have been absent in many of the early attempts of psychiatry or psychology to work with any of the medical subspecialty clinics.

An example may help to clarify this point. In many of the early writings on asthma in children, numerous authors, including French and Alexander (1941), stated very clearly that the etiology of asthma was due to the suppression of an intense emotion, specifically, "a suppressed cry for the mother." For years the dominant theme among psychosomatic researchers was that psychological variables played an etiologic role in asthma. More recently, Alexander (in press) has stated that although psychological factors might influence the appearance or severity of symptoms on any particular occasion, the influence is so small that there is no clinical significance to be attached to the mechanisms involved. Alexander provides substantial data showing that asthma is predominantly a physical illness that is best managed by the physician well trained in the treatment of asthma. The behaviorist can contribute substantially to this management, through his knowledge of procedures for enhancing compliance as well as through behavior therapy procedures that can be used in conjunction with appropriate medical management. Therein lies the very reason for the growth of behavioral medicine—true collaborative involvement in both research and patient care.

The methodological issues described in this chapter are intended to be representative, not exhaustive. Clearly there are issues that have not been addressed here, or that could have been addressed in more detail. The basic point is that behavioral pediatrics should not allow scientific rigor to be compromised. By maintaining rigorous scientific standards, behavioral pediatrics can continue to gain recognition as a legitimate area of interest within pediatrics. This rigor, and a sensitivity to the most pressing problems faced by the pediatric health care provider, can combine to strengthen the foundation of behavioral pediatrics.

REFERENCES

Alexander, A. B. Behavioral medicine in asthma. In R. B. Stuart (Ed.), *Compliance, generalization, and maintenance in behavioral medicine.* New York: Brunner/Mazel, in press.

Azrin, N. H., & Foxx, R. M. *Toilet training in less than a day.* New York: Simon & Schuster, 1974.

Azrin, N. H., Sneed, T. J., & Foxx, R. M. Dry bed: A rapid method of eliminating bedwetting (enuresis) of the retarded. *Behavior Research and Therapy,* 1973, **11,** 427–434.

Baer, D. M., Wolf, M. M., & Risley, T. R. Some current dimensions of applied behavior analysis. *Journal of Applied Behavior Analysis,* 1968, **1,** 91–97.

Barnard, J. D., Christophersen, E. R., & Wolf, M. M. Patient-mediated treatment of children's self-injurious behavior using overcorrection. *Journal of Pediatric Psychology,* 1976, **1**(3), 56–61.

Becker, M. H., & Maiman, L. A. Sociobehavioral determinants of compliance with health and medical care recommendations. *Medical Care,* 1975, **13,** 10.

Bernal, M. E. Behavioral feedback in the modification of brat behaviors. *Journal of Nervous and Mental Diseases,* 1969, **148**(4), 375.

Bernard, C. *An introduction to the study of experimental medicine.* New York: Dover, 1957. (Originally published 1865.)

Brazelton, T. B. Anticipatory guidance. *Pediatric Clinics of North America,* 1975, **22,** 533–544.

Campbell, D. T., & Stanley, J. C. *Experimental and quasi-experimental designs for research.* Chicago: Rand McNally, 1963.

Cerulli, M. A., Nikoomanesh, P., & Schuster, M. M. Progress in biofeedback conditioning for fecal incontinence. *Gastroenterology,* 1979, **76,** 742–746.

Christophersen, E. R., & Gyulay, J. Parental compliance with car seat usage: A positive approach with long-term follow-up. *Journal of Pediatric Psychology,* in press.

Davidson, M. Constipation and fecal incontinence. *Pediatric Clinics of North America,* 1958, **5,** 749–757.

Drabman, R. S., & Jarvie, G. Counseling parents of children with behavior problems: The use of extinction and time out techniques. *Pediatrics,* 1977, **51,** 78.

Engel, B. T., Nikoomanesh, P., & Schuster, M. M. Operant conditioning of rectosphincteric responses in the treatment of fecal incontinence. *New England Journal of Medicine,* 1974, **290,** 646–649.

Forehand, R., Flanagan, S., & Adams, H. E. A comparison of four instructional techniques for teaching parents the use of time-out. *Behavior Therapy,* 1979, **10,** 94–102.

Foxx, R. M., & Azrin, N. H. Dry pants: A rapid method of toilet training children. *Behavior Research and Therapy,* 1973, **11,** 435–442.(a)

Foxx, R. H., & Azrin, N. H. *Toilet training the retarded.* Champaign, Ill.: Research Press, 1973.(b)

French, T. M., & Alexander, F. Psychogenic factors in bronchial asthma. *Psychosomatic Medicine Monograph,* 1941, **4,** 2–94.

Gordis, L. Conceptual and methodologic problems in measuring patient compliance. In R. B. Haynes, D. W. Taylor, & D. L. Sackett (Eds.), *Compliance in health care.* Baltimore: Johns Hopkins University Press, 1979.

Green, M. The pediatric model of care. *Behavior Therapist,* 1980, **3**(3), 7–8.

Hersen, M., & Barlow, D. H. *Single-case experimental designs: Strategies for studying behavior change.* New York: Pergamon Press, 1976.

Kohlenberg, R. J. Operant conditioning of human and sphincter pressure. *Journal of Applied Behavior Analysis,* 1973, **6,** 201–208.

Levine, M. D., & Bakow, H. Children with encopresis: A treatment outcome study. *Pediatrics,* 1976, **58,** 845–852.

Matson, J. L., & Ollendick, T. H. Issues in toilet training normal children. *Behavior Therapy,* 1977, **8,** 549–553.

McKenney, J. M. The clinical pharmacy and compliance. In R. B. Haynes, D. W. Taylor, & D. L. Sackett (Eds.), *Compliance in health care.* Baltimore: Johns Hopkins University Press, 1979.

Olness, K. The use of self-hypnosis in the treatment of childhood nocturnal enuresis. *Clinical Pediatrics,* 1975, **14,** 273–279.

Patterson, G. R. Interventions for boys with conduct problems: Multiple settings, treatments and criteria. *Journal of Consulting and Clinical Psychology,* 1974, **42,** 471–481.

Rapoff, M. A., & Christophersen, E. R. Compliance of pediatric patients with medical regimens: A review and evaluation. In L. A. Hamerlynck (Ed.), *Compliance, generalization, and maintenance in behavioral medicine.* New York: Brunner/Mazel, in press.

Risley, T. R. Behavior modification: An experimental-therapeutic endeavor. In L. A. Hamerlynck, P. O. Davidson, & L. E. Acker (Eds.), *Behavior modification: An ideal mental health service.* Calgary, Alta., Canada: University of Calgary Press, 1970.

Sackett, D. L. Methods for compliance research. In R. B. Haynes, D. W. Taylor, & D. L. Sackett (Eds.), *Compliance in health care.* Baltimore: Johns Hopkins University Press, 1979.

Wright, L. Handling the encopretic child. *Professional Psychology,* 1973, **4,** 137–144.

Wright, L., Schaeffer, A. B., & Solomons, G. (Eds.). *Encyclopedia of pediatric psychology.* Baltimore: University Park Press, 1979.

6

Pediatric Neuropsychology: Status, Theory, and Research

Greta N. Wilkening
and
Charles J. Golden

Pediatric neuropsychology is the study of brain-behavior relationships in children. Though a variety of professionals have been interested in the effects of brain damage on child development for some time, it is only recently that pediatric neuropsychology has become an important, distinct area of investigation.

Despite increased interest in child neuropsychology, this field of investigation and practice remains very much the stepchild of adult neuropsychology. The marked increase in the study of neuropsychological functioning, as indicated by the publication of many new books, the development of workshops and courses, and the establishment of a division within the American Psychological Association, has focused mainly on the adult. A recent survey by us of available postdoctoral fellowships in clinical neuropsychology revealed that only 2 of 16 programs reported training emphasis on child neuropsychology, and of the remainder only one program even included children as a population worthy of special study.

Such a disparity in level of activity is a reflection of the very difficult problems inherent in completing research with children. The lack of any premorbid state that can be confirmed by objective data makes child neuropsychology distinctly different from adult neuropsychology. This is particularly true if one wishes to look at damage thought to occur at or around the time of birth.

An additional barrier is posed by the role of experience in childhood development. Though most adults who are living independently can be expected to have a certain minimal level of experience and skill gained through school attendance and related activities, this is not so for children, especially preschool-aged children. For example, verbal development is related to language experience and stimulation. Children may fail to develop adequate language either because they have not had adequate stimulation or as the result of factors secondary to cortical injury. The same holds true for other areas of development.

Research with children also presents difficulty in terms of eliciting cooperation. Though cooperation can be established with most adult subjects (and those who cannot or refuse to cooperate may be excluded from research programs), noncooperative behavior is prevalent among children and is even the norm among pre-school-aged children.

These complications in completing research have discouraged the emergence of many active research programs in the area of pediatric neuropsychology. Those studies that have been completed have most often been a direct outgrowth of work with adults, and are a limited reflection of what has been learned about the results of brain damage on adult behavior. This is true despite the awareness that brain-behavior relationships in children are not isomorphic with patterns seen in adults (Rudel & Teuber, 1971).

In spite of the relative paucity of long-term research programs in pediatric clinical neuropsychology, perusal of the literature in the field loosely defined as the "psychological effects of brain damage in children" reveals a startlingly diverse array of articles. This work has been completed by professionals with a variety of backgrounds and interests, including psychology, neurology, pediatrics, speech pathology, and education. Though one result of such diversity has been the emergence of creative and fascinating approaches, there has been a failure to organize this information so that it is useful to the clinician or to those planning research programs.

Difficulties in integrating the results of child neuropsychological investigation reflect, in part, the different emphases of various research programs. The purposes of neuropsychological research fall broadly into three major areas:

1. Research focused upon the development of tools for investigation of brain-behavior relationships.
2. Research focused upon the study of discrete disorders using neuropsychological tools to identify and describe the pathological processes.
3. Development of a theoretical approach to brain-behavior relationships.

The first area of interest includes such studies as those investigating the capability of individual instruments to discriminate "brain-damaged" from "non-brain-damaged" children. Typically, though the choice of which instrument to study has been theoretically derived, the instruments themselves were not based upon a theoretical understanding of the development of brain-behavior relationships in children. Under this paradigm an instrument is considered successful if it can reliably separate those children who are brain-damaged from those who are not.

A more sophisticated approach to tool development has been the attempt to elaborate instruments that would not only allow for the dichotomization of brain-damaged from normal children, but would also investigate more fully the child's functioning over a variety of higher cortical skills and provide information for remedial programs. The work of Boll and Reitan (Boll, 1974; Reitan, 1974b) on the use of the children's versions of the Halstead Battery is an example of this form of investigation.

The second area of inquiry into brain-behavior relationships in childhood has been the use of neuropsychological tools to answer questions about pathological brain states. This research is typified by studies examining recovery from meningitis or closed head trauma, or those projects that have attempted to look at whether specific treatments (e.g., central nervous system irradiation) are related to deficits in higher cortical functioning. Attempts to identify underlying skill deficits in the learning-disabled and retarded populations are other areas of exploration where neuropsychology has been used as a tool.

The third area of investigation is that of theory development. At times this type of research fuses with the second category, since researchers have most often used brain-damaged populations to help them understand brain-behavior relationships, and to analyze developmental aspects of neuropsychological functioning. For example, comparisons of the neuropsychological skills of children receiving central nervous system irradiation prior to three years of age with those older than three years at the time of treatment not only help us understand the possible iatrogenic effects of such treatment, but also contribute to our knowledge of the developing brain. Clearly this area of research cannot be totally divorced from either tool development or identification of clinical states. It is evident that a theoretical understanding of what happens as cognitive functions develop is necessary in order to wisely choose tests to investigate, to establish batteries, and to make sense of the results obtained from clinical research programs.

Within this chapter an extensive, but by no means complete, review of these three areas of neuropsychology will be presented. Finally, our theoretical approach toward child neuropsychology and the battery that has grown from this orientation will be described.

THE NEUROPSYCHOLOGIST AS A TOOL DEVELOPER

A great deal of energy and time has been devoted to the development of tools to be used in studying the effects of brain damage. Often these have focused on the use of single tests to discriminate brain-damaged from non-brain-damaged children. However, single tests used for categorization are inadequate for evaluation that is being conducted for the purposes of remediation or program planning.

The choice of a single test to diagnose brain damage in children is predicated on two beliefs: that all children with brain damage will present with a skill deficit in the area measured by that test; and that all brain-damaged children will present with unitary and consistent deficits regardless of the time of onset, localization, or extent of the damage. For instance, research with the Bender Gestalt to discriminate brain-damaged from normal children assumes that all children with brain damage will have some form of impairment in visual perceptual or motor difficulties. Though such research is based on a hypothesis about the nature of brain damage, it is not based upon a developmental neuropsychological theory.

The belief that all brain damage in children will present in a similar fashion reflects traditional teaching about the characteristics of brain-damaged children. Classically these children have been described as demonstrating consistent attributes irrespective of the multiple factors contributing to etiology. Brain-damaged children are said to be distractible and hyperactive, to have coordination difficulties, and to demonstrate affective lability. Some authors state that brain-damaged children have deficits in problem-solving skills. Poor intellectual functioning is often considered to be a concomitant factor, though discrepant patterns between strengths and weaknesses are sometimes seen as indicative of brain damage. Typically, authors have noted that the psychological effects of brain damage in children tend to be general, in contrast to adults, in whom the neuropsychological deficits are more discrete.

Such a unitary conceptualization of brain damage in chidlren has been maintained despite methodological problems in the research literature. Representative problems include patient populations limited to those with congenital brain damage or subjects whose brain damage was severe enough to warrant institutionalization. Many studies attempting to differentiate brain-damaged from normal children fail to identify the age of onset of the disorder, thus establishing groups heterogeneous in reference to what is believed to be a major variable in the manifestation of cerebral dysfunction in children.

One example of the failure to recognize the heterogeneity in brain-damaged children and of the inappropriateness of using a single test to diagnose and describe impairment is the literature on distractibility and attention span. It is widely asserted that brain-damaged children have short attention spans. This is then used as a diagnostic criterion, despite consistent findings that such children do not always present with this symptomatology. Rubin (1969) found that as a group brain-damaged children do-not differ from normal controls or familially retarded children in attending to relevant stimuli on figure-ground tasks. Kasper, Millechap, Backus, Child, and Schulman (1971) found that the distractibility of brain-damaged children was related to the nature of the stimulus and was not consistent across situations, although brain-damaged children were more distractible than the controls. However, Diaz (1971) found that brain-damaged children were no more distractible than normal controls. Rutter (1977) suggested that distractibility and impulsiveness were more closely related to psychiatric disorder, a frequent concomitant of brain damage, than they were to the organic damage itself.

The relationship between intelligence and distractibility has been confounded in many studies. Kasper et al. (1971) found that brighter brain-damaged children were less distractible than their less intelligent brain-damaged cohorts. Fisher (1970) also found IQ to be related to differential patterns of distractibility in a brain-damaged group.

Czudner and Rourke (1970) did find that brain-damaged children have a deficit in the ability to develop and maintain attention. However, they noted an age trend, with older brain-injured children being less distractible. They posited that brain-damaged children may learn to adapt to this deficit. This introduces yet another factor in evaluating the assumption of a unitary nature to brain damage in children.

Despite fairly convincing evidence that not all brain-damaged children present with similar behavioral patterns, the use of single tests to screen patients or to identify the presence of organic features remains a prevalent pattern. There has been extensive research with both publicly available and experimental tests in regard to the reliability with which they can discriminate brain-damaged from normal children.

Visual Spatial Tests

The *Bender-Gestalt* is frequently used in diagnostic work with children. Koppitz (1964) has developed scoring criteria that are commonly used both to assess the child's developmental level and to differentiate brain-damaged from emotionally disturbed children. Oliver and Kronenberger (1971) reported that when scores fell within the abnormal range, the developmental indicators derived from the Koppitz scoring system were successful in discriminating brain-damaged, emotionally disturbed, and normal adolescents, though the "emotional" indicators were unsuccessful at this same task. McConnell (1967) reported that the developmental scores were successful in discriminating substantially brain-damaged children from emotionally disturbed children in the five-to-ten-year-old range. These scores also discriminated minimally brain-damaged children from children who were diagnosed as having situational disorders and borderline psychoses. However, the developmental scores did not differentiate the neurotic or characteriologically disordered children from brain-damaged children, nor could nonorganic psychotic children be successfully discriminated from organic psychotics.

Bosaeus (1978) used the scoring system of Koppitz for children less than 10 years 11 months of age, and that of Pascall and Suttell with the protocols of older children. She found the Bender to have too many false positive results to be clinically useful. Seventy-one of 222 normal children (32 percent) were identified as brain-damaged using Koppitz's indicators for all subjects.

An adaptation of the Bender, the Background Interference Procedure, was developed by Canter (1970). The discriminative capacity of this form of the Bender has been supported by some studies (Adams, Peterson, Kenny, and

Canter, 1975; Kenny, 1971). However, the results of these studies have not been cross-validated, nor have the comparison groups been well defined.

It is obvious that results using the Bender, including variations of the Bender, have been inconsistent. Denson and May (1978) attribute this lack of consistency to the low test-retest reliability of the measures commonly used in scoring the Bender. Other discrepancies in research results are attributable to poorly defined criterion groups (Mordock, 1969). The Bender successfully discriminates brain-damaged from entirely normal children, but it is not as successful when emotionally disturbed children are included. Though the former discrimination is successful, this is not the distinction that is clinically relevant. Most often the clinician is being asked to discriminate between children who have functional disorders and those with organic damage. The Bender does not appear accurate or inclusive enough to be used alone as a screening tool. The skills measured by the Bender are important areas of neuropsychological functioning, however, and they should be assessed as part of a complete evaluation (Golden, 1981a).

Verbal Tests

The Illinois Test of Psycholinguistic Abilities (ITPA) was developed by Kirk, McCarthy, and Kirk (1961) as a means of measuring verbal skills in children, and was based upon a theoretical model of language processing. Though widely used in learning disabilities programs for assessing discrepant performance between areas of verbal and visual skill, research with this instrument has been disappointing (Golden, 1981a). The subtests do not assess separate abilities, but appear to yield only a measure of general verbal ability (Hallahan & Cruikshank, 1973). In terms of using the test as a neuropsychological instrument, Zaidel (1979) found the subtests do not reflect "natural hemispheric divisions. The functions measured by the ITPA are thought to be too complex to provide adequate measures of neuropsychological skills, and fail to reflect underlying linguistic skills.

Test Batteries

Because a unitary hypothesis in regard to neuropsychological sequelae of brain damage need not be posited, test batteries are thought to provide a more adequate description of neuropsychological functioning. Use of a battery allows for a description of a child's strengths and weaknesses and is more appropriate for designing rehabilitation and educational programs.

Though the *Wechsler Intelligence Scale for Children* (WISC) and its revised form (WISC-R) are considered single tests, they are composed of a variety of subtests and yield both a performance and a verbal IQ level, in addition to a full scale IQ. The subtests measure a number of different skills and have been thought of as providing a comprehensive assessment of cognitive development that can be used for neuropsychological assessment. Though the WISC-R has replaced the WISC in common clinical use, most of the neuropsychological research has used the older form of the test. The two forms do not yield equivalent results; the WISC-R tends to give somewhat lower IQs than the WISC.

Clinical neuropsychological interpretation of the WISC has been based upon patterns seen in the adult brain-damaged population, though the applicability of these assumptions has not been borne out by empirical research. Intertest scatter on the WAIS, the adult Wechsler scale, has typically been thought to be indicative of organic impairment. Similar interpretation of WISC profiles has proven to be fallacious. The WISC subtests are more sensitive to early brain lesions than are the WAIS subtests. Brain-injured children show more of an overall decrease on WISC IQs than on any other measures (Reitan, 1974a). Simensen and Sutherland (1974) reported that the research on WISC performance does not support use of intertest scatter in the diagnosis of organic impairment, though McIntosh (1974) reported successful discrimination of brain-damaged from normal children using a ratio of scores suggested for use with adults by Russell, Neuringer, and Goldstein (1970).

There has been a great deal written about the significance of differences between verbal and performance IQs in the diagnosis of brain damage in children. Though large differences in favor of the verbal IQ are diagnostically significant, smaller differences or differences in favor of the performance IQ are common in the normal and the brain-injured population (Bortner & Birch, 1969; Simensen & Sutherland, 1974). Reed and Reitan (1969) and Woods and Teuber (1973) found that when verbal and performance differences do exist they are not in the direction that would be anticipated based upon adult neuropsychological theory. These researchers found that children with both unilateral left and unilateral right hemisphere lesions tend to have lower performance than verbal IQs.

The discrepancies and confusion in the literature over the utility of the WISC in the diagnosis of brain damage are related to a variety of methodological issues. In particular, most research has failed to consider or control for age of onset of the disorder, though this appears to be an important variable in how brain damage is expressed behaviorally. Woods (1980) found that early lesions (onset prior to age 1 year) appear to produce overall declines in IQ with little marked intertest scatter or verbal versus performance IQ differences. Later left hemisphere lesions (mean age of onset 5.7 years) produced similar results, though later right hemisphere lesions (mean age of onset 6.4 years) showed only performance decrements. The later right hemisphere group was the only one to demonstrate significant verbal-performance discrepancies. Interpretation of WISC performance as assessing neuropsychological functioning obviously must attend to considerations of age of onset of neurological condition. Interpretation of verbal scale decrements as indicative of organicity should be done with extreme caution!

Halstead-Reitan Batteries

The most prevalent batteries currently in use for the neuropsychological evaluation of children are the Halstead-Reitan tests. There are two forms of the battery; the *Halstead Neuropsychological Test Battery for Children* aged 9 to 14 (Reitan, 1969) and the *Reitan-Indiana Neuropsychological Test Battery for Children* (Reitan, 1969) designed for ages 5 to 8 years. Both batteries are modeled after the adult Halstead-Reitan Neuropsychological Battery, with modifications from the adult tests primarily reflecting changes in the level of difficulty. Typically the batteries are administered so as to include measures of motor and tactile-perceptual functions, academic skills, verbal ability, visual spatial and sequential skills, immediate alertness, cognitive flexibility, reasoning skills, and incidental memory. The age-appropriate Wechsler test is generally included as a part of the exam. The batteries are designed to allow for interpretation using a pathognomonic sign approach, an evaluation of level and pattern of performance, and the presence of lateralized effects, as recommended by Reitan (1974a).

Though there has been less experimental investigation of the children's batteries than of the adult form, those completed indicate that the battery is effective in discriminating brain-damaged from normal children (Boll, 1972, 1974; Boll & Reitan, 1972; Klonoff & Low, 1974; Reitan, 1971, 1974b). Klonoff, Robinson, and Thompson (1969) report hit rates between 80 percent in five-year-olds to 96 percent in eight-year-olds. Klonoff and Low (1974) found overall hit rates of 80 percent in normal children and 75 percent in brain-injured patients less than nine years of age. When effectiveness with children over nine years of age was investigated Klonoff and Low (1974) reported a hit rate of 90 percent in normals and 80 percent in brain-damaged children. All these studies used discriminative analysis to determine hit rates. Recently Selz and Reitan (1979) developed a system of 37 rules that discriminated normal, learning-disabled, and brain-damaged children with 73 percent accuracy. These rules were based upon the four methods of inference as suggested by Reitan.

As would be anticipated, the patterns of sensitivity to brain damage among the tests comprising the battery are not identical to those observed in the adult population. On the Reitan-Indiana Neuropsychological Battery the most sensitive measures (excluding the WISC variables) are those of tactile perception (tactile form recognition, tactile finger recognition), reasoning and conceptual flexibility (progressive figures), and motor speed (marching test). It should be noted that the subjects used for this study were matched for sex and chronological age. IQ level was not considered. This is reflected in the finding that full scale WISC IQ was the most effective portion of the battery in differentiating the two groups.

When older children are evaluated on the Halstead Children's Battery, the most effective tests (excluding the Wechsler variables) are those of visual problem solving (trail-making test), motor speed (finger oscillation test— nondominant hand) and auditory perception (speech sounds perception test) (Boll, 1974). The less effective measures were those considered to be more sensitive in the adult: the tactual performance test and the category test. WISC measures were the most effective discriminators of brain damage in older children.

Selz and Reitan (1979) clearly point out that the discrimination between brain-damaged and normal children, though it is frequently asked for for diagnostic, legal, and heuristic reasons, is often not the most important issue. In order to be most useful, test batteries must provide a description of strengths and weaknesses that can be used to design remedial programs. The Reitan-Indiana Neuropsychological Test Battery and the Halstead Neuropsychological Test Battery for Children, though effectively discriminating brain-damaged and normal children, do so by utilizing tests of relatively high complexity. This may make it difficult for psychologists to design effective remedial strategies based upon a developmental understanding of the ontogenesis of cognitive functions.

INVESTIGATION OF SPECIFIC DISORDERS USING NEUROPSYCHOLOGICAL TOOLS

Neuropsychologists have been instrumental in assisting other professionals in the investigation of questions germane to the understanding and treatment of pathological conditions. In these instances neuropsychologists provide a tool that is used for evaluating the effectiveness of specific treatment programs (e.g., assessment of the effectiveness of the PKU diet or a specific protocol in the treatment of meningitis), predicting outcome subsequent to the CNS insult (e.g., follow-up studies of victims of traumatic head injury), assessing the presence of brain damage as a result of presumably non-CNS disease processes (e.g., assessment of the cortical functioning of cystic fibrosis patients), or evaluating possible iatrogenic effects of treatment for medical disorders (e.g., effects of CNS irradiation). Investigation of specific neurological syndromes using neuropsychological measures is another area in which neuropsychologists have been active and in which the tests previously described have been used as tools. It should be emphasized that the goal of these studies is not the further refinement or elaboration of neuropsychological instruments. The validity and reliability of the instruments are assumed.

There are many areas in which neuropsychological testing can be applied in order to elucidate some aspects of the pathological process. This section will review some of those applications in the areas of prognostication, evaluation of iatrogenic effects, and understanding of discrete neurological diseases.

Neuropsychology as a Tool: Neuropsychological Sequelae of Severe Head Trauma

The outcome of severe head trauma secondary to accidental and nonaccidental head injury has been investigated using neuropsychological tools. In general these studies have focused on children who have sustained injuries resulting in prolonged periods of unconsciousness. Neurosurgeons and pediatricians have been especially interested in establishing prognostic indicators for these children to give parents accurate information regarding likely outcome and to permit treatment decisions to be judiciously formulated. Prognostic indicators that have been examined are length of coma, computed tomography (CT) results, age at the time of insult, and family socioeconomic status. In some cases outcome criterion measures other than performance on neuropsychological tests have been used.

Length of coma has consistently been shown to be related to outcome. Heiskanen and Kaste (1974) found that children who were unconscious for more than two weeks rarely had full recovery, as assessed by normal school progress. Brink, Garrett, Hale, Woo-Sam, and Nickel (1980) related that children who were comatose for less than three months had better outcomes when this was evaluated by a criterion of return to independent ambulation. Lange-Cosack, Wider, Schlesener, Grumme, and Kubicki (1979) found that the frequency and severity of the sequelae increased as the duration of the coma lengthened. Levin and Eisenberg (1979) evaluated both length and severity of coma and found that the subsequent deficits, as measured by an extensive neuropsychological battery, were related to the severity of the coma. They found memory deficits to be the most consistent residual effects of a severe closed head injury, with half of their sample demonstrating impairments in verbal learning and memory, or continuous recognition, or both. Length of coma was significantly related to residual visual-spatial defects, which were present in 25 percent of the children evaluated. It should be noted that considerable neuropsychological impairment was evidenced even in children with intact or mildly abnormal neurologic findings.

Brink et al. (1980) found ventricular enlargement on CT scans to be associated with poor prognosis, when this is defined by failure to recover mobility and self-care skills. Levin and Eisenberg (1979), however, found no association between CT scan changes and neuropsychological deficits postinjury when CT abnormalities were considered as a group. They did find, however, that when children who showed left temporal damage on CT scan were considered as a separate group these children had significant verbal memory deficits. Other localization-behavior relationships between CT results and test results were nonsignificant.

Age at onset may be an important variable in prognosis. Levin and Eisenberg (1979) found that older children (between 13 and 18 years of age, as opposed to the group between 6 and 12 years of age at the time of injury) were more vulnerable to memory deficits subsequent to injury. Brink et al. (1970) and Lange-Cosack et al. (1979), however, found that long-term sequelae were more severe in children who were younger at the time of their injury. This discrepancy may be explained by the differences in the ages of those children composing the younger groups or in testing procedures. Lange-Cosack et al. considered their "young" children to be those less than five years at the time of their injury. Woo-Sam, Zimmerman, Brink, Uyehara, and Miller (1970) corroborated the finding that young children are more vulnerable to the effects of traumatic brain damage. In their sample children less than eight years of age incurred more deficits, as measured by standard tests of intelligence. Klonoff and his coworkers (Klonoff, Low, & Clark, 1977; Klonoff & Paris, 1974) found a different pattern of rate of recovery in children who were less than nine years at the time of trauma than was evident in children older than nine years when their head trauma was incurred. Despite differential rates of recovery the majority of the patients in both age groups had made marked recovery on neuropsychological tests by the end of five years.

Woo-Sam et al. (1970) found socioeconomic status to be unrelated to posttrauma neuropsychological performance. Time between injury and evaluation is a significant factor in assessing the amount of recovery that will occur. Though the largest increments of improvement occur during the first year postinjury (Brink et al., 1970), changes in functioning continue to occur for at least five years (Klonoff et al., 1977).

Though there are some well-established indicators of prognosis subsequent to acute and severe head trauma, some considerations have not been accounted for in the studies currently completed. A glaring concern is the failure to account for etiologic differences. Brink et al. (1980) reported that children who sustained head injury subsequent to nonaccidental trauma had worse outcomes than those who were injured in accidents. This further confounds interpretation of the results of previous studies because it appears that there is an unequal distribution of etiologic patterns across the age ranges. Young children more often sustain nonaccidental head trauma than older children (Lange-Cosack et al., 1979).

Neuropsychology as a Tool: Neuropsychological Sequelae of CNS Infections

The literature on the neuropsychological effects of central nervous system infections is difficult to interpret due to methodological differences between studies and problems in research design. Many articles do not specify the type of infection the child sustained. Socioeconomic status is most often not controlled for. Perhaps most problematic is that the time from onset of symptoms to initiation of treatment is not described. Those studies that have reported on the long-term outcomes of children with specified CNS infections are reviewed here.

Matthews, Chun, Grabow, and Thompson (1968) studied children one to six years after their illness with California encephalitis, a relatively mild viral illness of the central nervous system (Weil, 1980). Using the WISC mazes, Ravens Progressive Matrices, the category test of the Halstead-Reitan, the wide range achievement test, the finger tapping test, the Purdue pegboard, and a behavior rating checklist, they found no significant neuropsychological sequelae of the illness. There was no relationship between neuropsychological performance or rated level of residual neuropsychological impairment and the child's age at the onset of illness, or the time between the illness and testing. These findings were supported by Rie, Hilty, and Cramblett (1973), though in this study the control group was composed of children who had been evaluated for psychiatric disturbances, a group that may not be an adequate comparison.

Sabatino and Cramblett (1968) also studied the neuropsychological sequelae of California encephalitis. Using a battery including the WISC, the draw-a-man test, the Bender-Gestalt, a test for auditory perception, a test of motor accuracy, the wide range achievement test, a test of oral reading, and the Quay and Peterson Behavior Checklist, they assessed children seven months to two years posthospitalization for treatment of their acute illness. It is not clear how old the children were at the time of illness. They found no identifiable impairments in higher language skills. There were indications of impairment in the perception of basic visual and auditory information, and symptoms of "organic" hyperactivity. If there are consistent patterns of neuropsychological dysfunction subsequent to this mild form of encephalitis these deficits are not clearly based on the research currently available.

Several researchers have evaluated the neuropsychological sequelae of *Hemophilus influenzae (H. influenzae)* meningitis. Wright and Jimmerson (1971) compared the performance of ten children considered by physicians to be "unscathed" by their illness to ten controls matched for age, race, and family income. The children who had had *H. influenzae* were 5 to 14 years old at the time of their illness. The WISC, the Bender, and the Frostig were administered to both groups. They found no differences between groups on Bender and Frostig performance. They found significant differences favoring the controls on comprehension, similarities, picture completion, and block design and coding, as well as on performance IQ, verbal IQ, and full scale IQ. They concluded that these "unscathed" children had indeed sustained some impairment in higher cortical functioning secondary to their illness.

Sells, Carpenter, and Ray (1975) used the WISC to evaluate the functioning of children who had had *H. influenzae* meningitis. Most of these children were less than three years of age at the time of illness. All were less than five years at the onset of illness. The mean full scale IQ was 84. The correlations of IQ with age at onset, interval between onset, and treatment and medical complications were nonsignificant. The performance of nine of the children was compared with that of a sibling. Two of the nine children performed over one standard deviation below the performance of their sibling. They concluded that in this group of young children there were residual neuropsychological handicaps subsequent to *H. influenzae* meningitis.

Sells et al. (1975) studied 19 children who had been ill between 1 and 64 months of age (median age of onset 7 months) with CNS enterovirus. The performance of these children was compared with that of a control group matched for age, sex, and socioeconomic status. There was, however, no attempt to assure that the children in the control group were indeed normal. Fifteen percent of the postinfection children had severe neurological findings, including seizure disorders, spastic quadriplegia, and delayed speech and language development. Twenty-six percent had possible impairment, as indicated by IQs in the 70–85 range, or speech delay or serious behavior problems with an IQ of greater than 90. The mean head circumference of the children whose illness occurred during the first year of life was significantly less than that of the control group. Most of the deficits in psychological testing and speech and language were exhibited in those children who had been ill during their first year of life.

Sell, Webb, Pate, and Doyne (1972) studied children who had had bacterial meningitis when they were two months to three years of age. They found significant IQ differences between postmeningitic children and their sibling controls.

Fitzhardinge, Kazemi, Ramsay, and Stern (1974) reported upon the neuropsychological functioning of 30 children who had had neonatal meningitis. The children were one year to ten years eight months of age at the time of testing. No control group was utilized. Almost half of the children had been less than 38 weeks gestational age at the time of their birth. Mean IQ at follow-up was 90. Shaffer (1973) in a review of the literature reported that lasting neurological or intellectual handicaps subsequent to encephalitis or meningitis is most likely when the infection occurs during the first two years of life.

This brief review of the literature on the neuropsychological sequelae of CNS infections indicates that there are some predictable patterns of sequelae subsequent to such illnesses. It appears that the younger the child at the time of illness the more likely he or she is to sustain damage. In older children the less mature cortical areas are more vulnerable to damage.

Neuropsychology as a Tool: Neuropsychological Sequelae of Leukemia and Its Treatment

Research with children who have leukemia indicates that there are three sources of CNS disturbance associated with this illness. There are acute neurological disorders unrelated to treatment (Hanefeld & Riehm, 1980). In addition there are acute, short-term neurologic iatrogenic effects of leukemia treatment, including seizures, transient encephalopathies, myelo(radiculo)pathy, polyneuro(myo)pathy syndrome, and methotrexate-induced encephalopathies (Hanefeld & Riehm, 1980).

Of greatest concern are the long-term neuropsychological sequelae of leukemia treatment in children who have had CNS prophylaxis (CNS irradiation) and (sometimes) intrathecal methotrexate (that is, introduction of the chemotherapeutic agent methotrexate into the CSF via lumbar puncture). These deficits do not seem to become apparent when all ages of children are considered as one group. Soni, Marten, Pitner, Duenas, and Powazek (1975) found no differences between children with acute lymphocytic leukemia (ALL) treated with irradiation and children with solid tumors treated with irradiation to other parts of the body on measures of intelligence, academic achievement, or visual motor functioning. Soni and her coworkers did note, however, that the WISC performance scores of the controls improved over the repeated testings, though the scores of the leukemics did not. Both groups had received chemotherapy. In the same study the performance of children with ALL who had received CNS prophlaxis was compared to children with ALL who did not receive irradiation. Again there were no differences.

Eiser and Lansdown (1977) and Goff, Anderson, and Cooper (1980) found that when leukemic children who had received CNS irradiation were broken into younger and older age groups (on the basis of time of diagnosis) the younger children demonstrated deficits. Eiser and Lansdown (1977) found that children who were diagnosed as having leukemia between two and five years of age and were treated with CNS irradiation showed significant deficits when compared with controls matched for age, sex, and socioeconomic status. There were no deficits in the group of children treated with CNS irradiation who were older than five years at the time of diagnosis. Eiser and Lansdown did note, however, that there were no signs of gross intellectual impairment in either group.

Goff et al. (1980) compared the performance of long-term survivors of leukemia who were less than eight years old at the time of diagnosis and who had received CNS prophylaxis to patients with newly diagnosed leukemia who had received chemotherapy but had not yet received CNS irradiation. They found that the mean IQs of the newly diagnosed patients were significantly superior to those of the long-term survivors. The largest and most consistent differences were on the digit span and arithmetic scales of the WISC. On the Halstead Battery and the long-term survivors demonstrated an impairment on the speech sounds perception test. Eight of the long-term survivors had had CNS leukemia. There were no differences between these children and those long-term survivors who had not had CNS leukemia.

Ch'ien, Rhomes, Stagner, Cavalla, Wood, Goff, Pitner, Hustu, Seifert, and Simone (1980) found signs of CNS impairment (EEG abnormalities and deficits in neuropsychological testing) in children who had had the somnolence syndrome subsequent to CNS irradiation. He noted that children who receive cranial irradiation with 2,400 rads or more of ^{60}Co are at high risk to develop learning disabilities.

Neuropsychology as a Tool: Aphasia in Children

There are three forms of aphasia in children:

1. developmental aphasia
2. acute acquired aphasia
3. acquired aphasia with gradual onset

The child with *developmental aphasia* is marked by a failure to acquire language skills and functions. These children demonstrate severe dysfunction in both the reception and expression of language. Though rudimentary language may develop, it is likely to be characterized by lack of conventional grammar, deviation from developmental language norms in terms of both achievement of skills and order of acquisition, and an atypical relationship in the comprehension-production ratio. Behaviorally such children are likely to be emotionally labile and hyperactive and demonstrate perseveration and inconsistent performance. These children may have an auditory acuity deficit, but the magnitude of the language handicap is disproportional to the acuity loss. A majority of the children present with abnormal neurological findings and EEG results that implicate the left cerebral hemisphere. Developmentally aphasic children approximate the norm in terms of intellectual functioning when nonverbal tests of intelligence are utilized (Eisenson, 1968, 1969).

Most authors (Eisenson, 1968, 1969; Tallal & Newcombe, 1978) currently see the major defect as being in the child's ability to deal with linguistic sequences. Though the aphasic child appears to be able to adequately discriminate phonemes in isolation, she or he cannot make these same discriminations when the phonemes are incorporated into the complex linguistic structures of speech, and these distinctions must be made very quickly. Eisenson relates this to A. R. Luria's theory of neuropsychological functioning, noting that the secondary divisions of the auditory cortex, as well as the postcentral kinesthetic area of the cortex, are involved in these tasks.

The prognosis of children with developmental aphasia is more like that of adult aphasics than like that of children with acute acquired aphasia. Progress is slow and requires extensive intervention.

Acquired aphasia, acute onset, in children refers to language disorganization occurring during childhood subsequent to a focal cerebral injury. Unlike developmental aphasia, acquired aphasia represents a regression from previously achieved levels of psycholinguistic skill. Acquired aphasia in children is seen as being different in important features from acquired aphasia in adults.

Unlike that of adults with acquired temporal aphasia, the speech of children with this disorder is notable for the reduction of expressive language. Even elicited speech is severely reduced (Alajouanine & Lhermitte, 1965; Hécaen, 1976). There is rarely logorrhae (increased verbalization marked by lack of content), semantic or phonemic paraphasias (substitutions of one word for another based on their belonging to the same conceptual sphere [semantic], e.g., teamaker for coffeepot, or based on the sound similarities of the words [phonemic], e.g., ox for axe), or perseveration. Alajouanine and Lhermitte (1965) also found that the written language of children with acquired aphasia was more disturbed than their oral language. Receptive disorders are not consistently observed (18 out of 32 children had receptive disorders in Alajouanine and Lhermitte's group, 1965; Hécaen, 1970, stated that over one-third of his sample had receptive disorders). Alajouanine and Lhermitte noted that their older childhood aphasics (10-to-15-year-olds) were more like adult aphasics than younger childhood aphasics (5-to-9-year-olds). The older aphasics demonstrated semantic and phonemic paraphasias, while the younger children did not. They attribute this to the relative absence of automatic language functions in the younger child. Acalculia (inability to complete mathematical calculations), both written and oral, was a frequent symptom (Hécaen, 1976).

Acquired aphasia in childhood is different from adult aphasia in that recovery appears to occur rapidly. Alajouanine and Lhermitte found favorable progress in two-thirds of their patients (1965). Hécaen (1976) found recovery in children with acquired aphasia, acute onset, to be more striking than that seen in adults. There are long-term deficits, however. Mild deficits, particularly in written language, remain (Hécaen, 1976). Alajouanine and Lhermitte (1965) found that none of their subjects followed a normal course in school, and that these children encountered difficulty in learning new data.

Acquired aphasia with a gradual onset and EEG abnormalities is an unusual condition of childhood that has been recognized since 1957, when it was described by Landau and Kleffner. Unlike childhood acquired aphasia with acute onset, the course of this syndrome is characterized by gradual failure to comprehend or respond to verbal stimuli, followed by loss of expressive speech (Gascon, Victor, & Lombroso, 1973; Mantovani & Landau, 1980; McKinney & McGreal, 1974; Peterson, Koepp, Solmsen, & Villiez, 1978; Shoumaker, Bennett, Bray, & Curless, 1974; Van Harskamp et al., 1974; Victor, Gascon, Goodglass, & Lombroso, 1972; Worster-Drought, 1971). Unlike the acute form of childhood aphasia, which is marked by expressive deficits, this form of aphasia is notable for the severe receptive defects that develop (Mantovani & Landau, 1980; Shoumaker et al., 1974). Another distinctive feature is the association of convulsive activity, which most often is reported as beginning after the loss of language skills. Even in the absence of overt seizure activity abnormal EEGs are uniformly present. Most often the EEGs of children with this disorder are marked by bilateral spike and slow waves, with highest voltage occurring posteriorly (Gascon et al., 1973; Shoumaker et al., 1974, Victor et al., 1972). Typically no neurological abnormalities other than aphasia are present (Mantovani & Landau, 1980; Shoumaker et al., 1974; Van Harskamp, Van Dongen, & Loonen, 1978; Victor et al., 1972). Reportedly nonverbal intelligence is within normal limits even when the aphasic symptoms are most prominent (Gascon et al., 1973; Shoumaker et al., 1974; Van Harskamp et al., 1978; Worster-Drought, 1971).

The course of this disorder is not clear, though it is agreed that restitution of language skills occurs more slowly with this form of aphasia than it does with acquired aphasia, acute onset (Mantovani & Landau, 1980; Shoumaker et al., 1974). Most authors feel that seizure control is readily achieved (Shoumaker et al., 1974; Victor et al., 1972; Worster-Drought, 1971), though the relationship between convulsive activity, EEG abnormalities, and language deficits is not well established. The majority of the reports suggest a relationship between the degree of EEG abnormality and language disturbance (Gascon et al., 1973; Shoumaker et al., 1974; Walters, 1974) though Van Harskamp et al. (1978) found no relationship between EEG improvement and the diminution of aphasic symptoms.

The course of the disorder is reported to fluctuate, with periods of exacerbation and remission (Mantovani & Landau, 1980; McKinney & McGreal, 1975). Improvement is usually slow (Gascon et al., 1973; Victor et al., 1972; Worster-Drought, 1971) and not always complete, though some instances of complete improvement have been reported (McKinney & McGreal, 1974; Mantovani & Landau, 1980; Peterson et al., 1978; Shoumaker et al., 1974). Spontaneous speech is reported to recover prior to receptive skills (Victor et al., 1972) and the ability to understand written speech reportedly precedes comprehension of oral material (Gascon et al., 1973).

The rarity of this disorder (roughly 50 cases have been reported since 1957) appears to have precluded adequate research. There are only a few studies using standard psychological batteries. Most reports utilize a case history format.

Etiology of this disorder is currently unknown. It has been suggested that the disorder may be caused by viral illness or an autoimmune encephalitis. Others have pointed to a subcortical process or a degenerative process of the peripheral, as opposed to the central, nervous system. It has been noted that the receptive deficits and the prognosis are similar to those seen in developmental aphasia, and suggested that this disorder represents one variant of that pathological process.

Mantovani and Landau (1980) did a follow-up study of seven patients 10 to 28 years after the onset of the disorder. Their data suggested that when language is adequately reestablished there is a decrement in visual spatial functioning. They hypothesized that language recovery may occur at the expense of nonverbal functions.

NEUROPSYCHOLOGISTS AS INVESTIGATORS OF BRAIN-BEHAVIOR RELATIONSHIPS

The theoretical aspects of pediatric neuropsychology that are pertinent to this review are those that will help clinicians ask appropriate questions about the data they collect during clinical exams, and those that assist them in understanding the implications and import of what they observe. It has become increasingly clear that brain damage in children is not manifest in the identical way that it is in the adult population. In order to understand the results of the neuropsychological evaluation of children we must be able to resolve questions about the capacity of the human cortex to adapt to damage and about the constraints on that adaptability.

The "Kennard Principle," so named by Hans-Lukas Teuber (Schneider, 1979), resulted from Margaret Kennard's work on the effects of early lesions on the motor cortex of baby monkeys. This principle stated that the behavioral effects of cortical lesions vary with the age at which they are inflicted. These differences pointed to a pattern of greater sparing of functions the earlier the lesion was incurred.

This principle was generalized to clinical neuropsychology as meaning that the effects of cerebral damage in young children would be less devastating than those accompanying brain damage in the adult. This argued for greater adaptability of the cerebral cortex based upon three possible mechanisms:

1. Functional organization is unspecific in the younger brain and areas are initially equipotential for the development of cortical functions.
2. Functions are represented in a more diffuse, widespread manner initially, and become more specific and localized with age and experience.
3. Active reorganization of the cerebral cortex occurs subsequent to cortical damage (Teuber & Rudel, 1962).

The possibility that the young brain is functionally equipotential, that representation is more diffuse, or that idiosyncratic, anomalous reorganization can take place subsequent to brain damage in the young child has been supported by a variety of observations. Reports of childhood aphasia subsequent to right hemisphere damage gave credence to the notion that the left hemisphere is not a unique substrate for language development. The rapid and radical recovery of children from traumatic aphasia was supportive of this idea, as was the development of language in left hemidecorticate children. Additional support was given by studies revealing that children with early lesions of the parietal lobe do not develop disturbances of sensory detection, as are uniformly seen in adults with similar lesions (Rudel, Teuber, & Twitchell, 1974).

Tasks of dichotic listening have suggested that when early brain damage occurs, anomalous but effective patterns of cortical reorganization occur.

Netley (1972) compared the performance of children with congenital infantile hemiplegia to those with later unilateral injuries (mean age of onset 17 months) and a group of normal controls on a task of dichotic listening. Testing was completed when the children were about 14 years of age. The recall scores of the late brain-injured groups for material presented to the ear contralateral to the operation site were significantly poorer than the recall scores of the early brain-damaged group. These data suggested the possibility for functional reorganization.

Though children do not seem to have the same behavioral sequelae of brain damage as do adults, and though there appears to be the capacity for alternate patterns of cortical organization subsequent to brain damage when it occurs early in life, there is evidence that there is not complete adaptability of the brain to insult and that some patterns of behavioral sequelae are consistent between adult and child. Rudel, Teuber, and Twitchell (1974) found that though children with early brain damage demonstrated no deficits on tasks of simple tactile sensation, performance on more complex sensory tasks involving more than one modality were impaired. These children demonstrated deficits in discrimination without an impairment in detection. These patterns of symptoms indicate that though early injuries may be less disabling to certain primary functions than later injuries, they are more disruptive of complex skills. It appears that development interacts with the results of brain damage to produce different patterns of test performance.

Dennis and Whitaker (1977) stated that the capacity for language acquisition in children who have had surgical removal of the left hemisphere subsequent to infantile hemiplegia (i.e., children who are now hemidecorticate) does not in itself argue for equipotentiality at birth. They point out that the argument for equipotentiality or complete plasticity is tenable only if it can be demonstrated that the pattern of language development in children with early left hemisphere damage is identical to that seen in normal children. The preponderance of the evidence does not support this hypothesis.

Dennis and Whitaker (1977) studied the language performance, at age nine, of three children who had hemispherectomies antedating the acquisition of speech. Though children with both left and right hemispherectomies developed speech, there were distinct differences in their performance on the Illinois Test of Psycholinguistic Abilities and on the token test. The right hemidecorticate patient demonstrated poorer performance on the visual closure test of the ITPA, as compared with the left hemidecorticate patients. Although all three children were able to manage the informational complexity of the earlier parts of the token test, the left hemispherectomy patients had difficulty with tasks requiring use of complex syntactic structures and in understanding sentences in which the surface word order was not identical to the temporal order of action. Full right hemisphere control of language results in delayed acquisition of understanding of word relationships, though superficially language functioning appears normal. These data indicate that there is some cortical restitution after damage, but not complete plasticity of function. The patterns of deficit presented by these children are congruent with adult patterns of impairment subsequent to brain damage. Similar conclusions have been drawn from work with aphasic children. Research with children who have had traumatic aphasia indicates that though oral speech is recovered there remain subtle language deficits. These children have difficulty in learning language-based academic skills (Alajouanine & Lhermitte, 1965).

Other research completed with children with early unilateral brain damage also suggests that the development of these children is detrimentally affected by the damage they have sustained. Woods (1980) compared the performance of children with early unilateral lesions (before one year of age) to the performance of their sibling controls and to children with unilateral lesions occurring during later childhood. Performance on the WISC or the Wechsler-Bellevue was utilized to assess neuropsychological status. Children with early lesions of either the left or right hemisphere performed more poorly than their sibling controls and the population mean. Verbal-performance IQ differences in this group were nonsignificant, regardless of the lateralization of the lesion. Unilateral left hemisphere lesions occurring at a mean age of 5.7 years produced an effect that was different from the anticipated effect of such a lesion in an adult population. These children, like the children in the early onset group, demonstrated both verbal and performance deficits, with no significant superiority in "right hemisphere skills." The late right hemisphere group (mean age of onset 6.4 years) demonstrated an interesting and significant pattern of performance. Unlike the three other groups (early left hemisphere, early right hemisphere, and late left hemisphere), this group had a statistically significant difference between verbal and performance scores, with mean performance IQ depressed and mean verbal IQ within normal limits.

This research suggests that though there is some capacity for atypical lateralization, and some reorganization subsequent to early unilateral brain damage, such adaptation is not complete. Language may develop subsequent to early left hemisphere damage, but neither verbal nor visual spatial skills are within normal limits. When left hemisphere brain damage occurs later in childhood there continue to be some apparent shifts in lateralization so that the right hemisphere assists in language performance, but again this is at a cost, and overall performance is below the population mean. The only group that follows the model that would be expected based on experience with adults who have incurred brain damage is the late right hemisphere group. Apparently in late right hemisphere injuries of childhood there is no change over typical patterns of lateralization to preserve visual spatial skills.

Age constraints upon the capacity for functional reorganization are also suggested by Netley's (1972) research on dichotic listening performance, which has been previously cited. Though the recall scores of the normals, late brain-damaged, and early brain-damaged groups did not differ when the stimuli presented to the remaining or dominant hemisphere were compared, the recall scores for material presented to the ear contralateral to the operation site or to the nondominant hemisphere were significantly different. The early hemispherectomy group performed significantly better than the late hemispherectomy group (mean age of onset 17 months), but significantly more poorly than the controls.

These data suggested that as early as 17 months children, by virtue of the acquisition of some linguistic skills, have established certain patterns of lateralized functional control and that the capacity of this group to develop alternative patterns of cortical organization has been limited. Although there is apparently some capacity to provide atypical functional patterns, increased age and experience with language set limits on this potential.

As was previously noted, another argument for early equipotentiality of function has been the belief that right hemisphere lesions in children are as frequently associated with acute acquired aphasia as left hemisphere lesions. Careful scrutiny sheds doubt upon this conception. Hécaen (1976) found a language disorder to be present in 88 percent of his patients with left hemisphere lesions, but in only 33 percent of his patients with right hemisphere lesions. Woods and Teuber (1978) found that aphasia is more often linked to clinical indications of left hemisphere pathology. In their sample of 26 patients, 2 of the 11 children with right hemisphere lesions had aphasic symptoms, while 10 of the 15 children with left hemisphere lesions were aphasic. Their review of the literature, indicating that aphasia occurs in children after right hemisphere damage with frequency equal to its occurrence after left hemisphere lesions, demonstrated that this historical understanding may have been based upon subjects with bilateral rather than unilateral pathology. They noted that many of the studies reporting aphasia secondary to right hemisphere damage were completed during the late 1930s and early '40s prior to the use of antibiotics or other modern medical treatments. They conclude that many of the subjects in earlier studies had had systemic infectious disorders and that the brain damage was not strictly unilateral, accounting for the emergence of aphasic symptoms with left hemiparesis.

The research as a whole supports a position that early childhood lesions do not produce the same pattern of deficits in higher cortical functions seen in later childhood or adult brain damage, that there is language development in the face of left hemisphere damage in children, but that there are consistent patterns of deficits that remain and are in some senses similar to those seen in brain-damaged adults. Such patterns of neuropsychological functioning do not support the view that the human cerebral cortex possesses, at birth, complete plasticity or equipotentiality, but suggest that to some degree anomalous reorganization occurs subsequent to damage. There are, however, constraints on such plasticity, with age and experience limiting reorganization. Unusual organization occurs at a cost, often with visual spatial skills being sacrificed to provide for more adequate language development.

Some investigators have interpreted this to mean that though early brain damage spares elementary functions it limits learning. Milner (1969) demonstrated that early unilateral brain damage results in persistent intellectual retardation. Reitan (1974b) found that the effect of brain damage to the young child is the limitation of the potential for normal development, which results in a generalized depression of skills. Teuber and Rudel (1962), in a study utilizing normal and adult onset brain-damaged adults and normal and early onset brain-damaged children, demonstrated the need to consider the process of normal development in attempting to delineate the effects of early brain damage. They investigated the ability of four tasks to discriminate brain-damaged individuals from normal controls. The subjects were studied over a ten-year period in order to assess longitudinally the effect of early brain damage on the later acquisition of skills.

These authors noted three possible patterns of the manifestation of brain damage when a developmental view was maintained. These are:

1. behaviors that develop more slowly as a result of brain damage, but show continued progression;
2. behaviors in which there will be an impairment at all ages;
3. behaviors in which there is an immediate and obvious effect that disappears as development proceeds.

In their longitudinal research Teuber and Rudel (1962) demonstrated that all three patterns were possible. The first task, one of setting a sound source to an overhead position, followed the first pattern. Neither normal nor brain-damaged children were able to complete successfully the task when young. With increasing age both brain-damaged and normal children could complete the task, but the normal children performed more and more like normal adults, so that after 11 years of age the task could be used to discriminate brain-damaged from normal children. This finding was particularly interesting developmentally in that performance on a visual analogue of this task (on which the pattern of the children's performance was identical to their performance on the auditory task) did not discriminate between normal and adult onset brain-damaged adults when individuals were chosen irrespective of the locus of injury. The test did, however, discriminate adults with anterior brain damage from normals and posterior brain-damaged adults. This task was then particularly sensitive to focal brain damage in the adult population but insensitive to brain damage in children less than 11 years of age.

The second task, that of adjusting a sound source under conditions of body tilt, followed the second pattern. This task discriminated the brain-damaged population from normals across the age range. On this task brain-damaged adults performed more like children. Children with severe brain damage performed more poorly than did children with mild brain damage.

The third task, that of righting oneself after body tilt, followed the third pattern. The task effectively discriminated brain-damaged from normal children up to about 13 years of age. Subsequent to this the task no longer was sensitive to the effects of brain damage, and normal and early onset brain-damaged children performed equivalently. The task did not discriminate normal and late onset brain-damaged adults.

This research suggests reasons for the apparent discrepancies in the literature. It emphasizes that the similarities and differences between adult and childhood brain damage that are observed are to a large degree a reflection of the questions being asked (Teuber & Rudel, 1962). The effects of early brain damage will be seen differentially depending on what task or test is chosen, and on the normal developmental pattern of performance for that task. In fact, it seems probable that at different developmental levels the same task is done in different ways. Although the final behavior may be the same, the psychological processes utilized to produce that behavior may be entirely different. This points to the necessity that neuropsychological theory be developmentally oriented and that any test used for the assessment of children be based upon a strong developmental theory.

Rudel and Teuber's research also emphasizes that there are some tasks on which the effects of brain damage on children's behavior are not immediately apparent, though performance on the same task at a later age will give evidence of impairment. If a skill is acquired later in life it makes little sense to assume that a task employing this skill will differentiate normal from brain-damaged children prior to the normal developmental emergence of this skill. This research supports the notion that there are behavioral similarities between brain-damaged children and adults that are observable when appropriate tasks are utilized, and that these congruent findings exist despite apparent dissimilarities in presentation.

DEVELOPMENTAL NEUROPSYCHOLOGY: THE LURIA-NEBRASKA NEUROPSYCHOLOGICAL BATTERY—CHILDREN'S REVISION

In order to be useful, a developmental neuropsychological theory must explain in a consistent manner the reported results that have been obtained in work with brain-damaged children. In particular, the theory must address the similarities and differences between the behavioral results of brain damage in children and in adults, and between children impaired at different ages.

Traditionally there have been two approaches to neuropsychological theory: localization theory and equipotential theory. Localization theory posits that the cerebral cortex is a highly differentiated structure with complex mental functions localized to specific areas or centers of the brain. Initially this was based on the observations that damage to discrete cortical areas produced consistent deficits between individuals. For example, Broca found that damage to the frontal lobe of the left hemisphere produced deficits in expressive speech. Subsequent to this there were numerous attempts to provide "maps" of the human cortex, and higher cortical functions such as reading and singing were localized to specific anatomic structures on the basis of clinical evidence. A strict localization model of cortical functioning implies that different structures of the brain provide a unique substrate for the completion of different cognitive processes, and that damage to these areas produces a deficit in specific skills while leaving all other functions intact.

Clearly such a model is insufficient for understanding cortical functioning in the child. It is difficult to explain how children who have undergone surgical removal of the left hemisphere could develop speech and language skills using localization theory. In additon, such a conceptualization does not account for the general depression in development that is observed in children who have sustained discrete localized damage.

The equipotential conceptualizaton of neuropsychology suggests that for all human behavior all areas of the brain participate on an equal basis. The cortex is regarded as an undifferentiated, homogeneous mass, and anatomic or psychological distinctions within the cerebrum are thought to be largely irrelevant to the understanding of behavior. The behavioral effects of brain damage are regarded as being mediated by the amount of tissue destroyed rather than the localization of the damage. Brain tissue is thought of as being highly plastic, with recovery of functions possible if there is a great enough mass of tissue remaining.

This conceptualization of cortical functioning does not adequately account for the results of some of the research that has been done with children who have sustained brain damage. Milner (1974), as reported by DeRenzi and Piercy (1969), has shown that right hemisphere lateralization of language subsequent to childhood onset brain damage occurs only when specific areas of the left posterior brain are damaged. The equipotential theory cannot consistently explain the patterns of deficits seen in children that are related to lateralization of injury.

The Russian neurologist A. R. Luria (1966, 1980) has contributed a third and different theory of neuropsychological functioning. This theory accounts for the consistencies between both localization and equipotential theories and research and clinical results without creating the discrepancies between theory and observation that are problematic in these other models. Luria's theoretical approach provides a developmental model for the understanding of brain-behavior relationships.

Luria's theory conceptualizes overt behavior as the result of the synchronous and interactive performance of a chain of brain areas. These chains of cortical activity are called functional systems. No one area of the cortex is responsible for any overt behavior, though each area plays a specific and constant role in any given chain and in all the functional systems in which it is involved.

For example, the postcentral area of the cortex is involved with tactile sensation. Damage to this area will be evidenced in deficits of simple sensation. In addition, all cortical functions in which sensation plays a role will be disturbed. Because afferent feedback is important for the accuracy of motor movement, the functional systems for movement may be disturbed when the postcentral area is damaged. Articulation is also highly dependent upon the adequacy of kinesthetic feedback. Damage to the postcentral area of the cortex may be evidenced as deficits in expressive language, such as slowness of speech, or substitution of similarly articulated sounds for one another. The postcentral area is not conceptualized as being the critical area for either motor movement or speech; however, the functions mediated by that area provide an important role in these and a variety of other higher cortical functions.

Cortical areas are pluripotential. Any specific area of the brain is involved in a multiplicity of functional systems. The cortex then is viewed by this theory as a highly differentiated system whose parts are considered to be responsible for specific and distinct aspects of the whole of behavior. The mediation of any overt behavior is based upon the coordinated working of constellations of anatomically distinct ganglion cells (Luria, 1980).

Luria does not posit that there is only one functional system for any given behavior. Functional systems are not considered to be unique. The same behavior may be completed in several alternate fashions and, though the overt behavior is identical, the cortical processes utilized to complete that task may be different. For example, oral reading, which is an immensely complex behavior, may be completed by the sequential recognition, phonemic analysis, association, and linking of a series of letters. This chain involves auditory association, kinesthetic feedback, the association of visual and verbal stimuli, spatial orientation, and adequate articulatory movement as the minimum number of links. Oral reading, however, can also be completed as a verbal response to a single optic stimulus. The reader observes the word, recognizes it as a sight word, and says it without recourse to phonetic analysis. Though the processes differ and alternate cortical areas are involved, the overt behavior is the same.

Not only is it possible to complete tasks utilizing different functional systems but, according to Luria, it is also anticipated that at different stages in the ontogenetic development of higher-level cognitive functions the cortical constituents of the functional system will be altered. Complex functional systems of conjointly working cortical areas are not present at birth. Rather they are established gradually as the child develops in the process of social interaction and educational activity. Initially these patterns of cortical coordination are based upon relatively elementary sensory and motor processes. With the emergence of language this system begins to be the basis for higher cognitive skills. With practice many tasks become automatized and complex behaviors can be completed without recourse to basic sensory functions. For instance, the labored, drawn writing of the young child is the product of a different functional system than the fluid, rapid and smooth writing of his adolescent sibling. The change in cortical relationships composing higher-level functions throughout is regular and predictable (Luria, 1980).

The idea that functional systems are not unique, and that they are expected to change, has significant theoretical implications. An important implication for those interested in child neuropsychology is that the effects of a cerebral lesion on higher cortical functions will vary with the developmental status of the individual. Disturbances of relatively basic sensory and integrative processes in childhood will have a devastating effect upon the development of higher cognitive functions, as these more basic skills serve as the foundations for the development of more complex skills. Luria (1966) stated that subsequent to the development of higher functional systems disturbances of elementary sensory and integrative processes will have a more limited effect and may be compensated for by other previously elaborated functional systems.

This theoretical approach adequately accounts for the general decline in overall functioning that has regularly been observed in children who have suffered early brain damage. Young children have not yet elaborated multiple functional systems and do not have an array of methods to choose from in order to complete a task. When one part of the unique functional system is impaired subsequent to an injury, they do not have alternative chains of cortical processes. In addition, when elementary functions are damaged the child lacks the foundation for the elaboration of more complex functional systems. General impairment occurs because these essential links in the chain are not available.

Luria's theory also accounts for the sparing of lower level skills when early brain damage occurs. The research demonstrates that when early brain damage is incurred cortical functions do develop, though there are continuing patterns of deficits indicative of the failure to engage in more complex integrative tasks or to understand more syntactically complex verbal material. Luria's theory would predict that though development will occur more slowly in such children, alternate functional systems will develop. These systems may be less efficient or accurate and may require unusual adaptations, but because complex skills are completed by the conjoint activity of multiple cortical units behavioral patterns will be elaborated.

This theory also accounts for the observation that children with brain damage demonstrate patterns of behavioral deficits similar to those seen in adults. Luria's theory would predict that all functional systems requiring input from a particular cortical area should be impaired when damage to that anatomical area occurs. Although alternate functional systems may be elaborated, behaviors cortically dependent upon the function mediated by that area will not develop. In these cases the deficits of a child with early onset brain damage will resemble those of an adult when higher level skills are assessed.

Finally, the notion that the effect of a lesion of a particular part of the brain will differ depending upon the stage in the ontogenesis of the behavior during which the lesion occurs is useful in understanding why children who incur damage when they are young present different symptoms than those who are damaged when they are older. Once the child has developed the second signal system of language, there is less reliance upon elementary sensory functions and damage will result in less pervasive deficits. The presentation of symptoms depends upon the number and type of functional systems that have been established prior to the time the damage is incurred.

Luria's approach to neuropsychological development is useful in understanding the behavior of children because he has also developed a scheme for describing progressive neurological development based upon physiological and functional data (Luria, 1966). Neurological development in a neuropsychological sense is the result of several processes; myelinization, dendritic and neuronal growth, establishment of pathways among cells, in addition to perhaps as yet unrecognized physical and biochemical events (Golden, 1981b). We do not at present adequately understand the relationship between physical cortical development and psychological maturation. Further research is necessary to more accurately discern deviant or unusual patterns.

Luria's theory would predict that there are five stages in neuropsychological development. These stages correspond to the emergence of functions of various cortical areas. The first stage involves maturation and operation of the reticular system and those structures necessary for the maintenance of optimum levels of arousal and attention. This system is normally mature and operational early in the first year of life, although development of this unit is dependent upon time since conception, rather than time from birth. This system is most vulnerable to damage during the perinatal period, when it is being formed.

The second stage of neurological development occurs concurrently with the first stage. It involves the development of the three primary sensory areas (simple visual, tactile, and auditory perception) and the motor unit. These are highly differentiated cortical areas, and are geographically organized. Myelinization of these areas occurs early in cortical development (Van der Vlught, 1979). Behaviors mediated by the primary areas appear to have had some survival function, are genetically determined, and do not develop as the result of learning. These behaviors drop out as more integrated functional systems emerge.

During stage three, which begins concomitantly with the first two stages but continues through the preschool period, the unimodal association areas and the secondary areas of the cortex become functional. Skills such as coordinated movement, visual and auditory recognition and discrimination, and the association of words and objects develop. Although there is cross-modal learning, this usually represents the result of rote memory; integrative problem solving does not generally occur.

Stage four in neuropsychological development concerns primarily the area around the tertiary parietal cortex, that area of the brain responsible for the integration of multimodal sensory integration. This area is a relatively new one phylogenetically and is thought to mature later than the primary and secondary areas of the cortex. The tertiary parietal area is not thought to be active until about five to eight years of age (Golden, 1981b). Tertiary area performance is involved in the acquisition and enactment of most educational skills. Reading, arithmetic functioning, understanding of complex grammatical structures, analogic reasoning, categorization, etc., all depend upon the integrity of this area of the cortex. When this area does not function adequately, secondary to damage or to slower developmental progress, academic learning is seriously impeded. Standard instruments of intellectual functioning usually measure tertiary parietal, stage four skills.

The fifth stage of neuropsychological development involves elaboration of the prefrontal area of the cortex. The area is phylogenetically and ontogenetically the last to develop. The prefrontal divisions of the cerebral cortex, as the newest areas, are the most vulnerable to damage. This cortical unit has rich and complex connections with the subcortical area and the more posterior portions of the cerebrum. Stage five development is not thought to occur until adolescence. The prefrontal areas are involved in the maintenance of intention and planning, the evaluation of behavior, impulse control, and cognitive flexibility.

This theoretical progression in neuropsychological development is useful in understanding an individual child's performance and in making sense of research results. This approach to development implies that there are qualitative differences between cortical functioning at different ages. The type of performance that is expected of a child at stage four cannot be appropriately expected from a child who is not yet functioning at this level. It is not just that the types of functions mediated by the tertiary parietal area are harder, but also that they are qualitatively different. This is true of the differences between all stages. This understanding has important implications, since it implies that higher-level tasks will not differentiate brain-damaged from normal children when both are young and cannot be expected to be functioning at the higher level. For example, tasks demanding skills mediated by the tertiary parietal area will not discriminate normal three-year-olds from three-year-old brain-damaged children, since neither group can realistically be expected to have reached the stage four level of development. This may explain the pattern of performance Teuber and Rudel (1962) found on their first task, setting a sound source to an overhead position, which failed to discriminate young normals from brain-damaged subjects, but effectively discriminated them at later chronological ages. A similar pattern has been reported for alternation behavior (Van der Vlught, 1979). Alternation behavior is not observed before four years of age. Prior to age four, perseveration occurs in both brain-damaged and normal children; subsequent to this alternation behavior is expected for normals, though perseveration, indicating a dysfunction of the hippocampal system, may continue in brain-damaged children.

Although it is possible for children who are functioning at a stage three secondary association area level to produce the same overt behaviors in response to a question that may also be completed using stage four skills, Luria's theory predicts that their approach to the task will be qualitatively different. They have used different functional systems to arrive at the same overt behavior. For example, math problems may be solved by learning math facts by rote (stage three), or a child may have an active understanding of the spatial and quantitative nature of arithmetic processes (stage four). While the overt behavior is identical, the cortical areas engaged in the functional systems are different.

The understanding that the same overt behaviors can be completed using different functional systems at different ages implies that in completing neuropsychological evaluations the tasks chosen must be as simple and unitary as possible. We must control to as large an extent as we can the makeup of the functional systems utilized to complete an item. By using simple tasks and by varying the presentation and the mode of response we can control how tasks are completed.

Luria's approach to clinical assessment grew from his theoretical understanding of neuropsychological development. He used simple tests that focused on as specific as possible brain-based behavior. This helped him both to identify the link in a functional chain that was not intact and to minimize the number of false positive responses normals produced.

Luria employed multiple items to identify areas of deficit. By varying tasks so that as few links as possible were changed, he was able to identify which step in a complex process (i.e., which cortical areas) were not functioning adequately. For example, if an individual could perform the complex chain of cortical functions a-b-c-d-e adequately but failed on a task requiring a-b-c-d-e-f, then Luria would have predicted that all tasks requiring step f would be impaired. If through further assessment this was shown to be so, then Luria would have concluded that the cortical area responsible for function f was somehow impaired.

This form of syndrome analysis was completed by Luria on a clinical, unsystematized, and unquantified basis. The adult form of the Luria-Nebraska Neuropsychological Battery (Golden, Hammeke, & Purisch, 1980) provides a standardized, quantified, and structured exam that makes use of Luria's approach. This research has indicated that the test can be used to complete the three functions of neuropsychology (see Golden, 1981a, for a partial review of this research):

1. Statistically discriminating brain-damaged from normal adults, and describing patterns of neuropsychological strength and weakness to assist in localization, prediction, and rehabilitation.
2. Studying the nature of specific neurological diseases.
3. Extending our theoretical knowledge of brain-behavior relationships.

Recently a revision of the battery has been developed for use with children from 8 to 12 years of age. Cortical functioning in the areas of motor, rhythm, visual, receptive and expressive language, reading, writing, arithmetic, memory, and intelligence skills are assessed. Since the battery is not designed to be used with those individuals who have entered the fifth stage of neurological development, no measures of these functions are included.

Standardization data has been developed on 136 normal children. External validity data are currently being gathered. All items in this battery are simple enough for a normal eight-year-old to complete. Tasks have been chosen so that the component skills necessary for that task, i.e., the functional system, can be described. This allows us to assess skills in a methodical and analytic manner, providing a discrimination of brain-damaged from normal children. It also provides a structure for evaluating which basic skills are intact and which are impaired. By carefully defining patterns of success and failure we hope to be able to define which stage in neurological development a child has reached. This should permit us to plan rehabilitation strategies based upon the use of intact areas for the development of alternative functional systems. We hope this battery will prove useful in the investigation of pediatric neurological and other medical illnesses and for further investigation of brain-behavior relationships in childhood.

CONCLUSION

Pediatric neuropsychology is a new and dynamic field. It is a fascinating area because we have such a great deal to learn about normal cortical development and the effects of brain damage upon cerebral development.

With the emergence of new noninvasive means of measuring structural changes in the cortex we are beginning to investigate brain-behavior relationships with more adequate external criteria. Results of the CT scan and other physiological measures of cortical functioning (regional cerebral blood flow, PET scans) have been compared with the performance on neuropsychological test batteries, and we are slowly gaining an understanding of the intricate and subtle relationships between the physical changes in the brain and behavior in the adult population.

In the future these techniques may be applied to the pediatric population and will assist us in our study of brain-behavior relationships in children. We have yet to understand the schedule of structural cortical development and what variation may be considered normal. Although we recognize the plasticity of the human cortex and the options for the development of unusual functional systems and idiosyncratic patterns of lateralization and localization, we do not yet have data that describe or adequately define limits to this adaptability. Continued research with a variety of neuropsychological instruments, especially in conjunction with the newer, more revealing forms of physiological measures, will assist us in investigating these questions. This information can be used in the investigation of discrete clinical entities to aid in our understanding of the factors contributing to atypical development, to assist other clinicians in making decisions regarding treatment, and to help in understanding the results of cortical trauma.

REFERENCES

Adams, J., Peterson, R. A., Kenny, T. J., & Canter, A. Age effects and revised scoring of the Canter BIP for identifying children with cerebral dysfunction. *Journal of Consulting and Clinical Psychology,* 1975, **43**, 117–118.

Alajouanine, T., & Lhermitte, F. Acquired aphasia in children. *Brain,* 1965, **4**, 652–653.

Boll, R. Conceptual vs. perceptual vs. motor deficits in brain-damaged children. *Journal of Clinical Psychology,* 1972, **28**, 157–159.

Boll, T. J. Behavioral correlates of cerebral damage in children aged 9 through 14. In R. M. Reitan & L. A. Davison (Eds.), *Clinical neuropsychology: Current status and applications.* New York: Wiley, 1974.

Boll, T., & Reitan, R. M. Motor and tactile deficits in brain damaged children. *Perceptual and Motor Skills,* 1972, **34**, 343–350.

Bortner, M., & Birch, H. Patterns of intellectual ability in emotionally disturbed and brain-damaged children. *Journal of Special Education,* 1969, **3**, 351–369.

Bosaeus, E. The relationship between psychological test results and EEG patterns in healthy children. *Scandinavian Journal of Psychology,* 1978, **19**, 181–191.

Brink, J., Garrett, A. L., Hale, W. R., Woo-Sam, J., & Nickel, V. L. Recovery of motor and intellectual function in children sustaining severe head injuries. *Developmental Medicine and Child Neurology,* 1970, **12**, 565–571.

Brink, J. D., Imbus, C., & Woo-Sam, T. Physical recovery after severe closed head trauma in children and adolescents. *Journal of Pediatrics,* 1980, **97**, 721–727.

Canter, A. H. *The Canter Background Interference Procedure for the Bender-Gestalt Test: Manual for administration, scoring and interpretation.* Iowa City: Iowa Psychiatric Hospital, 1970.

Ch'ien, L. T., Rhomes, J. A., Stagner, S., Cavalla, K., Wood, A., Goff, J., Pitner, S., Hustu, H. O., Seifert, M. J., & Simone, J. V. Long-term neurological implications of somnolence syndrome in children with acute lymphocytic leukemia. *Annals of Neurology,* 1980, **8**, 273–277.

Czudner, G., & Rourke, B. Simple reaction time in "brain-damaged" and normal children under regular and irregular preparatory conditions. *Perceptual and Motor Skills,* 1970, **31**, 767–773.

Dennis, M., & Whitaker, H. A. Hemispheric equipotentiality and language acquisition. In S. S. Segalowitz & F. Gruber (Eds.), *Language development and neurological theory.* New York: Academic Press, 1977.

Denson, T. L., & May, D. C. The reliability of children's drawings as indicators of brain damage. *Educational Research Quarterly,* 1978, **3,** 45–48.

DeRenzi, E., & Piercy, M. The Fourteenth International Symposium of Neuropsychology. *Neuropsychologia,* 1969, **7,** 383–386.

Diaz, A. M. Effects of visual and auditory distraction on paired-associate learning of brain-injured and non-brain-injured children. *Dissertation Abstracts International,* 1971, **31,** 5231.

Eisenson, J. Developmental aphasia: A speculative view with therapeutic implications. *Journal of Speech and Hearing Disorders,* 1968, **33,** 3–13.

Eisenson, J. Developmental aphasia (Dyslogia): A postulation of a unitary concept of the disorder. *Cortex,* 1969, **4,** 184–200.

Eiser, C., & Lansdown, R. Retrospective study of intellectual development in children with acute lymphoblastic leukemia. *Archives of Diseases in Children,* 1977, **52,** 525–529.

Fisher, L. Attention deficit in brain damaged children. *American Journal of Mental Deficiency,* 1970, **74,** 502–508.

Fitzhardinge, P. M., Kazemi, M., Ramsay, M., & Stern, L. Long-term sequelae of neonatal meningitis. *Developmental Medicine and Child Neurology,* 1974, **16,** 3–10.

Gascon, G., Victor, D., & Lombroso, C. T. Language disorders, convulsive disorders, and electroencephalographic abnormalities: Acquired aphasia in children. *Archives of Neurology,* 1973, **28,** 156–162.

Goff, J. R., Anderson, H. R., & Cooper, P. F. Distractibility and memory deficits in long-term survivors of acute lymphoblastic leukemia. *Developmental and Behavioral Pediatrics,* 1980, **1,** 158–163.

Golden, C. J. *Diagnosis and Rehabilitation in Clinical Neuropsychology.* (2nd ed.) Springfield, Ill.: Charles C. Thomas, 1981. (a)

Golden, C. J. The Luria-Nebraska Children's Battery: Theory and Initial Formulation. In G. Hynd & J. Obrzut (Eds.), *Neuropsychological assessment and the school-age child: Issues and procedures.* New York: Grune & Stratton, 1981. (b)

Golden, C. J., Hammeke, T. A., & Purisch, A. D. *The Luria-Nebraska Neuropsychological Battery.* Los Angeles: Western Psychological Services, 1980.

Hallahan, D. P., & Cruickshank, W. M. *Psychoeducational foundations of learning disabilities.* Englewood Cliffs, N.J.: Prentice-Hall, 1973.

Hanefeld, F., & Riehm, H. Therapy of acute lymphoblastic leukemia in childhood: Effects on the nervous system. *Neuropädiatrie,* 1980, **11,** 3–16.

Hécaen, H. Acquired aphasia in children and the ontogenesis of hemispheric functional representation. *Brain and Language,* 1976, **3,** 114–134.

Heiskanen, O., & Kaste, M. Late prognosis of severe brain injury in children. *Developmental Medicine and Child Neurology,* 1974, **16,** 11–14.

Kasper, J. C., Millechap, J. G., Backus, R., Child, D., & Schulman, J. L. Study of the relationship between neurological evidence of brain damage in children and activity and distractibility. *Journal of Consulting and Clinical Psychology,* 1971, **36,** 329–337.

Kenny, T. J. Background interference procedures: A means of assessing neurologic dysfunction in school-age children. *Journal of Consulting and Clinical Psychology,* 1971, **37,** 44–46.

Kirk, S. A., McCarthy, T. J., & Kirk, W. D. *Illinois Test of Psycholinguistic Abilities.* (Exp. ed.) Urbana, Ill.: University of Illinois Press, 1961.

Klonoff, H., & Low, M. Disordered brain function in young children and early adolescents: Neuropsychological and electroencephalographic correlates. In R. M. Reitan & L. A. Davison (Eds.), *Clinical neuropsychology: Current status and applications.* New York: Wiley, 1974.

Klonoff, H., Low, M. D., & Clark, C. Head injuries in children: A prospective five year follow-up. *Journal of Neurology, Neurosurgery and Psychiatry,* 1977, **40,** 1211–1219.

Klonoff, H., & Paris, R. Immediate short-term and residual effects of acute head injuries in children: Neuropsychological and neurological correlates. In R. M. Reitan & L. A. Davison (Eds.), *Clinical neuropsychology: Current status and applications.* New York: Wiley, 1974.

Klonoff, H., Robinson, G. C., & Thompson, G. Acute and chronic brain syndromes in children. *Developmental Medicine and Child Neurology,* 1969, **11,** 198–213.

Koppitz, E. M. *The Bender-Gestalt Test for Young Children.* New York: Grune & Stratton, 1964.

Landau, W. M., & Kleffner, F. R. Syndrome of acquired aphasia with convulsive disorder in children. *Neurology,* 1957, **7,** 523.

Lange-Cosack, H., Wider, B., Schlesener, H. J., Grumme, Th., & Kubicki, St. Prognosis of brain injuries in young children. *Neuropädiatrie,* 1979, **10,** 105–127.

Levin, H. S., & Eisenberg, H. M. Neuropsychological impairment after closed head injury in children and adolescents. *Journal of Pediatric Psychology,* 1979, **4,** 389–402.

Luria, A. R. *The working brain.* New York: Basic Books, 1973.

Luria, A. R. *Higher cortical functions in man.* New York: Basic Books, 1966.

Luria, A. R. *Higher cortical functions in man.* (2nd ed.) New York: Basic Books, 1980.

Mantovani, J. F., & Landau, W. M. Acquired aphasia with convulsive disorder: Course and prognosis. *Neurology,* 1980, **30,** 524–529.

Matthews, C. G., Chun, R. W., Grabow, J. D., & Thompson, W. H. Psychological sequelae in children following California arbovirus encephalitis. *Neurology,* 1968, **18,** 1023–1030.

McConnell, O. L. Koppitz's Bender-Gestalt scores in relation to organic and emotional problems in children. *Journal of Clinical Psychology,* 1967, **23,** 370–374.

McIntosh, W. J. The use of a Wechsler Subtest Ratio as an index of brain damage in children. *Journal of Learning Disabilities,* 1974, **7,** 43–45.

McKinney, M. C., & McGreal, D. A. An aphasic syndrome in children. *Canadian Medical Association Journal,* 1974, **110,** 637–639.

Milner, B. Residual intellectual and memory deficits after head injury. In E. Walker, W. Caveness, & M. Critchley (Eds.), *The late effects of head injury.* Springfield, Ill.: Charles C. Thomas, 1969, pp. 84–97.

Milner, B. Hemispheric specialization: Scope and limits. In F. O. Schmitt & F. G. Worden (Eds.), *The neurosciences, third study program.* Cambridge: MIT Press, 1974.

Mordock, J. B. A procedural critique of "Bender-Gestalts of organic children: Accuracy of clinical judgement." *Journal of Projective Techniques and Personality Assessment,* 1969, **33,** 489–491.

Netley, C. Dichotic listening performance of hemispherectomized patients. *Neuropsychologia,* 1972, **10,** 223–240.

Oliver, R. A., & Kronenberger, E. J. Testing the applicability of Kopitz's Bender-Gestalt scores to brain-damaged, emotionally disturbed and normal adolescents. *Psychology in the Schools,* 1971, **8,** 250–253.

Peterson, U., Koepp, P., Solmsen, M., & Villiez, T. Acquired aphasia with electroencephalographic manifestaton in children. *Neuropädiatrie,* 1978, **9,** 84–96.

Reed, J. C., & Reitan, R. M. Verbal and performance differences among brain-injured children with lateralized motor deficits. *Perceptual and Motor Skills,* 1969, **29,** 747–752.

Reitan, R. M. *Manual for administration of neuropsychological test batteries for adults and children.* Indianapolis: Author, 1969.

Reitan, R. M. Trail making test results for normal and brain-damaged children. *Perceptual and Motor Skills,* 1971, **33,** 575–581.

Reitan, R. M. Methodological problems in clinical neuropsychology. In R. M. Reitan & L. A. Davison (Eds.), *Clinical neuropsychology: Current status and applications.* New York: Wiley, 1974. (a)

Reitan, R. M. Psychological effects of cerebral lesions in children of early school age. In R. M. Reitan & L. A. Davison (Eds.), *Clinical neuropsychology: Current status and applications.* New York: Wiley, 1974.(b)

Rie, H. E., Hilty, M. D., & Cramblett, H. G. Intelligence and coordination following California encephalitis. *American Journal of Diseases in Children,* 1973, **125,** 824–827.

Rubin, S. S. A reevaluation of figure-ground pathology in brain damaged children. *American Journal of Mental Deficiency,* 1969, **74,** 111–115.

Rudel, R. G., & Teuber, H. L. Spatial orientation in normal children and in children with early brain injury. *Neuropsychologia,* 1971, **9**, 401–407.

Rudel, R. G., Teuber, H. L., & Twitchell, T. E. Levels of impairment of sensorimotor functions in children with early brain damage. *Neuropsychologia,* 1974, **12**, 95–108.

Russell, E. W., Neuringer, C., & Goldstein, G. *Assessment of brain damage: A neuropsychological key approach.* New York: Wiley-Interscience, 1970.

Rutter, M. Brain-damage syndromes in childhood: Concepts and findings. *Journal of Child Psychology and Psychiatry,* 1977, **18**, 1–21.

Sabatino, D. A., & Cramblett, H. G. Behavioral sequelae of California encephalitis virus infection in children. *Developmental Medicine and Child Neurology,* 1968, **10**, 331–337.

Schneider, G. E. "Is it really better to have your brain lesion early?" A revision of the "Kennard Principle." *Neuropsychologia,* 1979, **17**, 557–583.

Sell, S. H., Merrill, R. E., Doyne, E. O., & Zimsky, E. P. Long term sequelae of Hemophilus influenzae meningitis. *Pediatrics,* 1972, **49**, 206–211.

Sell, S. H., Webb, W. W., Pate, J. E., & Doyne, E. O. Psychological sequelae to bacterial meningitis: Two controlled studies. *Pediatrics,* 1972, **49**, 212–217.

Sells, C. J., Carpenter, R. L., & Ray, C. G. Sequelae of central nervous system enterovirus infections. *New England Journal of Medicine,* 1975, **243**, 1–4.

Selz, M., & Reitan, R. M. Rules for neuropsychological diagnosis: Classification of brain function in older children. *Journal of Consulting and Clinical Psychology,* 1979, **47**, 258–264.

Shaffer, D. Psychiatric aspects of brain injury in childhood: A review. *Developmental Medicine and Child Neurology,* 1973, **15**, 211–220.

Shoumaker, R. D., Bennett, D. R., Bray, P. F., & Curless, R. G. Clinical and EEG manifestations of an unusual aphasic syndrome in children. *Neurology,* 1974, **24**, 10–16.

Simensen, R. J., & Sutherland, J. Psychological assessment of brain damage: The Wechsler Scales. *Academic Therapy,* 1974, **10**, 69–81.

Soni, S. S., Marten, G. W., Pitner, S. E., Duenas, D. A., & Powazek, M. Effects of central nervous system irradiation on neuropsychologic functioning of children with acute lymphocytic leukemia. *New England Journal of Medicine,* 1975, **293**, 113–118.

Tallal, P., & Newcombe, F. Impairment of auditory perception and language comprehension in dysphasia. *Brain and Language,* 1978, **5**, 13–24.

Teuber, H. L., & Rudel, R. G. Behavior after cerebral lesions in children and adults. *Developmental Medicine and Child Neurology,* 1962, **4**, 3–20.

Van der Vlught, H. Aspects of normal and abnormal neuropsychological development. In M. Gazziniga (Ed.), *Handbook of behavioral neurobiology,* Vol. 2. New York: Plenum Press, 1979.

Van Harskamp, F., Van Dongen, H. R., & Loonen, M. C. Acquired aphasia with convulsive disorders in children: A case study of a seven-year follow-up. *Brain and Language,* 1978, **6**, 141–148.

Victor, D., Gascon, G., Goodglass, H., & Lombroso, G. Proceedings: The syndrome of acquired aphasia, EEG abnormalities with or without convulsive disorder in children. *Epilepsia,* 1972, **13**, 349–350.

Walters, G. V. The syndrome of acquired aphasia and convulsive disorder in children. *Canadian Medical Association Journal,* 1974, **110**, 611–612.

Weil, M. L. Infections of the nervous system. In J. H. Menkes, *Textbook of child neurology.* Philadelphia: Lea & Febiger, 1980.

Woo-Sam, J., Zimmerman, I. L., Brink, J. D., Uyehara, K., & Miller, A. R. Socio-economic status and post-trauma intelligence in children with severe head injuries. *Psychological Reports,* 1970, **27**, 147–153.

Woods, B. T. The restricted effects of right hemisphere lesions after age one: Wechsler test data. *Neuropsychologia,* 1980, **18**, 65–70.

Woods, B. T., & Teuber, H. L. Early onset of complementary specialization of cerebral hemispheres in man. *Transactions of the American Neurological Associaton,* 1973, **98**, 113–117.

Woods, B. T., & Teuber, H. L. Changing patterns of childhood aphasia. *Annals of Neurology,* 1978, **3,** 273–280.

Worster-Drought, C. An unusual form of acquired aphasia in children. *Developmental Medicine and Child Neurology,* 1971, **13,** 563–571.

Wright, L., & Jimmerson, S. Intellectual sequelae of Hemophilus influenzae meningitis. *Journal of Abnormal Psychology,* 1971, **77,** 181–183.

Zaidel, E. Performance on the ITPA following cerebral commissurotomy and hemispherectomy. *Neuropsychologia,* 1979, **17,** 259–280.

7

The Assessment and Management of Pain in Children

J. Gerald Beales*

In recent years an increasing amount of research effort has been devoted to the subject of pain. But the great majority of investigations involving human subjects have looked exclusively at adults, and comparatively little direct study has been made of pain in children.

If pain were a straightforward and genetically determined process, this would not be a cause for concern. It is, however, a subjective experience much influenced by such psychological processes as cognition and attention. Differences in level of cognitive development produce differences in pain experience even within the pediatric age group, and an adequate understanding of children's pain cannot be gained by the simple application of results obtained from adult subjects.

No doubt the regrettable dearth of research into childhood pain experience is in part a consequence of the considerable methodological difficulties involved. The use of children in laboratory pain experiments poses substantial ethical problems. Published reports dealing with children refer almost exclusively to clinical rather than experimentally produced pain, and are based on clinical impression rather than scientific study. Hard, quantitative data are rare, and most of what are available refer to "psychogenic" pain in children. The pain produced by physical disease and trauma remains very much a neglected field.

Study of pain in very young children is also seriously hindered by problems of communication. Words like "pain" and "hurt" may be entirely absent from a preschool infant's vocabulary, or given a meaning quite different from that understood by an adult investigator. Crying can be easily misinterpreted—it does not always indicate physical discomfort (Illingworth, 1967). Conse-

*The author is at present financed by a grant from the Nuffield Foundation, and also wishes to express his appreciation and thanks to Dr. P. J. L. Holt, Dr. J. H. Keen, and Mrs. V. P. Mellor for their continuing encouragement and support.

quently, there remains a lack of knowledge about even such fundamental issues as the age at which an infant becomes capable of experiencing pain (Swafford & Allan, 1968). Meanwhile, some surgeons apparently continue to operate upon their youngest patients without anaesthetic, in the unsubstantiated belief that they have not yet developed the neural connections necessary for pain perception (Gross & Gardner, 1980; Poznanski, 1976).

Much of the treatment (or lack of treatment) of pain in children is, in fact, based on impression and assumption rather than adequate evidence. There is clearly a great deal still to be learned, and means of overcoming the substantial remaining methodological problems have to be found. However, what data are available do have significant practical implications for the assessment and management of pain in children, and indicate some important psychological factors that influence childhood pain.

THE INFLUENCE OF PSYCHOLOGICAL FACTORS ON CHILDHOOD PAIN EXPERIENCE

Particularly from the child's point of view, pain can seem to be a purely negative and undesirable phenomenon. But its value and importance for well-being are vividly demonstrated by the fate of those rare children born with a neurological defect rendering them incapable of pain experience. Cases have been reported of severe injury, destruction of joints, self-mutilation, and death resulting from congenital insensitivity to pain (Baxter & Olszewski, 1960; Melzack, 1973). Pain is clearly essential as a warning of tissue damage, and as a deterrent against self-destructive behavior. There is *not,* however, a direct and automatic relationship between tissue damage and pain. The degree of pain suffered by a child or adult is not an immediate and inevitable consequence of the nature and extent of injury sustained.

Under certain circumstances quite severe injury can occur without accompanying pain (Beecher, 1959; Melzack, 1973). On the other hand, a great many adults and children suffer repeated and prolonged pains of sufficient severity to interfere with normal life, which occur in the absence of demonstrable organic pathology.

Different individuals with similar pathology can experience quite different degrees of pain, and an injury or disease that may fail to produce pain on some occasions can, at other times, cause the same patient considerable discomfort.

There have been reports of younger children experiencing less severe pain than adolescents with similar injury or disease (Beales, in preparation; Swafford & Allan, 1968). And lower levels of pain have been found among children with juvenile chronic arthritis than among comparable adults with rheumatoid arthritis (Laaksonen & Laine, 1961; Scott, Ansell, & Huskisson, 1977). Indeed, many juvenile chronic arthritis patients apparently experience no pain from their inflamed joints (Beales, in preparation; Grokoest, Snyder, & Schlaeger, 1962).

The traditional concept of the pain process as involving direct transmission of "pain signals" from "pain receptors" along "pain pathways" to a "pain center" in the brain has been refuted by overwhelming evidence. It is now clear that nociceptive signals that are triggered by tissue damage are modulated at successive synaptic levels along their route to the brain, and that brain activities themselves exercise substantial control over the selection and abstraction of sensory inputs at lower levels of the central nervous system (Melzack & Casey, 1968; Melzack & Wall, 1965).

The human brain is incapable of consciously experiencing all the inputs available to it at any one moment from the body's many sensory receptors. Some form of filtering is essential, and pain-producing signals have to compete for conscious awareness with signals representing other sensory modalities. If pain is anticipated or feared, and the brain is on the lookout for it, nociceptive signals are much more likely to overcome the competition and give rise to actual pain experience. If attention is focused on some other event such nociceptive signals may be inhibited and most individuals have had the experience of being so engrossed in a particular activity that they were not immediately aware of having injured themselves in the process (Melzack, 1973; Melzack, Weisz, & Sprague, 1963).

Like thirst and hunger, pain motivates specific behavior, and the relative priority given to pain-producing signals may depend upon the kind of action most appropriate at the time. It has been observed in both man and animals that pain may be absent at the moment when severe injury occurs and for some time after. On such occasions the well-being or even survival of the organism requires that the highest priority be given to such behaviors as fighting, fleeing, and seeking aid, which pain would only inhibit. But once the immediate injury phase is ended, pain may occur to serve the valuable function of discouraging further activity and enforcing rest (Wall, 1979). Children whose clothing catches fire are frequently able to extinguish the flames with their bare hands, and run perhaps several hundred yards to reach home or some other place of comparative safety, without experiencing pain. Settled in a hospital bed, however, a severely burned child tends to display the kind of response seen commonly in sick or injured children—a preference for lying quiet and undisturbed, and a reluctance to move or allow affected areas to be touched (Beales, in preparation).

Interpretation of the source of nociceptive signals and the situation as a whole can apparently determine the ability of such signals to give rise to pain. If the signals are identified as having little sinister significance, and other events or activities are considered to be of greater importance at the time, the nociceptive input is more likely to be inhibited than if the signals are perceived to indicate serious threat (Beecher, 1959; Melzack, 1973; Pavlov, 1927, 1928).

A child has to learn what pain-producing signals mean or represent. Young children quickly learn to associate the experience of pain with visible damage to the body surface, but signals originating from beneath that surface have much less obvious meaning. An internal pain may be identified as a punishment inflicted by a parent, rather than perceived as a sign of pathology (Gross & Gardner, 1980). Fears of disability and death may well be absent. Studies among terminally ill children indicate that, in the earliest years, death either has no meaning or is seen as avoidable or reversible by an act of will. Understanding increases between the ages of 5 and 11, but it is only in adolescence that many children come to share the adult's appreciation of the inevitability and irreversibility of death, and to recognize it as a consequence of internal physiological malfunction (Burton, 1974; Easson, 1968; Green, 1967; Howarth, 1974; Nagy, 1959).

There have been very few investigations of children's concepts of health and illness (Campbell, 1975; Mechanic, 1964). However, a recent study (Bibace & Walsh, 1980) suggests that such concepts may develop in accordance with Piaget's stages of cognitive development (Piaget, 1930). Bibace and Walsh report that it is only with the development of formal-logical thinking, at around the age of 11, that children acquire a concept of their internal structure and interpret illness in "physiologic" terms. Children at the prelogical stage (aged 2 to 6 years) are said to be concerned essentially with the external surface of the body—the stomach, for example, being conceptualized as the outer surface of the abdomen.

Among children with juvenile chronic arthritis (JCA) it has similarly been found (Beales, 1980) that, whereas younger patients (up to the age of 11) are concerned about, and distressed by, visible damage to the skin surface, they are much less aware of the significance of internal pathology. Younger JCA patients tend to identify the body very much with its exterior. Older children, however (in the 12 to 17 age group), have a greater understanding of their internal structure, and a greater appreciation of the implications of internal disease. By this age, they rate the well-being of the "body beneath the surface" as at least as important as that of the visible exterior, if not more so.

The visual appearance of surface lesions reinforces pain experience. Children with cuts and abrasions often indicate that their injury "feels" particularly painful because it "looks painful." A child cannot see pathology beneath the body surface, but he can imagine what it looks like. In the case of JCA, fantasies about the internal appearance of damaged joints tend to be much more frequent among adolescents than among the younger patients. Children in the 6-to-11 age group are either concerned only with the external appearance of the joint (swelling or redness) or picture the subsurface situation in comparatively undisturbing terms. A 10-year-old girl, who attributed the swelling and restricted mobility of her knee joint to its being filled with a substance resembling cold mashed potato, was more amused than distressed by her fantasy. The teenagers generally imagine the state of their joints as being much more sinister, and are often significantly disturbed by fantasies that are gross exaggerations of medical fact and feature such things as splintered bone, lacerated blood vessels, internal hemorrhaging, and congealed blood.

Chronic internal disease tends also to have more serious implications for activities and ambitions among older than among younger children (Beales, in preparation; Tropauer & Dilgard, 1970). Because lifestyles and goals change with age, the same clinical condition can come to have very different significance for the child over the years. Younger patients tend to be primarily concerned with play, and as long as their disease does not greatly interfere with preferred play activities, or if alternative activities are available, they do not consider the condition as being of great personal importance. By the age of puberty patients begin to assess their condition in terms of its implications for physical attractiveness and social esteem, for ability to continue education and pursue a chosen career, for chances of finding a marriage partner, and (in the case of girls) for ability to have children and cope with a family. A chronic, disabling disease becomes recognized as much more of a disaster.

The same internally originating sensations therefore tend to be interpreted quite differently by children of different ages, and accorded different priority in the competition for attention. It seems likely that such age variation in the cognitive appraisal of nociceptive inputs has much to do with the lower levels of pain reported by 6-to-11-year-olds with juvenile chronic arthritis compared with patients aged 12 to 17. It probably also has much to do with the more severe pain reported by adults with rheumatoid arthritis in comparison with JCA patients as a whole. The closer the child comes to adulthood, and the adult's appreciation of illness, the closer his joint pain comes to the levels experienced by rheumatoid arthritis sufferers (Beales, Keen, & Holt, in preparation).

In chronic illness, a child's pain can consequently become more severe over a period of years even if there is no deterioration of the clinical condition. Not infrequently a patient complains of increasing pain despite undergoing an actual physical improvement, and clinicians who assume a simple and direct relationship between tissue damage and pain are likely to dismiss such complaints as exaggerated and mischievously meant. In fact, pain may increase not only because greater priority is given to pain-producing signals, but also because competition from other sensory inputs is reduced. As goals and interests change, and are increasingly interfered with, the patient becomes prone to more frequent bouts of boredom in which he has nothing else to do but anxiously contemplate his condition and look out for signals representing spread or worsening of the disease.

Interpretation of and sensitivity to pain-producing signals arising from internal tissue damage are very much related to age during childhood. But other factors also have a bearing here. Anxious parents, preoccupied with health and illness, can easily communicate their anxiety to their offspring, and cause even a young child to pay great attention to internally originating sensations. Such preoccupation with physical well-being, and transmission of anxiety from generation to generation, has been particularly associated with certain cultures (Zborowski, 1969), but it seems common enough in all societies. A great deal obviously depends upon the particular illness experience of the family. Parents are much more likely to look out for signs of ill health in their child, and encourage the child (deliberately or otherwise) to do the same, if they or other close close relatives have suffered serious illness. Parents are even more likely to do this if they believe (rightly or wrongly) that their child might have inherited a predisposition or vulnerability to a particular condition. A great many children who present with limb pains at juvenile rheumatology clinics, and who turn out to have no detectable physical pathology, have a parent or grandparent who suffers from rheumatoid arthritis or some other severe joint disease.

Parental anxiety appears to be an important causal factor not only in cases of psychogenic limb pains (often referred to as "growing pains"), but also in the headache and abdominal pain that afflict a great many children. In a large-scale study of a Scandinavian school population, limb pains were found among 15.5 percent of the children (Oster, 1972; Oster & Nielsen, 1972). The same study reported a 20.6 percent incidence of headache, and a 14.4 percent incidence of abdominal pain. Apley's pioneer investigation of children with abdominal pains (1975) reported that 10.8 percent of the school-age children studied had this symptom, and that an organic cause could be found in less than one-tenth of the cases.

Three complaints—nonorganic headache, limb pain, and abdominal pain—clearly have much in common, and frequently occur in combination in the same child (a fact recognized as long ago as 1933, when Wyllie and Schlesinger, 1933, coined the term "periodic syndrome" to describe this group of disorders). And although the precise etiology remains obscure, the majority of studies have found a high incidence of exaggerated concern about health, and of psychogenic pain, among the parents of these children (Apley, 1975; Berger, 1974; Green, 1967; Hughes & Zimin, 1978; Oster, 1972; Stone & Barbero, 1970). Sometimes the child's pain is similar to that afflicting a parent (Apley, 1975; MacKeith & O'Neill, 1951), but frequently it occurs in a different site, and the family displays a general "pain-proneness" rather than a common symptom (Oster, 1972). Rather than being a simple imitation of a parent's pain, the child's condition seems to have more to do with the transmission of anxiety and preoccupation with bodily well-being from generation to generation. Children with psychogenic pains are usually "worriers" themselves (Stone & Barbero, 1970), who fear that internally originating pain represents something sinister and uncontrollable—a fear frequently reinforced by the mother. Stone and Barbero (1970) have noted "a contagious, circular anxiety" in the parent-child relationship that seems to "heighten the pain and fear in the child."

Pain resulting from an initial, quite trivial muscle sprain or abdominal upset may be misinterpreted by parent and child. Having attributed exaggerated significance to the pain, the child is then likely to focus his attention upon the body part affected, and to assign an unduly high priority to sensory inputs originating from that source. Consequently, even when the underlying physical condition has resolved itself, weak nociceptive signals arising from what might be described as normal body wear and tear may be detected and augmented. Anxiety and emotional distress may themselves set up muscle spasms that add to the child's pain. And the more severe and prolonged the pain becomes, the more certain parents and child are likely to be that there is something seriously wrong. Insistence by the doctors to whom they turn that nothing organic can be found may only add to the sense of helplessness and despair. Anxiety and pain perpetuate each other in a particularly vicious circle.

It seems likely, however, that some children with nonorganic pains perceive the pains primarily as an advantage rather than as a sign of undesirable internal pathology. There can be few children who have not attempted to avoid some unwanted activity by reporting illness, and pain can undoubtedly be convenient on occasion—consequently, it is often invented. But pain that is convenient is not always imaginary. Priority can be given to internally originating sensations whether the significance attributed to them is of a positive or negative kind. The child may learn to look out for pain not because he fears signs of illness, but because he is keen to find them. Persistent school-refusers who experience initial pain as a result of muscle spasm or gastrointestinal upset caused by school-associated emotional distress are likely to enthusiastically focus their attention upon that pain, and to search for similar sensations when they are required (Apley, 1975; Berger, 1974). Young school-refusers without an anxious mother to expedite their understanding of illness may welcome subsurface pain as a bounty with no sinister significance, rather than be alarmed by fears of internal pathology.

By influencing the priority given to pain-producing signals, cognitive processes can therefore exert a substantial impact on the frequency, duration, and severity of pain experienced by a child, whether or not those signals have their origins in demonstrable, clinically significant, physical pathology. There is a second means, however, by which cognitive appraisal of the pain source can affect the level of suffering.

Pain is a complex experience. It comprises a combination of "feelings." It involves sensation, but not all somatic sensations constitute pain. At varying degrees of intensity, and in different circumstances, sensations of heat, pressure, and stretching, for example, can be either exceedingly uncomfortable or highly pleasurable. Sensory experience that is not unpleasant cannot be considered pain—pain only occurs when the affective "coloring" of sensation is negative. And the polarity and degree of affect attached to a sensation can be modified by learning.

This is generally recognized in respect to other sensory modalities. The extent to which a particular sight or sound, for example, evokes pleasant or unpleasant feelings depends upon what it is associated with. If the sensation indicates some desirable event in the external world, or the presence of a valued object, the sight or sound itself is likely to be experienced as pleasurable. If, through learning, the sensation comes to signify threat, its affective tone is more likely to be negative. A baby's cry may be music to its mother's ears, but a monstrous noise to anyone not emotionally attached to the infant.

Similarly with pain: the affective coloring of somatic sensations may be influenced by what the sensations are associated with. A slap may be experienced as pleasurable, or as painful and distressing, depending upon whether it is recognized by the child as a punishment or as a playful and affectionate gesture (Melzack, 1973). If a feeling of heat, pressure, or stretching somewhere inside the body is perceived as indicating disastrous pathology, the negative affect attached to the sensory experience is likely to be more extreme than if it is considered to have no such sinister meaning. According to the particular interpretation that a child makes of sensations originating beneath his body surface, he may experience those sensations as either pleasant or unpleasant— pain may be substantial or absent altogether.

In a study of pain among children with juvenile chronic arthritis (Beales, Holt, Keen, & Mellor, in preparation), it was found that although several of the younger patients denied joint pain altogether, and 6-to-11-year-olds generally reported lower levels of pain than did the 12-to-17-year-olds, patients in both age groups experienced very similar qualities of sensation from their joints. All the children in the sample—including those who said they had no pain— reported "burning," "sharp," or "aching" feelings. But the meaning that the 6-to-11-year-olds attributed to such sensations was very different from that attributed to them by the older age group.

The younger children, in fact, seemed to frequently view the joint sensations in isolation, not associating them with the chronic condition. And when such an association was made, because the disease was much less of a personal disaster for these younger patients it was not a particularly unpleasant one. Consequently, when the 6-to-11-year-olds were asked to rate how "nice" or "nasty" were the feelings they had in their affected joints, low values of "nastiness" were generally reported. Children who subsequently denied pain insisted that the sensations were not at all unpleasant, and one young boy asserted that the "burning" feeling in his knee was, if anything, quite "nice."

Among the 12-to-17-year-olds, however, things were markedly different. All the patients in this age group volunteered that the sensations in their affected joints "reminded them" of their disease and its personal implications. They clearly associated the joint sensations with the negative meaning their arthritis had for them, and feelings of burning, piercing, or whatever in the joint were more unpleasant because of the horrific physical damage they were imagined to be caused by. Teenagers spoke of any joint sensation provoking episodes of "depression" and "anxiety," during which their emotional distress contributed to the pain experience. Whereas the younger children tended to view joint pain philosophically, simply waiting until it disappeared, their older counterparts were plunged into an emotional response that exacerbated and prolonged suffering.

Younger children also found it much easier to distract themselves during bouts of pain, because the pain and its associations did not generate very much thought. The teenagers, however, were preoccupied with their joint symptoms and gave a great deal of thought to their implications—pain reminded the child of his predicament, which caused him to focus attention upon the pain source, which itself increased the prospect that nociceptive signals would overcome the competition and reach levels of conscious awareness. In fact external as well as internal events reminded JCA patients of the limitations imposed upon them by their disease, and several children reported that episodes of pain commenced when they started thinking about their joints as a result of seeing other children "doing things that I can't do."

The two mechanisms outlined here by which cognitive processes influence pain experience are therefore closely interrelated and reinforce each other. Their operation has advantages for the well-being of the individual, but they do not constitute a perfect system. They allow the fruits of childhood learning and experience about physical pathology to be put to use in modulating pain perception and consequent behavior. They relate pain and action to the perceived personal significance of an illness or injury, instead of restricting the human organism to a series of reflex responses to tissue damage. The greater the importance that comes to be attached to particular nociceptive signals, the more likely those signals are to produce conscious pain of sufficient severity to prompt the individual to devote time and effort to trying to remedy the pathology. If the signals are not identified as having much significance, they may be inhibited before they can interfere with other matters requiring thought or with other activities.

To an extent, the experience of pain can be restricted to those occasions when, according to the individual's understanding of the world and his own body, pain *ought* to be experienced. But because such understanding is incomplete even in the adult, mistakes can easily be made. Children who are in the process of learning about their own physical makeup and the implications of physical damage are particularly prone to errors of judgment. Pain can be augmented and prolonged because a child incorrectly believes it to indicate serious illness. On the other hand, a young patient who fails to appreciate the full implications of a chronic disease may consciously experience nociceptive inputs triggered by the pathology as affectively neutral sensation rather than as actual pain—and he may consequently defy all attempts by parents and clinicians to make him "take it easy." Because he attributes greater importance to his visible body surface, such a young patient may be caused more discomfort and distress by venepuncture or a grazed knee than by subsurface pathology that is of far greater physiological significance.

Furthermore, the rest and recuperation that pain motivates is not always a desirable response in cases of illness and injury. Nature's remedies are occasionally at odds with those developed by medical science. Movement of an injured limb may be clinically preferable to prolonged immobility. And where the disease is such that a return to full health is impossible, however much the child remains inactive, motivating the patient to get out of bed and lead as normal a life as he can is a prime concern. Vital as it is to well-being, pain can sometimes do the individual more harm than good.

Psychological factors, of course, do not exercise total control over the pain process. Events that occur at the site of tissue damage, and at lower levels of the nervous system, also have much to do with the degree of discomfort a child experiences. But the power of cognitive processes to influence the frequency, duration, and severity of pain is sufficient to indicate their value as a tool for management. Modifying a child's appraisal of his physical condition is potentially a useful means of relieving inappropriate and unnecessary pain, whether that pain is "psychogenic" or arises from manifest injury, acute illness, or chronic disease.

THE ASSESSMENT OF CHILDREN'S PAIN

Whatever analgesic methods are used, effective and efficient management of pain in children depends upon reasonably accurate assessment. But such assessment is by no means easy, and mistakes are often made. Not infrequently young patients are denied analgesia, and thereby caused unnecessary suffering, because their pain is not recognized by the adults responsible for their care. Genuine reports of pain are sometimes dismissed as attempts to gain attention or to avoid some unpleasant task. On other occasions, unnecessary drugs are administered because it is assumed that a child "must have" pain in view of his clinical condition, whether he indicates it or not.

The association of pain with tissue damage leads to a widespread tendency both inside and outside the medical professions to assess a child's level of pain by reference to the nature and extent of the physical insult. There is assumed to be a "proper" level of pain that a child is "entitled" to complain of for each injury, disease, or therapeutic procedure. Venepuncture, for example, is considered to produce its own specific amount of discomfort—if the perforated child complains less than the acceptable amount, he is praised for his bravery; if he claims more pain than he is allowed, he is accused of being deliberately troublesome or cowardly. And any improvement in a child's clinical condition, any healing of damaged tissue, is expected to be accompanied by a diminution of pain. A young patient who asserts that his pain is becoming more severe, despite the clinical improvement, is likely to be censured for attempting to deceive.

But because psychological and other factors play so large a part in the pain process, the degree of tissue damage incurred is a poor guide to the actual level of discomfort. Conversely, the amount of pain reported by a child is an unreliable indicator of physical pathology. Because young children can experience nociceptive signals as affectively neutral or even pleasant sensations, absence of reported pain does not always have diagnostic significance. Certainly the questioning of younger patients should not be restricted to actual pain—it may well be worthwhile asking a young child who appears to be ill, but who denies discomfort, if he nonetheless has any "funny" or unusual "feelings inside."

Another common rule-of-thumb method of assessing the true level of a youngster's pain is to make a comparison with the amount of pain expressed by other children. If one individual is not brought to tears as a result of incurring some physical insult, there seems to be no reason why any other child should be. Therefore, if one child in the family, school class, or hospital ward fails to make a lot of fuss, any of his peers who subsequently suffer similar damage, and who cry more than he did, may find themselves receiving more condemnation than sympathy.

Comparisons of this kind, however, are usually unfair. Even if the children concerned are of the same age, there are several reasons why one youngster may genuinely experience more pain than another with similar pathology. Because of differences in personal experience, even youngsters of similar years can attribute different meaning and significance to the same injury. And the child who failed to show much pain might have been fortunate in having other things available to distract his attention from his wound. The child who cried might have had nothing else to think about.

Differences in the availability of sources of distraction, and in other situational factors, also make it impossible to reasonably infer a child's actual level of physical discomfort by comparing present reports with the same child's previous expressions of pain. There is a widespread belief that each individual has a fixed "pain threshold," so that if an injection, for example, fails to evoke expression of discomfort on one occasion, it is considered incapable of causing the patient genuine pain on any subsequent administration—whatever the child might say. But the ability of nociceptive signals to give rise to conscious experience of pain is not simply dependent upon stimulus strength, and it therefore cannot be taken for granted that a procedure that does not hurt the first time it is performed upon a particular child must fail to do so when it is repeated.

Nor can it be assumed that a child who does not indicate pain despite serious internal pathology must have an unusually high pain threshold that renders him incapable of experiencing pain when, for example, venepuncture is performed. The significance a young patient attributes to surface, as opposed to internal, damage may cause him to suffer more real pain as a result of what is, objectively, a lesser physical insult.

Yet another quite common misconception is that children who suffer from chronic disorders somehow become "used" to physical discomfort, and are less susceptible to pain the longer their disease continues (Mennie, 1974). Not only are they believed to suffer less pain as a result of their chronic pathology, they are also sometimes assumed to have a raised threshold to pain from any source—so that long-standing patients are denied anesthesia or analgesia in circumstances in which it would be provided for newly diagnosed children. There is, of course, no evidence to support this belief, and a great deal that is incompatible with such a generalization.

If a child's report of pain is at odds with the level of pain anticipated according to the nature of the physical insult, it should certainly not be taken for granted that what the child says is untrue. Nor should it be assumed that if a young patient's account disagrees with that provided by a parent, the adult must inevitably know best—but that assumption is frequently made. And a doctor is particularly inclined to accept a mother's version as closest to the truth if she has success in intimidating the child into amending his story to comply more closely with hers—although this may have far more to do with the distribution of power in the mother-child relationship than with the true level of the child's physical discomfort.

Parents, in fact, are not always reliable reporters of their children's pain. There are particular reasons why their accounts are sometimes highly inaccurate, and may sometimes even be intended to deliberately deceive the doctor.

Parents tend to see pain as the prime indicator of physical pathology in their offspring, and they consider having a pain to be the most reliable sign of the existence of injury or disease. Therefore, they can often decide that the doctor will only take their child's case seriously if reasonable reports of pain are provided. Not infrequently, the parents of children with juvenile chronic arthritis are tempted to exaggerate their child's level of pain out of a misguided fear that otherwise the clinician will begin to lose interest in his patient.

The proper response to a parent who insists that her child has pain which the child himself denies may therefore not be to prescribe analgesics for the youngster, but simply to reassure the parent that the child's case is indeed being taken seriously.

Mothers and fathers are also anxious that their child should not be considered "soft," complaining of more pain than he should. If the child claims a greater degree of pain than the parent considers proper in view of his illness or injury, his parents may be shamed by his apparent cowardice, and may consequently attempt to deter him from giving the doctor what is in fact an accurate report.

But if the youngster reports less pain than is considered reasonable by the parents, they are likely to interpret this to the doctor as an indication of his bravery, and endeavor to convince the medic that the child is really suffering far more than he is admitting to.

The doctor should be extremely cautions about accepting from a parent a lower estimate of pain than a child is claiming. Taking the parent's word in such a case can have at least three unfortunate consequences: it can result in a failure to provide the patient with adequate analgesia, it can destroy the child's trust and faith in the doctor, and it can encourage the parents to go on censuring their offspring for making what they believe to be unnecessary fuss. At the worst, trusting the parent can have the further result of causing a wrong diagnosis to be made.

Conversely, before analgesics are prescribed parents who make repeated references to their youngster's stoicism and bravery should be asked to specify their reasons for believing that the child is experiencing more pain than he admits to. Parents of juvenile arthritis patients who insist that their child is suffering greatly will, when pressed, often admit that they believe "he must have a lot of pain" in view of his condition, but that he has never shown much sign of discomfort. The clinician has to guard against being pressured by parents into administering pain-relieving drugs that the patient simply does not need.

Reasonably accurate assessment of a child's pain requires direct questioning or observation of the young patient, or both. In very young children, whose vocabulary is limited or nonexistent, a reasonable amount can be ascertained by observing the patient's activities or obtaining a detailed account of these from parents. Because pain effectively motivates "recuperative" behavior, a child who persists in playing as normal can be assumed with a fair degree of certainty to have little pain. Reluctance to move or be touched, and an unwillingness to participate in normal activities, suggest that the child is suffering discomfort (Illingworth, 1967).

Obtaining an account of the child's behavior is of value in assessing pain not only in the youngest patient. It is useful as a check against verbal reports of pain made by older children. Adolescents who assert that they are in constant agony, but who manage to indulge in normal and energetic pastimes, may be reasonably considered to be exaggerating the frequenty, duration, or severity of their pain.

Although the patient's own description of his pain is essential to any adequate assessment, it has to be recognized that children do lie about their level of discomfort, and precautions have to be taken against deception. Of course, it is not possible to always detect where a deliberately false report is being offered by a child, but there are circumstances in which the adult concerned—doctor, nurse, or parent—should be particularly on guard.

Where the child obviously has something to gain by claiming pain, any such claim should certainly be scrutinized carefully, and compared with the child's behavior. A youngster in a hospital may pretend pain in order to gain attention and company. A young patient who whines constantly and demands repeated analgesics may simply be missing his parents or friends, and may believe that reporting a physical symptom is the only way of making the nurses pay any attention to him. Before accepting the pain as genuine, and providing pain-relieving drugs, it can be beneficial in such cases for nursing staff to first try fussing the child a little and spending a little more time with him.

If children in hospitals are sometimes inclined to exaggerate their pain, there are also occasions when they are motivated to untruthfully deny it. Associating pain with pathology, the young patient commonly assumes that unpleasant treatment will end, and he will be allowed to return home, only when he ceases to report any physical discomfort. So he may desperately attempt to convince the doctor that he is feeling better, even though an unwillingness to move and be touched indicates that he continues to have pain.

Unwillingness to attend school is a not-unusual cause of invented pain among children. But it has to be recognized that school-refusal is also often accompanied by genuine psychogenic pain. Learning to associate pain with gain can lead to an increased sensitivity to nociceptive inputs. It should not be taken for granted that if a child is obviously benefiting by reporting physical discomfort, the pain must inevitably be a pretense. The youngster's pain might, in fact, be not only genuine, but have a significant organic cause—an attack of appendicitis or otitis media can sometimes occur at a convenient time for a child.

Boys may be more likely than girls to deny pain through bravado, and children of Mediterranean origin may be more inclined to exaggerate their level of discomfort than youngsters of Anglo-Saxon descent (Zborowski, 1969). But such generalizations should not be assumed to apply in every individual case. The most frenzied performance of exaggerated pain the writer has so far witnessed was put on by a tall, well-built, white English 15-year-old boy with an inclination to physical violence. One of the most stoical patients seen to date was the small, shy, fragile-looking daughter of a Jewish family.

To complement a child's verbal report of pain, the visual analogue scale is arguably the most useful tool for assessment available at present—whether the purpose of that assessment be diagnosis, monitoring of treatment, or research (Huskisson, 1974). The visual analogue scale (VAS) is simply a ten-centimeter line with no gradations indicated upon it; the two extremes are described to the child as "no pain at all" and "the worst pain you can imagine." The child is asked to mark a point along the line representing his level of pain. Offering an infinite number of points, this method is preferable to fixed-choice questions or graded scales that present the child with a limited number of alternatives and force him to fit his pain experience into a "mild," "moderate," or "severe" category. Comparatively young children are not only able to use the VAS, they often seem to *enjoy* doing so. The scale has been successful in obtaining reliable and reproducible "pain scores" among children aged from 5 to 17 years (Scott et al., 1977; Beales, in preparation). It has its limitations, however. The point at which a child indicates his pain along the line depends upon what his imagination offers in the way of the most severe pain possible. A young child, with limited direct and indirect experience of human pain and suffering, may be inclined to believe that his own pain, which is in reality quite mild, comes close to the upper limit. Another child who has witnessed extreme pain in, for example, a relative with terminal cancer, may consider his own substantial discomfort to be slight in comparison. For this reason, therefore, the VAS is more effective in recording changes in pain severity in the same child than in comparing the pain of one youngster with that of another. The scale should not be administered in the presence of a parent, for parents often attempt to intervene and influence their child's judgement when given the opportunity (Scott et al., 1977; Beales, in preparation).

In addition to assessing the severity of pain, it is also important to elicit its sensory quality—to establish whether the pain is sharp and piercing or dull and aching, or hot or cold, for example. The McGill pain questionnaire (Melzack 1975) offers a list of sensation items for administration to adult subjects, but the inclusion of such words as "lancinating" prevents its use among children with limited vocabulary. On the basis of interviews with children aged 6 to 17, the writer has devised a simple questionnaire that has been administered successfully to young patients with a variety of pain-producing conditions. This questionnaire includes 11 items of sensory quality, and the child is asked if his pain feels like "an ache," or as if the body part concerned has been "cut," "bumped," "burned," "grazed," "pricked," "pinched," "smacked," "given an electric shock," "squeezed," or "pulled."

There is, however, no perfect method of assessing a child's pain, and never can be. All methods must be approximate and prone to error. But for the sake of research and more effective management of pain in children, less imperfect means of quantifying this complex, subjective experience must be developed. Meanwhile, the avoidance of simplistic and erroneous assumptions about children's pain, a greater willingness to listen to the child—albeit with a critical ear—and use of the visual analogue scale in conjunction with a "sensory quality" questionnaire may together allow adults responsible for the care of sick and injured children to make a more accurate and sympathetic assessment than is often the case at present.

THE MANAGEMENT OF CHILDREN'S PAIN

The management of pain in children is not simply a matter of providing appropriate drugs or other physical treatment. Nor does it lie exclusively within the province of professional medical personnel. Because psychological processes play so important a part in the perception of pain, there is considerable scope for pain prevention and relief by the use of sociopsychological techniques. Such techniques can often be used effectively by parents and other nonprofessional adults concerned with the care of a sick or injured child. And since the words and actions of parents and other family members can greatly exacerbate or ameliorate a child's pain, it is almost invariably necessary to involve the family as a whole in any formal, professional pain management program.

Either alone or in conjunction with other methods of achieving analgesia, sociopsychological techniques are of potential value whether a child's pain is psychogenic or arises from demonstrable physical insult associated with chronic disease, acute illness or injury, or therapeutic procedure.

The Pain of Chronic Disease

The child's appraisal of his disease may have significant consequences for pain by influencing the relative priority given to pain-producing signals, and by determining the degree of negative affect linked with sensations triggered by tissue damage. In some cases, therefore, it may be possible to markedly reduce the patient's level of physical discomfort by modifying his perception and assessment of his condition.

Understanding of disease and its implications tends to come with age, so that chronically ill children generally perceive their condition in increasingly gloomy terms as they get older. It is obviously undesirable to discourage a young patient from acquiring a progressively more realistic appreciation of the seriousness of his disease and its likely effects. But chronically ill children of all ages quite often come to see their condition as more of a personal disaster than it need be, and counseling of both the patient and the family can do much to remedy this (Beales, 1979, in preparation).

The majority of young chronically ill patients seem to perceive their illness primarily in terms of its implications for activities: they deplore it to the extent that it prevents them from "doing what they want to do." Among younger children play is the prime concern, and a chronic disease is seen as being of less significance if favorite play activities are not interfered with or if alternatives are available. But adults responsible for the care of such children—parents and medical staff—sometimes fail to properly appreciate this. They impose their own scale of values, and consider play to be something of an irrelevance when a child is seriously ill and the prognosis is perhaps grave. Counseling of the younger patient can suggest to him alternative play activities appropriate to his interests and physical condition; counseling of the parents can encourage them to appreciate the child's point of view and take steps themselves to minimize the impact of the disease upon play. Even where the future outlook is bleak, the child's present appraisal of his condition and his experience of pain may thus be favorably modified. Among older children leisure pursuits are still of concern, but attention is increasingly paid to implications for work and domestic activities. Timely advice and guidance on education, career, and coping with household tasks can favorably influence an adolescent's appraisal of a permanent disability or chronic illness.

Restriction of activities can not only exacerbate pain by causing the child to perceive his condition in gloomy terms—it can also have the effect of reducing competition to nociceptive inputs. Chronically ill children whose favorite pursuits are no longer available to them are prone to bouts of boredom in which they have little else to contemplate but their condition and symptoms. Providing adequate sources of distraction, and thereby discouraging the focusing of attention on the pain source, can make a worthwhile impact on the pain experience of many such young patients. Unfortunately, parents sometimes add to the restrictions that the disease itself may impose upon the child, by "overprotecting." Even if parents themselves recognize the importance of allowing their offspring to lead as normal a life as possible, they are often put under considerable pressure to impose unnecessary limitations on the child's activities by well-intentioned but misguided relatives and neighbors. Chronically ill children not infrequently suffer avoidable distress and pain as a result of pressure to further restrict their leisure pursuits exerted by kindly grandparents. Sociopsychological counseling of the family as a whole not only educates parents on the undesirable consequences that "overprotecting" has for the child, but also provides them with support to allow them to resist harmful advice and criticism from outside.

Counseling of the patient and the parents can help to raise the sick child's self-esteem, and reduce tensions that may develop in family relationships as a result of having a chronically ill youngster in the home. Formal counseling can also deal with misunderstandings about the nature and extent of the physical pathology. Older children particularly may have exaggerated fears of crippling and death. Their fantasies about the appearance of internal pathology may be more horrific and distressing than the clinical reality. Adolescent girls may mistakenly believe that their illness will prevent them being able to subsequently bear and care for children. By eliciting and influencing the child's beliefs and fears about his condition the psychologist working alongside the clinician and other medical personnel may have a significant effect on the interpretation of sensory inputs originating from areas of pathology, and therefore on the severity of pain experienced by a child with chronic illness.

But in addition to his own direct involvement with the child and the family, the psychologist can also guide medical staff in regard to what to say, and what not to say, to the young patient, for when a child acquires an unnecessarily gloomy view of his condition doctors and nurses are often responsible, in part at least. In attempting to reassure the young patient, members of the health care team can easily cause increased fear and distress if the explanation of the condition that they give to the child is inappropriate to his level of understanding. Careless words can be misinterpreted—particularly words that have more than one meaning. The doctor who smilingly informed his patient of "the way we operate in this clinic" unintentionally led the child to believe that his psychogenic abdominal pain was the result of some internal pathology that could only be cured by major surgery. The friendly nurse who habitually jokes with her young patients is sometimes prone to forget that children do not necessarily share an adult's sense of humor, and that casual remarks can have a devastating effect on a child's perception of his condition if he does not recognize that they were meant in jest (Whitt, Dykstra, & Taylor, 1979).

Effective psychological management of pain in a child with chronic disease involves counseling of the adults responsible for his care—both lay and professional—as much as it involves dealing directly with the child.

Pain in Acute Illness and Injury

Where the underlying organic cause of pain is of short duration, much relief can often be achieved simply by providing adequate distractions and by discouraging the child from focusing his attention upon the pain source. Psychological intervention of this kind requires more in the way of common sense than specialist expertise, and may be used effectively by parents coping with a sick or injured child at home, and by nurses dealing with young patients with, for example, postoperative pain in a hospital (Swafford & Allan, 1968). But just as it is easy to relieve a child's pain by such means, it is also easy to unintentionally make it worse.

A child is more likely to focus his attention on the source of his pain if he is anxious about its significance. Consequently, reassurance is required. Time has to be spent talking to the child, and dealing with his worries. But instead of dispelling a child's fears, understandably anxious parents not infrequently communicate their own anxiety to their offspring, and thereby aggravate his distress and pain.

Similarly, a surface injury is likely to be experienced as more painful the more "unpleasant" it is perceived as being. The appearance of the wound, its perceived "nastiness," can influence the degree of negative affect attached to sensations coming from the damaged area. And by indicating her own horror and distress at the sight of her child's injury, a mother can cause the child to reappraise the damage and see it as more unpleasant than he had originally. Parents can produce a useful analgesic effect by exercising control over their own emotions and playing down, within reason, the significance of a wound or illness.

In the case of injury to the body surface, it is often true that "out of sight is out of mind" as far as the child is concerned. Visual confirmation that damage has occurred makes it more likely that the youngster will expect pain. Hiding the injury from view facilitates distraction, and children usually prefer to have their wounds bandaged, reporting that they "feel better" when they can no longer be seen. A comparable situation exists in the case of internal illness, where there is less likelihood of pain being experienced if the child is able to "forget about" his condition. Caring parents who repeatedly ask their off-spring how he is feeling increase the likelihood that he will suffer pain.

A child is clearly more likely to "dwell upon" his illness or injury, and the pain it gives rise to, if he has nothing else to occupy his mind. When a youngster is sufficiently ill to be kept in his bed, parents and nurses can often do more to relieve his pain by ensuring that he is constantly entertained than by providing regular doses of pain-relieving medicine. Distraction is, on the whole, compar-atively easy to accomplish among children—young patients want to be enter-tained, and would rather engage themselves in some enjoyable pastime than reflect upon their physical condition. It is among adults that distraction is generally more difficult to achieve. Ill health in adulthood tends to have more serious implications for wage-earning and domestic life, and the patient is consequently more likely to be preoccupied with his condition and recovery—he may feel guilty and irresponsible if he succeeds in obtaining pleasure during a temporary incapacity that is causing problems for his family. Children do not share an adult's reluctance to enjoy themselves when ill.

The ability of distraction to relieve pain is indicated by the fact that many sick children at home and in the hospital only complain of discomfort at night when they are trying to get to sleep. During the day they may have been sufficiently occupied with other things to prevent nociceptive signals from reaching the levels of conscious awareness. In the dark, with severe curtailment of competing sensory inputs, the pain-producing signals are given more or less free passage. Rather than imposing a strict "lights out" and relying upon drugs to produce analgesia, it may well be preferable to allow distraction to continue right up to the moment of sleep. Older children can read themselves to sleep. Younger children can be read to, and even in the hospital, where staff may too hard-pressed to provide such a service themselves, this is the kind of task that parents and other visitors are generally willing to take on.

Pain During Therapeutic Procedure

For many sick and injured children, pain is associated more with clinical investigation and therapy than with the pathological condition itself. Many childhood conditions are not painful in their own right—it is the venepuncture, for example, that hurts. Children with severe burns are liable to experience their most excruciating pain when the damaged areas are disturbed in the course of treatment.

Unlike much of the pain produced by disease and injury, therapy pain is overwhelmingly undesirable and negative in its effect—it has no significant value. Apart from the suffering it inflicts upon the child, it can seriously interfere with treatment and recovery, it can badly damage the relationship between young patient and medical staff, and it can impose great emotional strain upon doctors and nurses who, trying to benefit the youngster, find themselves feared as little better than torturers (Bernstein, 1963, 1965; Long & Cope, 1961).

Fear and anticipation of pain frequently play a large part in determining the degree of pain actually experienced by a child during therapeutic procedure. Dealing with such factors, which focus the child's attention on the pain source, and providing distractions to compete with nociceptive inputs can do much to relieve or avoid physical discomfort. Sometimes, however, the words and actions of medical staff can unintentionally add to the young patient's anxiety and expectation of being hurt (Beales, 1980, in preparation).

Young children particularly associate recovery from illness or injury with immobility and rest. Treatment that involves disturbance and manipulation of tender areas may consequently be perceived by the patient as an unnecessary and harmful assault rather than as positively beneficial. And sensations produced by manipulation of damaged tissue are experienced as more painful the more unpleasant and threatening a meaning the child attaches to them.

Furthermore, in response to the perceived assault the child may resist doctors or nurses attempting to undertake the therapeutic procedure upon him, and the medical staff concerned may react to such resistance by physically restraining the child. The more helpless the child feels, however—like the victim in a torture chamber—the more afraid he is likely to be, and the more he is likely to concentrate attention upon what is being done to him.

Wherever possible the child should be psychologically prepared well in advance of any potentially painful therapeutic procedure, so that he comes to view it as less of a threat and recognizes its necessity for his own well-being. Such preparation is primarily a matter of reassurance and explanation. Studies of the value of hypnosis among children with severe burns (Bernstein, 1963, 1965) suggest that sophisticated techniques of this kind are of only marginal value in their own right—the greatest benefit accrues from a sympathetic adult being prepared to spend a little time talking to the child, pointing out the benefits of treatment and encouraging the patient to work with, rather than against, medical personnel.

When a treatment procedure is taking place, the patient should ideally be allowed some sense of control over what is being done to him. If a child begins to resist, and asks for a temporary halt, it is often better to accede to his request, hold up the procedure, and spend a few minutes calming him, rather than to resort to the use of restraint. By instilling a feeling of cooperation and control in the child—a sense of working for his own benefit—it is frequently possible to minimize pain even though the child's attention is, as a result, being focused upon the procedure. Adequate preparation of the patient can have a noticeably beneficial effect upon pain in children as young as four or five years of age. Giving the child a feeling of responsibility for, and control over, his own therapy can similarly reduce pain among young patients whose treatment requires regular injections. Young diabetics and hemophiliacs, for example, almost invariably report that injections hurt less when they administer them themselves than when the task is undertaken by a nurse or parent.

Where it is not possible to adequately prepare a child psychologically for a potentially painful treatment procedure (in an emergency situation, for example, where there is insufficient time, or where the child is simply too young) pain may often be reduced or eliminated by distracting the patient's attention from what is being done to him. It is important in such a situation to avoid inadvertently focusing the child's awareness on the procedure and augmenting fear and anticipation of pain by, for example, exposing him to the sight of instruments—but all too often the young patient is presented with the spectacle of a loaded instrument trolley, on which his imagination may work, several minutes before work upon his wound actually starts. When it does commence, treatment of the wound should, as much as possible, be shielded from the child's sight. A youngster who is allowed to watch sutures being inserted into his damaged tissue is clearly going to be on the lookout for pain with each insertion of the suture needle. (Sometimes a child will deliberately look away from what is being done, only to be exposed to the sound of a running commentary as the medical personnel discuss with each other the work they are undertaking.) In fact, it is advisable to avoid exposing the child to the sight of the wound even during those moments when it is not being specifically cleaned or treated. A child who knows that he has suffered a surface injury expects the damaged area to be painful when it is touched. The worse the injury looks, the more tender and sensitive he expects it to be—and the more pain he expects, the more pain he is likely to experience. Children who arrive in hospital casualty departments with their wounds temporarily bandaged often give an impression of minimal discomfort—it is when the dressings are removed, and they are visually reminded of the damage they have sustained, that they frequently show signs of distress and become apprehensive of being touched.

The importance of the visual appearance of the wound for a child's experience of pain is particularly demonstrated by the young patients with severe burns whose injuries have been left bandaged and undisturbed for perhaps several days following initial treatment soon after their admission to the burn unit. These children, understandably, expect that healing will have been taking place during this period and that, when the bandages are removed for subsequent treatment, the damage will look less unpleasant than it did when they were first admitted. In fact, because of the nature of burn injuries the wound often looks considerably more unpleasant after the first few days, and children who are allowed to see the wound when the dressing is taken down frequently exhibit real shock and distress, and substantially increased expectation of pain and reluctance to be touched. If a child with severe burns is to be reassured and motivated to cooperate with treatment procedures, psychological preparation must therefore include a warning of the possible appearance of the damaged area when dressings are removed, and explanation that a wound that is getting better does not necessarily look better initially.

Where distraction is being used to avoid or reduce pain, it is necessary to ensure that the distraction commences before the procedure starts and continues uninterrupted until the work is finished. This means that the distraction must be systematically organized in advance. Impromptu distraction, as when a nurse attempts to engage a child in conversation, cannot be relied upon unless the procedure is very brief—the nurse invariably runs out of things to say at a crucial moment in the proceedings, and once the child has been allowed to focus his attention on what is being done to him, and has felt pain, it is not always easy to quickly reestablish distraction. Stories suitable to the patient's age and sex can be prepared on tapes and played to the child through earphones. Music, perhaps coupled with the visual attraction of a moving toy, can be used with the youngest children.

Distraction appears to have a part to play even where the child is given a measure of responsibility for his own therapy and has to give attention to it. Some young diabetics and hemophiliacs who administer their own regular injections report that they deliberately "think of something else" at the moment when they insert the needle, in order to avoid pain.

Psychogenic Pain

In the majority of publications dealing with psychogenic headache, abdominal pain, and limb pain prognosis is described as generally poor. Apley (1975) has reported that children who experience such pains are likely to continue suffering psychogenic pain in adulthood. Only limited success has been reported (Apley & Hale, 1973) from counseling aimed at reassuring the patient and parents about the true nature of the pain and absence of organic pathology.

The greatest success can be expected where the child's pain is associated with some specific emotional problem—within the family or at school, for example. Guidance and support aimed at that problem may do much to reduce tension and relieve the pain. And where the child welcomes his pain as a means of avoiding school, and consequently seeks out internally originating sensations, good results may be obtained by dealing with the underlying reasons for the patient's reluctance to attend school. But in the majority of cases the pain has a more complex etiology and is far more intractable, and psychological counseling can only hope to be effective if it is conducted in depth over a considerable period of time, and if it involves the family as a whole.

The kind of anxiety that appears to be a major causal factor in much childhood psychogenic pain is not easily dispelled by small doses of sympathy and reassurance. It is a major feature of the child's family life, and parents and their offspring reinforce it in each other. If there is to be any prospect of convincing patient and parents that the pain has no sinister organic significance, it is almost always necessary to subject the child to an impressive catalogue of clinical tests and investigations. But even after a series of negative results has been presented, and the family has appeared to accept the true nature of the pain, the child and the parents may well continue to hold a secret suspicion that the doctors are hiding the grim truth from them, or that something significant has been missed. Once outside the consulting room, their apparently deferential attitude toward the clinician may turn to one of hostility, as they remind each other that doctors are not infallible and that serious diagnostic errors are made "all the time." And even if anxiety relating to one particular episode of pain is dispelled, and the pain is successfully terminated, it cannot be assumed that a permanent cure has been accomplished. The next time the child develops an internal pain—perhaps as a result of a minor illness, muscle sprain, or (most commonly) gas—the anxiety will probably reemerge, a serious and unpleasant meaning will be attributed to the symptom, attention will be focused upon it, and the "new" pain will in turn be augmented and prolonged.

Producing a major and lasting change in the child's appraisal of internally originating nociceptive inputs requires long-term, expert psychological intervention involving the entire family, rather than the kind of brief and superficial counseling that is most often undertaken in such cases.

CONCLUSION

Although there are comparatively little hard, quantitative data available concerning pain in childhood, it is evident that psychological factors play a significant part in influencing a child's experience of pain. Pain is not simply determined by the nature and extent of tissue damage—it depends very much upon a youngster's cognitive appraisal of the pain source, and upon the relative significance he attributes to competing sensory inputs. The greater the priority he accords to nociceptive inputs, and the fewer the distractions available to him, the more likely pain-producing signals are to reach levels of conscious awareness. The more unpleasant the associations linked with somatic sensations, the more negative the affective coloring likely to be applied to those sensations. The manner in which a child interprets signals capable of producing pain can in part determine whether or not sensations are experienced at all as a result of tissue damage, and, if they are experienced, whether or not they are sufficiently unpleasant to constitute actual pain.

There is considerable scope, therefore, for relieving a child's pain by modifying the youngster's appraisal of the pain source, and by properly utilizing distraction. Psychological techniques can complement or provide an alternative to other methods of treating pain. Parents dealing with a sick or injured child at home can use simple psychological techniques to reduce or eliminate their offspring's consumption of the kind of "mild" analgesic drugs that are available without a doctor's prescription and that are purchased these days in enormous quantities.

A professional psychologist working with a hospital-based child health care team can make a major contribution to pain management by providing appropriate counseling of children about to undergo potentially painful therapeutic procedures, and by dealing with whole families in cases of pediatric chronic illness and psychogenic pain. In addition to making his own direct contribution to pain relief, the psychologist working alongside doctors, nurses, and physiotherapists can guide his colleagues in their encounters with young patients so that their words and actions can have a beneficial rather than a worsening effect on pain. Although psychological factors can reduce pain, they can also augment it, and the pain experienced by sick and injured children is quite often needlessly exacerbated by the speech and behavior of adults responsible for their care. A great deal of research could be usefully undertaken in children's hospitals to identify areas in which situational and social factors contrive to increase a young patient's fear and expectation of being hurt, and encourage him to concentrate attention upon the source of pain.

Optimum management of pain in children requires adequate means of assessing a child's level of physical discomfort, and present imperfect methods of measuring pain need to be improved upon. There is a particular need for better means of assessing pain in very young children, for it is among these patients especially that management is at present determined more by unsubstantiated assumption than by adequate understanding of what the child is actually experiencing. But perhaps the greatest need is for more research into the area of children's concepts of health and illness, and their understanding and evaluation of their own body as a biological construct. For although it is evident that a child's experience of pain can be substantially influenced by his interpretation of body signals, and can be relieved by encouraging reappraisal of those signals, much remains to be discovered about how children of different ages do in fact perceive and interpret, in terms of physical pathology, sensory inputs originating within themselves.

REFERENCES

Apley, J. *The child with abdominal pains.* (2nd ed.) Oxford: Blackwell, 1975.

Apley, J., & Hale, B. Children with recurrent abdominal pain: How do they grow up? *British Medical Journal,* 1973, **3**, 7–9.

Barber, T. X. The effects of "hypnosis" on pain. *Psychosomatic Medicine,* 1963, **25**, 303–333.

Baxter, D. W., & Olszewski, J. Congenital universal insensitivity to pain. *Brain,* 1960, **83**, 381–393.

Beales, J. G. The effects of attention and distraction on pain among children attending a hospital casualty department. In D. J. Oborne, M. M. Gruneberg, & J. R. Eiser (Eds.), *Psychology and medicine.* London: Academic Press, 1980.

Beales, J. G. Factors influencing the expectation of pain among patients in a children's burns unit. In preparation.

Beales, J. G. Pain in children with cancer. In J. J. Bonica & V. Ventrafridda (Eds.), *Advances in pain research and therapy,* Vol. 2. New York: Raven Press, 1979.

Beales, J. G., Holt, P. J. L., Keen, J. H., & Mellor, V. P. Juvenile chronic arthritis: The patient's perception of the disease. In preparation.

Beales, J. G., Keen, J. H., & Holt, P. J. L. The child's perception of the disease and the experience of pain in juvenile chronic arthritis. In preparation.

Beales, J. G., Keen, J. H., Mellor, V. P., & Holt, P. J. L. Fantasies about the appearance of affected joints among children with juvenile chronic arthritis. *Annals of the Rheumatic Diseases,* 1980, **39,** 603.

Beecher, H. K. *Measurement of subjective responses.* New York: Oxford University Press, 1959.

Berger, H. G. Somatic pain and school avoidance. *Clinical Pediatrics,* 1974, **13,** 819–826.

Bernstein, N. R. Management of burned children with the aid of hypnosis. *Journal of Child Psychology and Psychiatry,* 1963, **4,** 93–98.

Bernstein, N. R. Observations on the use of hypnosis with burned children on a pediatric ward. *International Journal of Clinical and Experimental Hypnosis,* 1965, **13,** 1–10.

Bibace, R., & Walsh, M. E. Development of children's concepts of illness. *Pediatrics,* 1980, **66,** 912–917.

Burton, L. Tolerating the intolerable—the problems facing parents and children following diagnosis. In L. Burton (Ed.), *Care of the child facing death.* London: Routledge & Kegan Paul, 1974.

Campbell, J. D. Illness is a point of view: The development of children's concepts of illness. *Child Development,* 1975, **46,** 92–100.

Easson, W. M. Care of the young patient who is dying. *Journal of the American Medical Association,* 1968, **205,** 63–67.

Green, M. Care of the dying child. *Pediatrics,* 1967, **40,** 492–497.

Green, M. Diagnosis and treatment: Psychogenic, recurrent, abdominal pain. *Pediatrics,* 1967, **40,** 84–89.

Grokoest, A. W., Snyder, A. I., & Schlaeger, R. *Juvenile rheumatoid arthritis.* Boston: Little, Brown, 1962.

Gross, S. C., & Gardner, G. G. Child pain: Treatment approaches. In W. L. Smith, H. Merskey, & S. C. Gross (Eds.), *Pain: Meaning and management.* Lancaster: MTP Press, 1980.

Howarth, R. The psychiatric care of children with life-threatening illnesses. In L. Burton (Ed.), *Care of the child facing death.* London: Routledge & Kegan Paul, 1974.

Hughes, M. C., & Zimin, R. Children with psychogenic abdominal pain and their families. *Clinical Pediatrics,* 1978, **17,** 569–573.

Huskisson, E. C. Measurement of pain. *Lancet,* 1974, **2,** 1127–1131.

Illingworth, R. S. *Common symptoms of disease in children.* Oxford: Blackwell, 1967.

Laaksonen, A. L., & Laine, V. A comparative study of joint pain in adult and juvenile rheumatoid arthritis. *Annals of the Rheumatic Diseases,* 1961, **20,** 386–387.

Long, R. T., & Cope, O. Emotional problems of burned children. *New England Journal of Medicine,* 1961, **264,** 1121–1127.

MacKeith, R., & O'Neill, D. Recurrent abdominal pain in children. *Lancet,* 1951, **2,** 278–282.

Mechanic, D. The influence of mothers on their children's health attitudes and behaviour. *Pediatrics,* 1964, **33,** 444–453.

Melzack, R. *The puzzle of pain.* Harmondsworth: Penguin, 1973.

Melzack, R. The McGill pain questionnaire: Major properties and scoring methods. *Pain,* 1975, **1,** 277–299.

Melzack, R., & Casey, K. L. Sensory, motivational and central control determinants of pain: A new conceptual model. In D. Kenshala (Ed.), *The skin senses*. Springfield, Ill.: Charles C. Thomas, 1968.

Melzack, R., & Wall, P. D. Pain mechanisms: A new theory. *Science,* 1965, **150,** 971–979.

Melzack, R., Weisz, A. Z., & Sprague, L. T. Strategems for controlling pain: Contributions of auditory stimulation and suggestion. *Experimental Neurology,* 1963, **8,** 239–247.

Mennie, A. T. The child in pain. In L. Burton (Ed.), *Care of the child facing death*. London: Routledge & Kegan Paul, 1974.

Nagy, M. H. The child's view of death. In H. Feifel (Ed.), *The meaning of death*. New York: McGraw-Hill, 1959.

Oster, J. Recurrent abdominal pain, headache and limb pains in children and adolescents. *Pediatrics,* 1972, **50,** 429–436.

Oster, J., & Nielsen, A. Growing pains: A clinical investigation of a school population. *Acta Paediatrica Scandinavica,* 1972, **61,** 329–334.

Pavlov, I. P. *Conditioned reflexes*. Oxford: Milford, 1927.

Pavlov, I. P. *Lectures on conditioned reflexes*. New York: International Publishers, 1928.

Piaget, J. *The child's conception of physical causality*. London: Kegan Paul, 1930.

Poznanski, E. A. Children's reactions to pain: A psychiatrist's perspective. *Clinical Pediatrics,* 1976, **15,** 1114–1119.

Scott, P. J., Ansell, B. M., & Huskisson, E. C. Measurement of pain in juvenile chronic arthritis. *Annals of the Rheumatic Diseases,* 1977, **36,** 186–187.

Stone, R. T., & Barbero, G. J. Recurrent abdominal pain in childhood. *Pediatrics,* 1970, **45,** 732–738.

Swafford, L. I., & Allan, D. Pain relief in the pediatric patient. *Medical Clinics of North America,* 1968, **52,** 131–136.

Tropauer, A., Franz, M. N., & Dilgard, V. W. Psychological aspects of the care of children with cystic fibrosis. *American Journal of Diseases in Children,* 1970, **119,** 424–432.

Wall, P. D. On the relation of injury to pain. *Pain,* 1979, **6,** 253–264.

Whitt, J. K., Dykstra, W., & Taylor, C. A. Children's conceptions of illness and cognitive development. *Clinical Pediatrics,* 1979, **18,** 327–339.

Wyllie, W. G., & Schlesinger, B. The periodic group of disorders in childhood. *British Journal of Children's Diseases,* 1933, **30,** 1-21.

Zborowski, M. *People in pain*. San Francisco: Jossey-Bass, 1969.

8

Behavioral and Cardiovascular Activity During Interactions Between "High-Risk" Infants and Adults

Tiffany Field

Just as there are both harmonious and disturbed interactions between adults (Chapple, 1970), there appear to be harmonious and disturbed interactions between adults and infants (Field, 1977a, 1979b). Just as adults report that some interactions "turn them on" or "make their heart race" or "blood pressure rise," these effects can also be noted for infants during early interactions. Research on the reciprocal effects of adult and infant interaction behaviors has a fairly recent history (Bell, 1968; Lewis & Rosenblum, 1974). Research on cardiovascular correlates of these interaction behaviors has an even more recent history (Field, 1979b,c; Field, Sostek, Vietze, & Leiderman, 1980). While both the parent and infant may affect each other's behaviors during early interactions, their mutual influences may be particularly dramatic for the high-risk infant and parent. (Infants referred to as high-risk in this chapter include those who have experienced "reproductive casualties," such as the perinatal complications of preterm delivery and repiratory distress syndrome, or "caretaking casualties" such as being born to a low-income, teenage mother.)

Two commonly noted disturbances of interactions between adults have been termed "latency to respond" and "interrupting." In addition to the many anecdotal observations of these adult interaction disturbances, the stresses associated with these have been demonstrated in laboratory manipulations by Chapple (1970). In one experimental manipulation, the experimenter remained silent, unresponsive, or slow to respond, which was increasingly stressful for

*I would like to thank the infants and mothers who participated in these studies and the research assistants who assisted with data collection. This research was aided by a social and behavioral sciences research grant from the National Foundation–March of Dimes and by grants from the Administration of Children, Youth, and Families, HEW, OHD 0090C1-764-01 and 90-C-1964(2).

the subject, who continued to make initiations to the experimenter without response and ultimately became inactive. In another manipulation, the experimenter continued to make initiations to the subject without letting the subject "get a word in edgewise," an equally stressful situation for the adult subject that also eventuated in inactivity.

Similar manipulations have been tried with infants and mothers. A number of researchers have manipulated early interactions in various ways such as asking the mother to remain still or stone-faced (Fogel, Diamond, Langhorst, & Demos, 1979; Trevarthen, 1975; Tronick, Als, Adamson, Wise, & Brazelton, 1978). As in the nonresponsive-experimenter condition of the adult study by Chapple (1970), the infants were stressed by a nonresponsive partner, as evidenced by excessive gaze aversion and fussing. The mother, like the "slow to respond" experimenter in Chapple's study, was probably equally as stressed. Similarly, some have presented a "nonstop stimulating" mother to the infant by merely asking her to "keep her infant's attention" (Callaghan, 1980; Field, 1977a). The mother in this situation no longer attends to her infant's gaze signals and "interrupts" the activity of the infant, eventuating in infant gaze aversion and nonresponsivity.

Experiments in nature, or naturalistic observations of high-risk-infant–mother dyads and high-risk-mother–infant dyads suggest that these types of interactions occur naturally with some frequency. For example, mothers of preterm infants have been noted to be extremely active or controlling and their infants verbally inactive and gaze-averting during early interactions (Brown & Bakeman, 1979; DiVitto & Goldberg, 1979; Field, 1977a, 1979b; Goldberg, Brachfeld, & DiVitto, 1980). These interactions simulate the "interrupting" experimenter situation of Chapple (1970). Conversely, lower-class mothers have been observed to be extremely inactive (or slow to respond, as in the Chapple situation of latent responding) and their infants verbally inactive and gaze-averting during early interactions (Bee, VanEgeren, Striessguth, Nyman, & Lockie, 1969; Field, 1980b; Field, Widmayer, Stringer, & Ignatoff, in press; Tulkin & Kagan, 1972). During these interactions there appears to be not only a relationship between the observable behaviors of the mother and infant but also parallels between unobservable but measurable physiological responses, i.e., elevated heart rate and blood pressure levels, of both mothers and infants (Field, 1979b,c; Field et al., 1980), which suggests some aggregation or concordance of maternal-infant interaction style, blood pressure, and heart rate during these early interactions.

The objective of this chapter is to discuss the suggested relationships between maternal and infant behavior and cardiovascular activity during early interactions, the continuity of these relationships over early infancy, and the manipulability of infant activity level and cardiovascular activity through the alteration of maternal activity. A number of studies suggest that the development of infant behavior, heart rate, and blood pressure may be affected by the mother's behavior. Low or high levels of maternal activity during early interactions are associated with less optimal behavior of the infant (such as nonresponsivity, gaze aversion, and fussiness) and with elevated heart rate and blood pressure levels.

CONTINUITY OF INTERACTION BEHAVIORS

The importance of early social interactions has been highlighted recently by longitudinal studies of infants that suggest continuities between early interaction patterns and later social and language development (Beckwith, Sigman, Cohen, & Parmelee, 1977; Clarke-Stewart, 1973; Field, 1979b; Jones, 1980; Pawlby & Hall, 1980). In addition to suggesting continuity, these studies provide a developing picture of normative and disturbed interaction patterns. In contrast to studies of social development, longitudinal studies of the continuity or stability of heart rate and blood pressure from early infancy to early childhood have not been conducted. However, infant heart rate and blood pressure levels appear to stabilize and approximate childhood levels sometime during the first year of life (Levine, Hennekens, Gourley, Cassady, Klein, Briese, Jesse, & Gelband, 1978a: Lewis, Wilson, & Ban, 1970; Lipton, Steinschneider, & Richmond, 1966).

In most of the prospective studies of high-risk infants it is still too soon to determine whether interaction differences predict later interaction or developmental differences. Nonetheless, a number of recent studies suggest that the differences seen in high-risk infant interactions are not confined to the neonatal or early infancy periods.

Follow-up studies of preterm infants, for example, suggest that those who show interaction disturbances early in infancy experience difficulties later in infancy. In one longitudinal study, infants performing at lower levels on sensorimotor assessments at nine months had experienced less mutual gazing at one month and fewer interchanges of smiling during gazing and less contingent responses to distress at three months, as well as less general attentiveness and contingent responses to nondistress vocalizations at eight months (Beckwith, Cohen, Kopp, Parmelee, & Marcy, 1976). In the two-year longitudinal follow-up of this group of preterm infants, the best predictor of developmental status at two years was the pattern of interaction observed during the first few months (Sigman, 1980). Similarly, Bakeman (1978) reports that interactions as early as three months are significantly correlated with teacher ratings of peer interactions as late as three years.

Our data suggest that the mothers who were more active and less sensitive to their infants' gaze signals at four months issued more imperatives and were overprotective or controlling during interactions at two years. The preterm infants of these mothers showed more gaze averting and fussiness at four

months and manifested behavioral problems such as hyperactivity, short attention span, and language production delays at two (Field, 1979b) and three years
(Field, Dempsey, & Shuman, 1979). For other high-risk infants Jones (1980),
reporting on Down's syndrome infants, and Kogan (1980), reporting on cerebral palsied children, suggest similar continuities.

For lower-class children (Clarke-Stewart, 1973), continuities between early
interactions and later development have also been observed. Dunn (1977) has
suggested that mothers' speech to the infants at 13 months is positively associated with the children's IQ scores on the Stanford-Binet at four and a half
years. Further, Pawlby and Hall (1980) have reported significant correlations
between the frequency of early interactions between lower-class mothers and
infants and the three-year language and speech development of the infants.
Thus there is some disconcerting evidence for continuity between early interaction disturbances and later developmental delays.

CONTINUITY OF HEART RATE
AND BLOOD PRESSURE MEASURES

Although longitudinal studies on heart rate and blood pressure are only
currently in progress, some have suggested a moderate stability of mean heart
rate levels through at least the first year (Lewis et al., 1970; Lipton et al., 1966).
Similarly, some stability has been noted for the development of blood pressure
in infants and young children (Field et al., 1980; Field & Widmayer, 1980;
Hennekens, Jesse, Klein, Gourley, & Blumenthal, 1976; Jesse, Hokanson,
Klein, Levine, & Gourley, 1976; Klein, 1979; Levine, Hennekens, Klein, Gourley, Briese, Hokanson, Gelband, & Jesse, 1978b). These and other investigators
have studied blood pressure levels over time in infants and young children and
have described relationships between blood pressure levels in infants and their
siblings and between parents and both natural and adopted children. The
findings suggest the importance of both environmental and genetic effects on
the determination of blood pressure during early infancy, an observation that is
consistent with studies of older children and adults.

A small but significant correlation has recently been reported for mother-
neonatal blood pressures (Lee, Rosner, Gould, Lowe, & Kass, 1976). Data
from our own lab also suggest correlations of mother-neonatal blood pressures, but only for hypertensive mother-infant pairs (Field & Widmayer,
1979a). However, another investigation reported that the mean level blood
pressures of slightly older infants of pre-eclamptic and chronically hypertensive mothers were nearly identical to levels of infants of normotensive mothers
(Klein, Hennekens, Jesse, Gourley, & Blumenthal, 1975). A longitudinal follow-up by the same group (Levine, Hennekens, Gourley, Cassady, Klein,
Briese, Jesse, & Gelband, 1978) suggested no relationship between mother and

infant blood pressures during the first year of life. Beyond the first year of life another group showed significant correlations between blood pressures of parents and their biological children, but no correlation between parents and children adopted as early as one year of age (Biron, Mongeau, & Bertrand, 1974). Some of the variability of these findings may derive from differences in methodology as well as intervening variables known to affect blood pressure readings such as gestational and chronological age, birth weight, and sleep-wake states of the infant at the time of the blood pressure readings (Lee et al., 1976).

Studies on familial aggregation of blood pressure that is, the tendency for individual family members to be similar to each other on the blood pressure measure, have also extended to young sibships. A study of siblings from 2 to 14 years of age reported sibling-sibling (sib-sib) and mother-child blood pressure correlations, with those of sib-sib being higher (Zinner, Levy, & Kass, 1971). Sib-sib correlations have also been reported when young infants' blood pressures are used (Klein, Jesse, Hennekens, Gourley, & Blumenthal, 1975). A comparison between the blood pressures of neonates and their siblings suggested that the variance between sibships was not significantly greater than the variance within sibships. However, when one-month-old readings were substituted for neonatal readings, a significant aggregation was noted. In addition, this group reported stronger correlations between readings of infants and full sibs than between infants and half sibs. The work of Hennekens et al. (1976) also suggests that sibling aggregation first occurs at one month. A study of monozygotic and dizygotic twin infants (Levine, Hennekens, Briese, Robertson, Cassady, Gourley, & Gelband, 1978c) suggests that significant genetic variance for systolic blood pressure can be detected at six months of age.

Taken together, these data suggest that there is evidence for aggregation of blood pressure beginning in infancy and that sibling aggregation may be detected at one month of age. However, since the first appearance of significant genetic variance appears to occur after the detection of significant familial (i.e., sibling) aggregation, there is also suggestive evidence that environmental influences on infant blood pressure may exert their strongest effects during the first months of life. This raises the possibility that the early environment mediated primarily by interactions between parents and infants may have some influence on the early development of infant blood pressure.

BEHAVIORAL AND CARDIOVASCULAR ACTIVITY DURING EARLY INTERACTIONS

In all of the interaction studies to be reviewed, behavioral measures were recorded on film or videotape for both infant and parent, and, occasionally, heart rate or blood pressure was simultaneously recorded. In some of the studies only contemporaneous developmental measures were reported, while in others follow-up data enabled an assessment of continuities between early interaction measures and later development. Since the data converge to suggest some consistent patterns, we are taking the liberty of generalizing about normal and disturbed (or optimal and nonoptimal) interactions and their heart rate and blood pressure correlates. Generalizations that can be made from the data are that the interactions of preterm-infant–mother dyads and lower-class mother-infant dyads are quantitatively and qualitatively less optimal or at least different from those of non-lower-class, non-preterm-infant–mother dyads. Quantitative differences include high levels of maternal activity in the case of mothers of preterm infants, low levels of activity in the case of lower-class mothers, and elevated heart rates and blood pressures in both groups of mothers. Simultaneously, low levels of responsivity, considerable gaze aversion, and fussiness and elevated blood pressure and heart rate characterize both sets of infants. Although there are also qualitative differences (Field, 1978, 1979a, 1980a), for example in contingent responsivity, sensitivity to each others' communication signals, game playing, and so on, these are more subtle, more difficult to quantify and analyze than the quantitative behavioral frequencies, proportions, and conditional probabilities, and therefore have not been as frequently analyzed together with heart rate and blood pressure. Thus the following discussion will focus on *quantitative* differences identified for these groups.

There are several quantitative differences that have been noted for infants experiencing different medical complications and for infants whose parents come from different cultures and income groups. For example, lower-class black infants tend to be gaze averters and verbally unresponsive (Field, Widmayer, et al., in press), while their mothers also tend to be hypoactive in all modes—facial, auditory, tactile, and vestibular (Field, 1980b; Kilbride, Johnson, & Streissguth, 1977; Sandler & Vietze, 1979). Mothers of preterm infants are typically hyperactive in all modes during interactions, while their infants, like the lower-income infants, are gaze averters and verbally unresponsive (Brown & Bakeman, 1979; Field, 1977a, 1977b, 1979b; Goldberg et al., 1980). Although the direction of effects is not clear, hyper- or hypoactivity of the mothers appears to contribute to unresponsiveness of the infants, since manipulations of maternal activity, for example, increasing or decreasing these low or high levels of maternal activity, leads to more verbal responsiveness and visual attentiveness of the infant, as well as reductions of heart rate and blood pressure levels in the infant (Field, 1979b, 1979c; Field, Sostek, et al., 1980).

A MODEL OF EARLY INTERACTIONS:
AN INVERTED *U* ACTIVITY CURVE

A model that can be borrowed from the arousal level, information processing, or performance literatures to characterize these effects is that of an inverted *U* function. Maternal hypoactivity and hyperactivity are at the extreme ends of the inverted U function, with infant behaviors such as attentiveness and vocalizations varying on the y axis as a function of the amount of maternal activity (Field, 1980a).

There is a long history of mapping performance on an inverted U-shaped function. The independent variables, depending on the theory, have included drive, anxiety, or arousal level (Fiske & Maddi, 1961; Spielberger, 1966). The theory predicts that at high levels of drive, anxiety, or arousal a subject's performance becomes disrupted due to overresponding, often to irrelevant cues. At low levels a low rate of behavior occurs, and hence a low level of appropriate responding.

More recently a number of authors have described a *discrepancy hypothesis* in terms of an inverted U function (Kagan, 1971; McCall, Kennedy, & Applebaum, 1977; McCall & McGhee, 1977; Schaffer, 1974). The discrepancy hypothesis states that an event that cannot be assimilated produces a state of arousal. A moderate level of arousal will produce attention. The level of arousal predicted under the discrepancy hypothesis is believed to follow an inverted U-shaped function, with low discrepancy producing rapid assimilation and rapid habituation and very discrepant events producing either little attention or negative affect.

In adopting this model for early interactions, we were proposing that minimal or excessive maternal activity (hypoactivity or hyperactivity) contributes to less optimal interaction, possibly as a function of its effects on infant arousal levels. Maternal behaviors commonly reported as frequencies, durations, or proportions of interaction time (including talking, smiling, exaggerated facial expressions, head nodding, tapping, poking, caretaking, and game playing) can be plotted on the x axis. The frequently reported infant behaviors (including looking, vocalizing, smiling, cycling, squirming, and fussing) can be plotted on the y axis. Typically the quantity of positive infant behavior varies from high to low as the quantity of maternal behavior varies from moderate to the extremes of high or low. This relationship can be described as an inverted U function, plotting optimality of interaction or, more specifically, plotting commonly recorded infant behaviors such as gaze activity or vocalizations on the y axis. An illustration of the proposed relationship appears in figure 8.1.

Interaction Manipulations Supporting an Inverted U Activity Curve

Although mother and infant activity are simultaneous, reciprocal phenomena, rendering any statement about direction of effects mere speculation, interventions have focused on the easiest-to-teach partner, the mother. Experimental

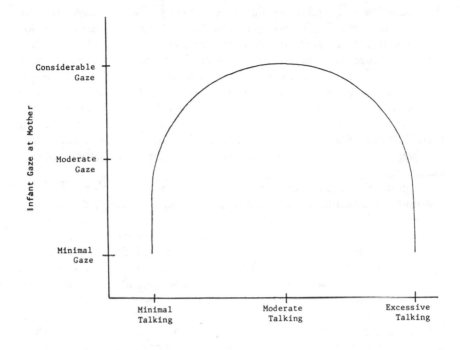

Fig. 8.1.   Proposed relationship between maternal talking and infant gazing at mother.

manipulations illustrate that interactions can be varied by altering the mother's activity level.

One manipulation that altered maternal activity involved changing the mother's visual stimulus (Trevarthen, 1975). Mothers began interacting with their infants, but suddenly were face to face with an adult appearing in a one-way mirror. The mothers altered the rate and pacing of their talking from the typically slow pace reserved for infants to more adult-paced verbal activity. This manipulation resulted in infant gaze aversion. Asking the mother to remain stone-faced in another manipulation invariably resulted first in active attempts by the infant to engage the mother, followed by waning interest and ultimate gaze aversion of the infant (Fogel et al., 1979; Tronick et al., 1978). A manipulation that had an opposite effect, namely that it increased infant gaze, involved asking the mother to "count slowly" while interacting (Tronick et al., 1978). This instruction effectively slowed down and diminished the activity of the mothers and enhanced infant attentiveness.

A series of manipulations that have been tried in our laboratory (Field, 1977a, 1979b, 1979c) was generally effective in modifying the amount of both the mother's activity and the infant's attentiveness and vocalization. An attention-getting manipulation, asking the mother to keep her infant's attention, dramatically increased the amount of her activity and decreased the amount of her infant's gaze and contented vocalizations. Conversely, asking the mother to imitate her infant's behavior effectively diminished maternal activity and elicited more infant gaze. An order effect, when using these two manipulations during the same session, suggested that mothers who were given the imitation instruction first learned that it was an effective attention-getting device and used it during the attention-getting situation. Thus the manipulations revealed an inverse relationship between maternal activity and infant attentiveness or gaze.

Other manipulations, including the mother's repetition of her phrases and the mother's silence during her infant's gaze aversion, also resulted in decreased maternal activity and increased infant attentiveness (Field, 1979b, 1979c). Similarly, during a feeding manipulation in which the mother was asked to remain silent during her infant's sucking periods, the infant also spent more time looking at her. These manipulations, however, were only effective in those dyads whose spontaneous interactions featured considerable maternal activity and infant inattentiveness, e.g., those of preterm infants and their mothers.

In the case of hypoactive mothers, e.g., lower-class mothers, we have manipulated activity level of the mother by simply giving her a nursery rhyme song to sing or teaching her a wordy version of some popular infant game such as "Tell me a story," "I'm gonna get you," "So big," "Itsy bitsy spider," "Peek-a-boo," or "Pat-a-cake" (Field, 1978, 1979a). Typically these mothers' verbal, tactile, and facial activity increased with these songs or games, and the infants' attentiveness and contented vocalizations correspondingly increased (Field, Sostek, et al., 1980).

The most observable, measurable effect of these manipulations is the variation in frequency of maternal and infant behaviors. An attention-getting instruction invariably elicits very high activity levels in the mother and very low activity and attentiveness or nonoptimal activity, such as gaze averting or fussing, in the infant. The extreme of that, the stone-faced, inactive mother, also elicits inattentiveness in the infant. If the mother's activity level tends to be high, an imitative instruction seems to lower her activity to a moderate level, and if her activity level is low, then giving her an infant game to play or song to sing facilitates a more moderate level of activity. In both cases, the infant engages in a greater amount of visual attentiveness and contented vocalizations. These manipulations of maternal activity and their effects on infant attentiveness can be superimposed on an inverted U curve, as in figure 8.2.

Cardiac Activity Data Supporting a Curvilinear Model

In the context of the arousal or activation model (Fiske & Maddi, 1961; Hebb, 1949), high or low levels of stimulation are considered to be arousing. High

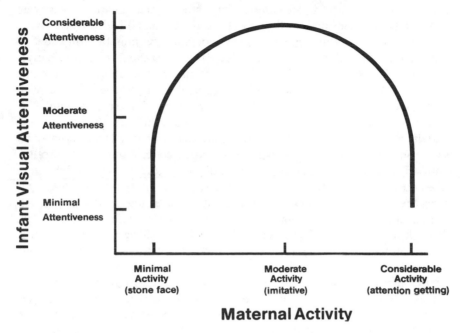

Fig. 8.2. Relationship between manipulated activity level of mothers during stone-face, imitative, and attention-getting interactions and infant visual attentiveness.

arousal levels in either an over- or underarousing situation are thought to be experienced as aversive. In an aversive situation we might expect to find elevated heart rate and elevated blood pressure (Frodi, Lamb, Leavitt, & Donovan, 1978; Frodi, Lamb, Leavitt, Donovan, Neff, & Sherry, 1978; Green, Stonner & Shope, 1975; Schachter, 1957).

In mother-infant interactions characterized by high activity level of the mother and low activity and gaze aversion of the infant, the arousal model would predict elevated heart rate, since the mother appears aroused and the infant shows considerable gaze aversion. To assess the physiological correlates of the already described interaction manipulations we simultaneously monitored heart rate activity. Since the mothers' and infants' behaviors occur with such rapidity during interactions that heart rate does not have sufficient time to return to baseline for a second-by-second analysis of heart rate, we used tonic heart rate or heart rate averaged across the interaction as compared to baseline heart rate.

The stone-faced manipulation of Tronick et al. (1978) and our attention-getting and imitative manipulations were used. Tonic heart rate of both the mother and infant paralleled their behaviors. In the case of the less active, imitative mother and more attentive infant interaction, heart rate was slightly below baseline heart rate levels for mothers and infants. And in the high-activity, attention-getting and low-activity, stone-faced situation, heart rate was significantly elevated for both mothers and infants (Field, 1979b).

Certainly the mothers' greater attentiveness during imitation (in order to observe the infants' behaviors to be imitated) and the infants' greater attentiveness in this situation (possibly due to the infants' greater ability to assimilate stimulus behaviors already in their own repertoires) may have contributed to more frequent decelerations, a heart rate parallel of attention (Graham & Clifton, 1966). Conversely, the higher activity level during attention-getting and the physical or emotional strain of remaining stone-faced in the no-activity situation may have contributed to heart rate accelerations of the mother. Similarly, the infant's head aversion, squirming, and fussing during those situations would elevate infant heart rate as a function of physical movement, such that heart rate would be artifactually elevated due to movement. Alternatively, or at the same time, the mother's overstimulation may have been difficult to assimilate or process and thus highly arousing or aversive for the infant, as reflected by the infant's frequent gaze aversion and elevated tonic heart rate. An infant behavioral-cardiac relationship has also been noted by Sroufe and his colleagues in stranger-approach situations (Sroufe, Waters, & Matas, 1974; Waters, Matas, & Sroufe, 1975). In turn, the infant's gaze aversion, squirming, and fussing may have been aversive for the mother, contributing to her elevated heart rate levels.

While videotapes of smiling and cooing infants have been shown to trigger only negligible changes in autonomic arousal of mothers (and fathers, but not the parents of the particular infants videotaped), videotapes of gaze-averting, fussy infants are perceived as aversive and elicit elevated heart rate and diastolic blood pressures and skin conductance increases in mothers and fathers (Frodi, Lamb, Leavitt, & Donovan, 1978). These increases were especially apparent when the infant being viewed was described as "premature" (Frodi, Lamb, Leavitt, Donovan, Neff, & Sherry, 1978). Unfortunately, Frodi and her colleagues observed these cardiac responses in mothers and fathers who were not parents of the videotaped infants and then did not simultaneously observe the behavioral responses of the parents. The picture is further confounded by the finding of cardiac deceleration responses to infant cries in the same situation with another sample (Donovan, Leavitt, & Balling, 1978) and the finding that cardiac deceleration characterized parents' responses to the cries of unfamiliar infants while cardiac acceleration occurred in response to the cry of the parents' own infant (Wiesenfeld & Klorman, 1978). Whether the heart rate elevations during our manipulations were a function of increased motor activity or increased arousal associated with the mutual aversiveness of maternal overstimulation and infant inattentiveness, they are suggestive of increased arousal in both mother and infant. If elevated heart rate and gaze aversion covary only when the system is highly aroused, as suggested by Lewis et al. (Lewis, Brooks, & Haviland, 1978), then it would appear that the infant at least was highly aroused during our manipulations. In any case, the heart rate levels measured in our study appear to conform to a curvilinear relationship or the U curve depicted in figure 8.3.

A comparison of preterm and term infant-mother dyads experiencing these manipulations revealed not only greater activity on the part of the mothers of preterm infants and greater gaze aversion on the part of the preterm infants (see figure 8.4), but also characteristically higher heart rate levels of both preterm infants and their mothers, despite equivalent baseline levels of the term and preterm dyads (Field, 1979b) (figures 8.5 and 8.6).

An interesting phenomenon emerging from these data was a parallel in infant and mother heart rate. As can be seen in figures 8.5 and 8.6, the directional heart rate change curves of the preterm infants and their mothers across interaction situations are parallel, as are those of term infants and their mothers.

A follow-up study was conducted with term and preterm infants to further investigate relationships between activity level of mother or amount of stimulation provided for the infant and the infant's behavioral and cardiac responses.

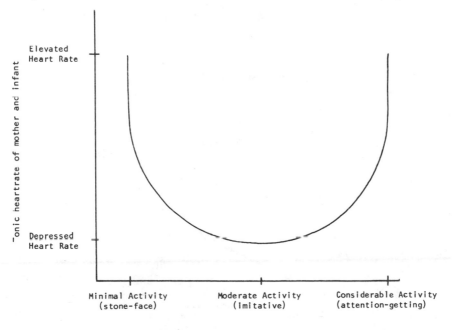

Fig. 8.3. Relationship between manipulations of maternal activity and mother and infant tonic heart rate.

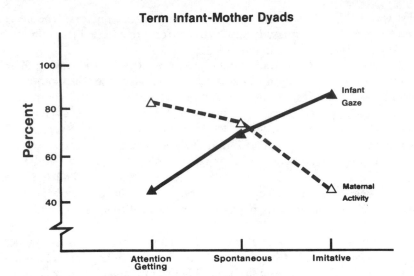

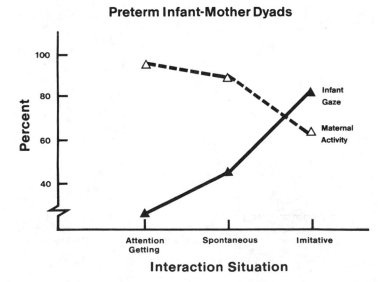

Fig. 8.4.   Inverse relationship between maternal activity and infant gaze in the term and preterm groups during attention-getting, spontaneous, and imitation interaction situations.

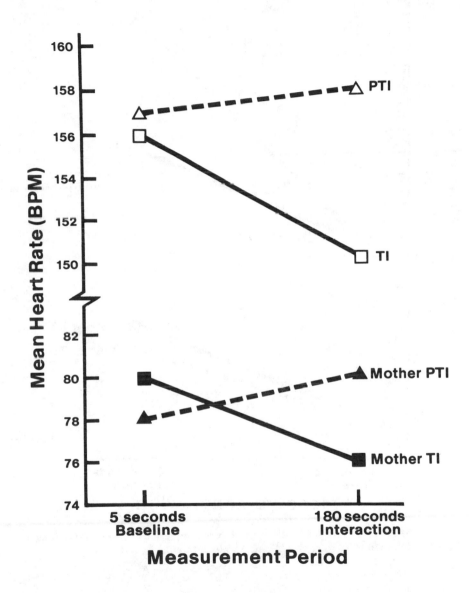

Fig. 8.5.   Mean heart rate for baseline and interaction periods of imitation situation
(PTI = preterm infant, TI = term infant).

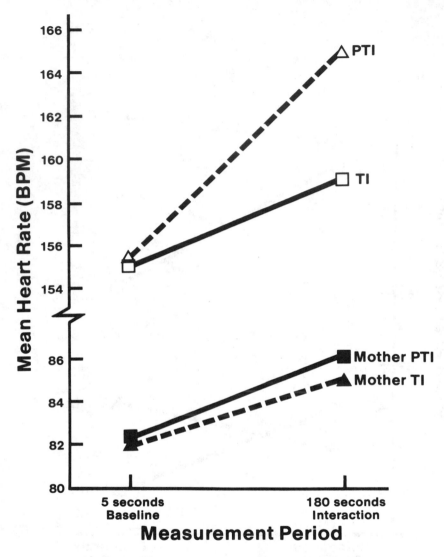

Fig. 8.6.   Mean heart rate for baseline and interaction periods of attention-getting situation (PTI = preterm infant, TI = term infant).

In this study both a live stimulus (the mother) and an inanimate stimulus (a Raggedy Ann doll) were used (Field, 1979c). Animation or activity level of these stimuli was altered; that is, for the more animated interaction situation the mother was invited to act spontaneously or naturally and for the less animated interaction situation she was asked to be imitative, since our previous work had suggested that her activity level would be lower in the imitative situation. For the more animated Raggedy Ann doll situation the head of the upright, suspended doll was automatically nodded and a tape recorded voice emanating from the direction of the doll slowly repeated the phrase, "Hi there, baby, how are you?" For the less animated Raggedy Ann doll situation, the doll (upright and suspended) remained silent and immobile. Thus, in increasing order of animation the faces were an inanimate and animate Raggedy Ann doll, a less animated and more animated mother. The looking data for the term and preterm infants can be seen in figure 8.7 and the heart rate data in figure 8.8.

As can be seen in these figures, looking levels were higher and heart rate levels lower for the less animated situations, and differences between term and preterm infants were only apparent during the mother situations. These data suggest either that the preterm infants are less able to process the information provided by more animate stimulation or to modulate arousal associated with animate stimulation, or that their mothers (who were more active than mothers of term infants) may be providing a stimulus overload or aversively high levels of stimulation that contributes to the infants' decreased looking and increased

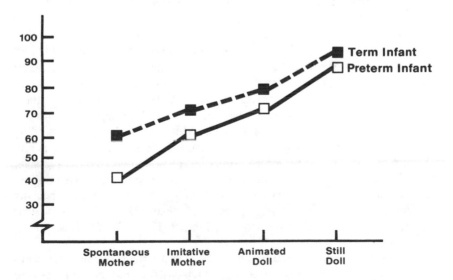

Fig. 8.7.   Percent of time that term and preterm infants engaged in looking during various animated and inanimate face situations.

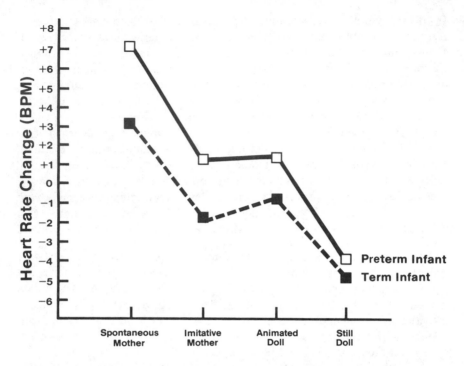

Fig. 8.8. Term and preterm infants' mean heart rate change (bpm) from baseline activity in response to the various animated and inanimate situations.

heart rate. Again, when the mother is invited to slow down (by imitation direction), infant looking (at mother) increases and heart rate levels are lower.

A small number of studies have incorporated the use of blood pressure as an index of physiological responsivity during early interactions. Frodi, Lamb, Leavitt, and Donovan (1978) showed mothers and fathers videotapes of term and preterm infants in situations where infants were smiling and situations where they were gaze-averting and fussy. While the videotapes of smiling infants triggered only negligible changes in autonomic arousal of mothers and fathers, videotapes of gaze-averting, fussy infants were perceived as aversive, and elicited elevated heart rate and diastolic blood pressures and skin conductance increases in the mothers and fathers. These increases were especially apparent when the infant being viewed by the mothers and fathers was described as "premature" (Frodi, Lamb, Leavitt, Donovan, Neff, & Sherry, 1978).

In our lab we have included blood pressure measurements during interaction observations of hypertensive, lower-class black mothers and their infants who were delivered by C-section. While activity levels, blood pressures, and anxiety scores of the hypertensive mothers were higher than those of the control group mothers, their infants were more responsive and showed lower blood pressure levels. The mothers' higher blood pressure levels may have been associated with greater amounts of physical activity during interaction (although they were not hyperactive like mothers of preterm infants, they also were not hypoactive, as many of the lower-class black control mothers were). Elevated maternal blood pressures may also have been associated with the higher state anxiety (Spielberger, 1966) scores of these women, or the anxiety over the surgical delivery of their infants (which appears to constitute a crisis for lower-class black women; cf. Field & Widmayer, 1980). The greater responsivity and lower blood pressure levels of their infants may have been related to the fact that they received more optimal stimulation (their mothers being neither hyperactive nor hypoactive, but more active than the hypoactive control mothers). In any case the greater responsivity and lower blood pressure levels fit with our proposed model: that moderate levels of maternal activity are paralleled by more optimal levels of infant responsivity and cardiovascular activity, possibly mediated by more optimal modulation of arousal.

A similar set of results was derived from a study in which we provided interaction coaching (manipulation of maternal activity levels) for lower-class black teenage mothers who were normotensive and their infants. While these typically hypoactive mothers became more active during the interaction coaching sessions, their state anxiety scores and blood pressure levels increased. At the same time, their infants became more responsive and blood pressure levels decreased (Field, Sostek, et al., 1980). While the effects on the infants would appear to be optimal, since the infants' developmental scores and interaction performance nine months later (at one year) were more optimal than those of the controls, we were concerned that a negative side effect of coaching lower-class mothers in "middle-class" interaction activity might be elevated state anxiety and blood pressure of the mother. These elevated levels noted at four months, however, were no longer observed at one year. The changes in these measures over time may have related to assessment situation differences between the two periods; that is, the mothers being instructed on interaction activity and then filmed when their infants were four months old were undoubtedly "uptight" about being instructed and filmed. Although we have noted lesser effects of videotaping on lower-class than on middle-class mothers when videotaping situations are compared to one-way mirror situations, there is nonetheless a resultant increase in maternal activity (Field & Ignatoff, 1980). The elevated cardiovascular activity levels may have been very temporary, relating to motor activity. Although recording of heart rate and blood pressure during interactions provides additional information on the state and arousal levels of the interactants, those measures are invariably affected by simple motor activity. Finally, in addition to considerable variability across mother-infant dyads, which cannot be overemphasized in the interpretation of group data, there may be considerable variability of cardiovascular activity levels over time. In the absence of longitudinal studies, the stability of behavioral and cardiovascular activity levels is unknown.

Spontaneous Interaction Data Supporting an Inverted U Activity Curve

Analogues of the previously described manipulated interactions are provided by "experiments in nature" or the more spontaneous, naturalistic interactions of high-risk-infant–mother dyads and high-risk-mother–infant dyads. The high-risk-infant–mother dyads, preterm infants and their mothers, are typically a hypoactive-infant–hyperactive-mother pair, each manifesting elevated heart rate and blood pressure levels during interactions. The high-risk-mother–infant dyads, lower-class mothers and their infants, are frequently hypoactive, but also manifest elevated heart rate and blood pressure levels during interactions.

Interactions of high-risk-mother–infant dyads. Among those infants who have been designated as being at risk for interaction problems because of high-risk mothers are those born to adolescent, less-educated, or lower-class mothers. In addition, some have viewed multiple-birth infants (e.g., twins) and later-born infants as having potential interaction problems. Frequently these infants are unresponsive, and their mothers are often hypoactive or hyporesponsive.

A study comparing the interactions of white middle-class and black lower-class adult and teenage mothers and their infants revealed a very low level of activity on the part of the teenage mothers (Field, 1980b). Teenage mothers were less active, less verbal, and less contingently responsive, and played "infant" games less frequently. This was observed for both white middle-class teenage mothers whose infants at birth received optimal interaction scores on the Brazelton Neonatal Scale (for responses to animate and inanimate stimulation) and for black lower-class teenage mothers whose infants were more developed motorically (based on the Brazelton motor items at birth and the Denver motor items at three months). Thus, without respect to their infants' initial social responsivity and initial (as well as contemporaneous) motor development, the teenage mothers were relatively inactive. Although these infants were not "difficult" neonates, by three or four months of age they engaged in less eye contact and emitted fewer contented vocalizations. Another study of lower-class black teenage mothers and their neonates suggested that during mother-neonate feeding interactions the teenage mothers were less verbal (Sandler & Vietze, 1979).

Social class comparisons of early interactions have frequently revealed that both lower-class infants and their mothers are less active, particularly verbally, than their middle-class counterparts. As early as the first month of life, lower-class infants received significantly less verbal stimulation from their mothers in both a lulling and chatting fashion, and their mothers cared for them without talking to them (Kilbride et al., 1977). Similarly, studies of older infants reveal less activity among lower-class mothers and infants than middle-class dyads. Lewis, Wilson, and Ban (1970) reported less smiling and vocalizing among the lower class infants and less contingent mother vocalization. In addition, Field (1980b) reported less activity, verbal interaction, and contingent responsivity and less frequent playing of infant games among lower-class black mothers than among middle-class white mothers.

A cross-cultural study comparing British working- and middle-class mothers with American lower- and middle-class mothers suggested that both in England and the United States the lower-class mothers engaged in less verbal and imitative behavior and less game playing during early face-to-face interactions (Field & Pawlby, 1980). Their infants were simultaneously less verbal, smiled less frequently, and engaged in less eye contact. Interactions of slightly older infants (ten months old) and their lower-class mothers also featured less verbal activity and fewer reciprocal vocalizations (Bee et al., 1969; Tulkin & Kagan, 1972). Similarly, less educated mothers are reported to talk less frequently, respond with less contingent vocalizations, and give less specific communications when engaging in face-to-face talk with both their one- and eight-month-old infants (Cohen & Beckwith, 1976).

Two other groups reported to receive either less eye contact or less verbal stimulation include multiple-birth infants (twins) and higher-birth-order infants. A few investigators have reported differential behavior on the part of mothers and their two twins. Stern (1971), for example, reported less maternal eye contact with one twin who later exhibited behavioral problems. Kubicek (1980) also reported less eye contact between one twin and his mother; in this case the twin experiencing less eye contact was later diagnosed as autistic. A study of monozygotic twins and their mothers by our group suggests that the mother is typically less active with the second-born twin (Field, Walden, Widmayer, & Greenberg, 1982). However, in the case of prematurely born twins or twins discrepant on birth weight, the mother was typically overactive with the twin who had the lower birth weight or who experienced the most perinatal complications. This was primarily noted in backward probability analyses, wherein the mothers' behaviors were analyzed as a function of the antecedent behaviors of the infants. In the case of the less developed or more fragile twin, the mother responded to weak signals, e.g., she vocalized to a half-turn of the infant's head toward herself as opposed to her typically waiting for a full head turn and eye contact of the stronger twin before talking. Thus she always appeared to be "jumping the gun" with the fragile twin, leaving him very little space to fully respond or emit a behavior prior to her ("interrupting") response.

The factors contributing to lesser maternal activity and stimulation in these groups is unclear. In some of the studies, neonatal assessments as well as developmental assessments made at the same time as the interaction assessments of these infants (e.g., Field, 1980b) revealed no particular lags in development or interactive deficits that might contribute to the less responsivity of their mothers. The mother's condition itself, for example, depressed socioeconomic status or multiple children to care for, may leave the mother with less time and energy for interaction. Many of these mothers appeared "depressed" or had "flattened affect" during face-to-face interactions. This may be a manifestation of being "anxious" about being filmed (Field & Ignatoff, 1981) or may simply reflect that their face-to-face interaction "repertoire" is more limited since this is not their "typical style of interaction" with infants. In non-face-to-face interaction situations, for example, the lower-class mothers tended to "jostle" their infants or provide more vestibular stimulation. Their infants, accustomed to more rigorous, physical stimulation, may have developed higher thresholds to stimulation and thus may have been unresponsive when their mothers were more "subdued" and less active during face-to-face interactions. A similarly simple explanation for the lesser amount of activity of teenage and less-educated mothers may be a limited interaction repertoire due to less experience or exposure to infants, and less knowledge about appropriate infant stimulation. Whatever the cause, the low levels of face-to-face stimulation are disconcerting, given the reports that mothers of infants and children who were later diagnosed as schizophrenic or autistic engaged in less eye contact during early interactions (Massie, 1978) and that mothers of abused infants engaged in less verbal interactions with their infants (Dietrich & Starr, 1980).

Interactions of high-risk-infant–mother dyads. In terms of activity levels, the interactions of preterm infants and their mothers are frequently characterized by hypoactivity or hyporesponsivity of the infant and hyperactivity of the mother. In these dyads the infant is often described as being less active and responsive, and the mother as exerting more effort or appearing to try harder to engage her infant (Beckwith & Cohen, 1980; Brown & Bakeman, 1979; DiVitto & Goldberg, 1979; Field, 1977a,b, 1979b; Goldberg et al., 1980). Comparisons between term and preterm infants suggest the the preterm-infant–mother dyad experiences more difficulty interacting than the term-infant–mother dyad. For example, a study on early feedings of preterm and term infants revealed that the preterm infants were more distractible during feeding and their mothers less sensitive to infant feeding behaviors and rhythms (Field, 1977b). The mothers of preterm infants, unlike those of term infants, stimulated their infants continuously, failing to reserve their stimulation for the nonsucking periods when the infant was otherwise unoccupied and free to interact. Although some have suggested that sensitive mothers reserve stimulation for these periods (Kaye & Brazelton, 1971), the constant stimulation by the mothers of preterm infants may have reflected their attempts to organize their distractible infants and encourage milk ingestion. Their infants appeared to be less responsive and less organized in their feeding behavior, and elicited more coaxing or "stimulation to feed" behavior from their mothers. The increase in maternal stimulation in response to infant unresponsiveness, however, seemed to be counterproductive inasmuch as it appeared to enhance rather than diminish the infants' unresponsiveness.

Another study of feeding interactions of both term and preterm infants reported that the "more difficult to rouse" infants received a high level of functional stimulation during feedings, and those who were unresponsive to auditory stimulation received more auditory and tactile stimulaton during feedings (DiVitto & Goldberg, 1979). Mothers of the preterm infants were more active and invested more effort interacting with their infants with notably less success than parents of full-term infants.

Brown and Bakeman (1979) and Field (1980b) report similar findings. Unlike the samples of middle-class white mothers of the Field (1979b) and DiVitto and Goldberg (1979) studies, the Brown and Bakeman (1979) and Field (1980b) samples were comprised of lower-class black mothers and their preterm infants. Of the early feeding interactions, they reported that preterm infants (versus term infants) were less active and were viewed as less responsive. Mothers of the preterm infants were generally more active and, in particular, were more persistent and more likely to initiate and continue behavioral episodes than the lower-class black mothers of full term infants. They exerted more effort and their interactions were more stereotyped or less varied. As noted by Brown and Bakeman (1979), the burden of maintaining the interactions fell disproportionately on the mothers of the preterm infants.

Not unlike the feeding interactions, the face-to-face interactions of preterm infants during the first few months of life have also been characterized by hypoactive, hyporesponsive infants and hyperactive mothers (Field, 1977b, 1979b). In our studies of face-to-face interactions the preterm infants were less responsive and showed more aversive behaviors (gaze aversion, squirming, and fussing) and their mothers were more stimulating in all modes (visual, tactile, auditory, and vestibular) during both the infants' eye contact and gaze aversion periods. Similarly, the mothers of postterm infants, who also gaze-averted, squirmed, and fussed, were typically hyperactive or overstimulating. A follow-up of these infants at two years (Field, 1979b) suggested that the mothers who were overactive during early face-to-face interactions were overprotective and overcontrolling during later interactions with their infants. The infants who were visually inattentive during the early interactions were verbally unresponsive and showed language delays during the two-year interactions (Field, 1979b) and less developed language skills and behavior problems at three years (Field, Dempsey, & Shuman, 1979).

Floor play interactions of eight-month-old and one-year-old preterm infants and their parents studied by Goldberg et al. (1980) featured less playing and smiling and more fretting by the preterm infants. The parents of the preterm infants spent more time being close to, touching, and demonstrating toys to their infants than did parents of term infants. Similar observations of twelve-month floor play have been noted (Field, Sostek, et al., 1980).

The picture that emerges from these analyses of different types of interactions (feeding, face to face, and floor play) at different stages during the first two years of life among preterm infants and their parents is a vicious circle: the infant is relatively inactive and unresponsive and the parent tries to engage the infant by being more and more active or stimulating, which in turn leads to more inactivity and unresponsivity on the part of the infant. Although the parent's activity appears to be directed at encouraging more activity or responsivity of the infant, that strategy is counterproductive inasmuch as it leads to less instead of more infant responsivity.

Other groups for which similar phenomena have been observed include the Down's syndrome infant, the deaf infant, and the child with cerebral palsy. Analyses of interactions between Down's syndrome infants and their mothers suggest that the infants engaged in less eye contact and initiated fewer interactions (Jones, 1980) and smiled and vocalized less frequently than normal infants (Buckhalt, Rutherford, & Goldberg, 1978). Their mothers were simultaneously noted to be more active and directive during these play interactions (Jones, 1980) and talked at a faster rate (Buckhalt, Rutherford, & Goldberg, 1978). Similarly, deaf infants (Wedell-Monnig & Lumley, 1980) and cerebral palsied infants (Kogan, 1980) have been noted to exhibit fewer interactive behaviors, and their mothers are more active and controlling during interactions.

The above authors have speculated about the frequently observed hyperactivity of the mothers of unresponsive infants labeled "at risk" due to perinatal complications or handicapping conditions, or both. The vaguest interpretation suggests that the "frustration" of receiving minimal responses from the infant leads to a kind of "aggressivity" on the part of the mother. Berkowitz (1974) has suggested that aggressivity often occurs in an aroused person who is presented with an aversive stimulus or a stimulus perceived to be aversive. The relative unresponsiveness of the preterm infant, his relatively less developed repertoire of coos and smiles, his frequent gaze aversion and fussiness may be perceived as aversive by the mother, as might the often-noted "fragile" features of the preterm infant. In addition, the "difficult" temperaments of these infants (as evaluated by the parents; cf. Field, Hallock, Dempsey & Shuman, 1978) may have contributed to a parental perception of these infants as being somewhat aversive. All of these aversive factors may be generalized by the parents to even those situations when the infant is not displaying aversive behaviors such as gaze aversion or fussiness. Thus, infants viewed as aversive may simply elicit more aggressive behaviors from their parents. Another notion is that the mothers are more active to compensate for the relative inactivity of their infants, perhaps "to keep some semblance of an interaction going." A third interpretation posits that the mother wants her child to perform like his agemates and attempts to encourage performance by more frequent modeling of behaviors. Still another explanation offered is that the mothers view their infants as fragile and delayed and, as a result, tend to be overprotective. Overprotectiveness in the extreme is construed as overcontrolling behavior. Since these infants appear to be less responsive than their normal counterparts, parents may need to work harder at generating responses such as attention, smiles, and contented vocalizations. The problem relates to finding the optimal level of stimulation, since low levels do not seem to arouse or elicit responses from these infants while high levels eventuate in gaze aversion and fussiness. Because of the seemingly higher thresholds to stimulation noted in preterm infants (Field, Dempsey, Hatch, Ting, & Clifton, 1979), Down's syndrome infants (Cicchetti & Sroufe, 1978), and retarded infants (Kogan, 1980), the stimulation requirements may be greater for these infants than for normal infants. But since these infants are also more difficult to console once thresholds are exceeded (and fussing and crying ensues), the parent may be dealing with a more limited zone of optimal stimulation than are the parents of the normal infant. Although direction of effects or causality cannot be derived from these studies of early interactions, the data have evoked considerable concern, since the behaviors of these dyads appear to persist beyond the period of early interactions.

OTHER FACTORS THAT MAY AFFECT EARLY INTERACTION ACTIVITY, HEART RATE, AND BLOOD PRESSURE

Additional factors that may affect early measures of interaction activity, heart rate, and blood pressure in both mother and infant are maternal perceptions, attitudes, and anxiety and infant temperament. Therefore some of the literature pertaining to these factors will be discussed.

Theories of anxiety distinguish between state anxiety, which is relatively temporary and situational, and trait anxiety, which is a more or less permanent anxiety-proneness (Spielberger, 1966). Spielberger and his colleagues (Spielberger, Gorsuch, & Lushene, 1970) developed the State-Trait Anxiety Inventory (STAI) with separate subsections to measure state anxiety and trait anxiety. Anxiety has been generally viewed as a drive or motivation. For complex tasks, drive theory predicts an inverted U relationship between anxiety and performance, similar to that inverted U relationship already posited for maternal and infant activity level. At high levels of anxiety a subject's performance may become disrupted due to overresponding, often to irrelevant cues, leading to a high level of activity, much of which is irrelevant or inappropriate. At low levels of anxiety a low level of activity occurs, and thus a low number of appropriate behaviors. Although this relationship has not been assessed in early infant-mother interactions, it is probable that a high or low anxiety state of the mother may contribute to a high or low level of maternal activity, resulting in the disturbed interaction behaviors and elevated heart rate and blood pressure levels already discussed.

Data relevant to the question of maternal anxiety effects are: (1) higher state anxiety on the State-Trait Anxiety Inventory was accompanied by elevated blood pressure in the lower-class black teenage mothers in the interaction coaching study already discussed (Field et al., in press), and others have reported relationships between trait anxiety and blood pressure (Cattell & Scheier, 1958); (2) maternal anxiety may contribute to infant colic (Lakin, 1957), since highly anxious mothers have been noted to have more colicky babies than normal anxious mothers (Brown, 1961); (3) although we did not independently assess "depression" of these mothers, those "state anxiety" mothers appeared "depressed" during interactions with their infants.

Although direction of effects or even simple relationships between maternal anxiety-depression and infant measures such as gaze aversion or colic or between maternal anxiety-depression and infant temperament are unclear, there is increasing evidence that infant temperament is highly correlated with behavior during early interactions. In a number of studies by our group (Field, 1977a,b, 1979b; Field, Dempsey, Hallock, Shuman, 1978; Field et al., 1980) infant temperament, as perceived by the mothers, was highly related to inter-action behaviors such as fussiness and gaze aversion, with more of these behaviors and elevated heart rate appearing in those infants classified as having "difficult" temperaments. This relationship between temperament and interaction behavior persisted over the first year of life, and temperament ratings were an efficient predictor of later infant performance (Field, Dempsey, & Shuman, 1979).

It is not clear whether infant temperament was in fact more "difficult" or was merely a misperception of the mother, since all of the infant temperament studies to date have employed only parental perceptions as an index of infant temperament and have not compared those perceptions to ratings by independent observers. In addition, validity of parental perceptions may be highly variable. For example, we have noted fairly reliable and valid parental perceptions when comparing mother assessments of neonatal and infant behavior on the MABI (an adaptation of the Brazelton scale, 1973, for parents) with independent examiner ratings on the Brazelton (Field, Dempsey, Hallock, & Shuman, 1978). However, these results, based on a sample of white middle-class mothers, did not hold for samples of black lower-class mothers (Field, 1980b; Field et al., in press; Widmayer & Field, 1980).

An interesting phenomenon that emerged from the MABI data provided by lower-class black mothers was that they assigned optimal ratings to their infants on the motoric process items of the Brazelton at the neonatal stage, unlike the examiners' ratings of the same babies. As if in a self-fulfilling prophecy, the black lower-class infants at four months were motorically more developed. And their prevideotaping interactions, while reflecting less verbal, facial, and eye-contact activity, appeared more physical, as if these mothers valued different types of interaction behavior than did white middle-class mothers and had different attitudes toward or expectations for the interactions. Thus ethnic differences may contribute to early interaction activity differences as well as to developing heart rate and blood pressure differences. Just as the activity levels of lower-class black mothers and their infants are notably lower during early interactions, heart rate (Sameroff, Bakow, Mc-Comb, & Collins, 1978; Schachter, Kerr, Wimberly, & Lakin, 1974) and blood pressure levels (Field et al., in press) are notably more elevated in lower-class black infants.

Ethnic or cultural relativity of parent perceptions, attitudes, and activity during early interactions cannot be overlooked (Field, Sostek et al., 1981). Examples from American Indian (Callaghan, 1981; Chisholm, 1981; Fourcher & Freedman, 1981), African (Dixon, Keefer, Tronick, & Brazelton, 1981), South Pacific (Martini & Kirkpatrick, 1981; Zaslow, Sostek, Vietze, Kreiss, & Rubinstein, 1981) and British, which shares similar language and child-rearing patterns (Field & Pawlby, 1980), cultures suggest considerable variations in early interaction patterns across cultures.

Thus although the current measures we have for maternal anxiety-depression and infant temperament are somewhat subjective, there are some data suggestive of their predictive validity. In any case, since both maternal anxiety and infant temperament may interact with or independently affect early interaction activity level and cardiac measures, they should be closely monitored and assessed in a study of these relationships.

To summarize:

1. There are data that suggest that maternal activity levels are high in the case of mothers of preterm infants and low in the case of lower-class black mothers.

2. These high and low levels of maternal activity appear to bear a curvilinear relationship to (a) elevated heart rate and blood pressures in the mothers and (b) nonoptimal interaction behaviors and elevated heart rate and blood pressures of the infants.

3. In addition, these behavioral and cardiovascular activity relationships can be manipulated by altering maternal activity levels.

4. Since infant blood pressures show a familial aggregation at least to sibling blood pressures by the end of the first year, there is reason to suspect that the early development of infant blood pressure may be affected by maternal behavior.

5. Since infant interaction behaviors are correlated with later social development, there is reason to believe that maternal behavior during early interactions may have some enduring effects on the development of infant behavior.

6. Additional factors that may interact with or independently relate to infant and maternal interaction activity, heart rate, and blood pressure levels include infant temperament and maternal anxiety, perceptions, and attitudes that may vary by context and culture.

All of these points are speculative, since the supporting data are sparse. Further studies might focus on the relationships between maternal and infant interaction activity, heart rate, and blood pressure levels in groups who are at risk or appear to experience nonoptimal interactions (high and low levels of interaction activity and elevated cardiovascular activity), and the effects of manipulating those activity levels as well as the effects of other intervening factors (maternal anxiety, attitudes, and perceptions and infant temperament). Studies of this kind might elucidate some of the important factors affecting the early development of infant interaction and cardiovascular activity.

REFERENCES

Bakeman, R. High-risk infant: Is the risk social? Symposium presented at the meeting of the American Psychological Association, Toronto, May 1978.

Beckwith, L., & Cohen, S. E. Interactions of preterm infants with their caregivers and test performance at age two. In T. Field, S. Goldberg, D. Stern, & A. Sostek (Eds.), *High-risk Infants and children: Adult and peer interactions.* New York: Academic Press, 1980.

Beckwith, L., Cohen, S. E., Kopp, C. B., Parmelee, A. H., & Marcy, T. G. Caregiver infant interaction and early cognitive development in preterm infants. *Child Development,* 1976, **47,** 579–587.

Beckwith, L., Sigman, M., Cohen, S. E., & Parmelee, A. H. Vocal output in preterm infants. *Developmental Psychobiology,* 1977, **10,** 543–554.

Bee, H. L., VanEgeren, L. F., Streissguth, A. P., Nyman, B. A., & Lockie, M. S. Social class differences in maternal teaching styles and speech patterns. *Developmental Psychology,* 1969, **1,** 726–734.

Bell, R. Q. A reinterpretation of the direction of effects in studies of socialization. *Psychological Review,* 1968, **75,** 81–95.

Berkowitz, L. Some determinants of impulsive aggression: Role of mediated associations with reinforcements for aggression. *Psychological Review,* 1974, **81,** 165–176.

Biron, P., Mongeau, J., & Bertrand, D. Familial aggregation of blood pressure in childhood is hereditary. *Pediatrics,* 1974, **54,** 659–660.

Brazelton, T. B. *Neonatal Behavioral Assessment Scale.* National Spastics Society Monograph. London: Heineman, 1973.

Brazelton, T. B., Koslowski, B., & Main, M. The origins of reciprocity: The early mother-infant interaction. In M. Lewis & L. Rosenblum (Eds.), *The effect of the infant on its caregiver.* New York: Wiley, 1974.

Brown, M. Attitudes and personality characteristics of mothers and their relation to infantile colic. Unpublished Ph.D. dissertation, Vanderbilt University, 1961.

Brown, J. V., & Bakeman, R. Relationships of human mothers with their infants during the first year of life: Effect of prematurity. In R. W. Bell & W. P. Smotherman (Eds.), *Maternal influences and early behavior.* New York: Spectrum, 1979.

Buckhalt, J. A., Rutherford, R. B., & Goldberg, K. E. Verbal and nonverbal interaction of mothers with their Down's syndrome and nonretarded infants. *American Journal of Mental Deficiency,* 1978, **82,** 337–343.

Callaghan, J. Face-to-face interaction styles: A comparison of Anglo, Hopi and Navajo mothers and infants. In T. Field, A. Sostek, P. Vietze, & A. Leiderman (Eds.), *Culture and early interactions.* Hillsdale, N.J.: Lawrence Erlbaum, 1981.

Cattell, R. B., & Scheier, I. H. The nature of anxiety: A review of thirteen multivariate analyses comprising 814 variables. *Psychological Reports.* 1958, **4,** 351–388.

Chapple, E. D. Experimental production of transients in human interaction. *Nature,* 1970, **228,** 630–633.

Chisholm, J. Residence patterns and the environment of mother-infant interactions among the Navajo. In T. Field, A. Sostek, P. Vietze, & A. Leiderman (Eds.), *Culture and early interactions.* Hillsdale, N.J.: Lawrence Erlbaum, 1981.

Cicchetti, A., & Sroufe, A. An organizational view of affect: Illustration from the study of Down's syndrome infants. In M. Lewis & L. A. Rosenblum (Eds.), *The Development of affect.* New York: Plenum Press, 1978.

Clarke-Stewart, K. A. Interactions between mothers and their young children: Characteristics and consequences. *Monographs of the Society for Research in Child Development,* 1973, **38,** entire volume.

Cohen, S. E., & Beckwith, L. Maternal language in infancy. *Developmental Psychology,* 1976, **12,** 371–372.

Dietrich, K. N., & Starr, R. H. Maternal handling and developmental characteristics of abused infants. In T. Field, S. Goldberg, D. Stern, & A. Sostek (Eds.), *High-risk infants and children: Adult and peer interactions.* New York: Academic Press, 1980.

DiVitto, B., & Goldberg, S. The effects of newborn medical status on early parent-infant interaction. In T. Field, A. Sostek, S. Goldberg, & H. H. Shuman (Eds.), *Infants born at risk.* New York: Spectrum, 1979.

Dixon, S., Keefer, C., Tronick, E., & Brazelton, T. B. Face-to-face interaction among the Gusii. In T. Field, A. Sostek, P. Vietze, & A. Leiderman (Eds.), *Culture and early interactions.* Hillsdale, N.J.: Lawrence Erlbaum, 1981.

Donovan, W. L., Leavitt, L. A., & Balling, J. D. Maternal physiological response to infant signals. *Psychophysiology,* 1978, **15,** 68–74.

Dunn, J. Changes in styles of mothering. In *Parent-infant interaction.* London: Ciba Foundation Symposium (new series), 1977.

Field, T. Effects of early separation, interactive deficits and experimental manipulations on infant-mother face-to-face interaction. *Child Development,* 1977, **48,** 763–771. (a)

Field, T. Maternal stimulation during infant feeding. *Developmental Psychology,* 1977, **13,** 539–540. (b)

Field, T. The 3 Rs of infant-adult social interactions. Rhythms, repertoires and responsivity. *Pediatric Psychology,* 1978, **3,** 131–136.

Field, T. Games parents play with normal and high-risk infants. *Child Psychiatry and Human Development,* 1979, **10,** 41–48. (a)

Field, T. Interaction patterns of high-risk and normal infants. In T. Field et al. (Eds.), *Infants born at risk.* New York: Spectrum, 1979. (b)

Field, T. Visual and cardiac responses to animate and inanimate faces by young term and preterm infants. *Child Development,* 1979, **50,** 188–195. (c)

Field, T. Interactions of high-risk infants: Quantitative and qualitative differences. In D. Sawin et al. (Eds.), *Current perspectives on psychosocial risks during pregnancy and early infancy.* New York: Brunner/Mazel, 1980. (a)

Field, T. Interactions of infants born to black, lower class teenage mothers. In T. Field et al. (Eds.), *High-risk infants and children: Adult and peer interactions.* New York: Academic Press, 1980. (b)

Field, T., Dempsey, J., Hallock, N., & Shuman, H. Mothers' assessments of the behavior of their infants. *Infant Behavior and Development,* 1978, **1,** 156–167.

Field, T., Dempsey, J., Hatch, J., Ting, G., & Clifton, R. Habituation of cardiac and behavioral responses to tactile and auditory stimulation by preterm and full-term infants during the neonatal period. *Developmental Psychology,* 1979, **15,** 406–417.

Field, T., Hallock, N., Dempsey, J., & Shuman, H. Mothers' assessments of term infants and preterm infants with respiratory distress syndrome: Reliability and predictive validity. *Child Psychiatry and Human Development,* 1978, **9,** 75–85.

Field, T., Dempsey, J., & Shuman, H. Developmental follow-up of pre- and post-term infants. In S. Friedman & M. Sigman (Eds.), *Preterm birth and psychological development.* New York: Academic Press, 1981.

Field, T. & Ignatoff, E. Videotaping effects on play and interaction behaviors of low income mothers and their infants. *Journal of Applied Developmental Psychology,* 1981, **2,** 227–236.

Field, T., & Pawlby, S. British and American working and middle-class mother-infant interactions. *Child Development,* 1980, **51.**

Field, T., Sostek, A., Vietze, P., & Leiderman, A. (Eds.) *Culture and early interactions.* Hillsdale, N.J.: Lawrence Erlbaum, 1981.

Field, T. & Widmayer, S. Developmental follow-up of infants delivered by Caesarean section and general anesthesia. *Infant behavior and development,* 1980, **3,** 253–264.

Field, T., Walden, T., Widmayer, S. & Greenberg, R. The early development of preterm, discordant pairs: Bigger is not always better. *Infant behavior and development,* 1982, in press.

Field, T., Widmayer, S., Stringer, S., & Ignatoff, E. Teenage, lower class mothers and their preterm infants: An intervention and developmental follow-up. *Child Development,* 1980, **51,** 426–436.

Fiske, D. W., & Maddi, S. R. *Functions of varied experience.* Homewood, Ill.: Dorsey Press, 1961.

Fogel, A., Diamond, G. R., Langhorst, B. H., & Demos, V. Alteration of infant behavior as a result of "still-face" perturbation of maternal behavior. Paper presented at the Society for Research in Child Development, San Francisco, 1979.

Fourcher, B., & Freedman, D. Maternal rhythmicity and mother-infant interaction among United States Black, Caucasian, and Navajo. In T. Field et al. (Eds.), *Culture and early interactions.* Hillsdale, N.J.: Lawrence Erlbaum, 1981.

Frodi, A. M., Lamb, M. E., Leavitt, L. A., & Donovan, W. L. Father's and mothers' response to smiles and cries. *Infant Behavior and Development,* 1978, **1,** 187–198.

Frodi, A. M., Lamb, M. E., Leavitt, L. A., Donovan, W. L., Neff, C., & Sherry, D. Fathers' and mothers' responses to the faces and cries of normal and premature infants. *Developmental Psychology,* 1978, **14,** 490–498.

Goldberg, S., Brachfeld, S., & DiVitto, B. Feeding, fussing and play: Parent-infant interactions in the first year as a function of early medical problems. In T. Field et al., (Eds.), *High-risk infants and children: Adult and peer interactions.* New York: Academic Press, 1980.

Graham, F. K., & Clifton, R. K. Heartrate change as a component of the orienting response. *Psychological Bulletin,* 1966, **65,** 305–320.

Green, R. G., Stonner, D., & Shope, G. L. The facilitation of aggression by aggression: Evidence against the catharsis hypothesis. *Journal of Personality and Society Psychology,* 1975, **31,** 221–226.

Hebb, D. O. *Organization of behavior.* New York: Wiley, 1949.

Hennekens, C. H., Jesse, M. J., Klein, B. E., Gourley, J. E., & Blumenthal, S. Aggregation of blood pressure in infants and their siblings. *American Journal of Epidemiology,* 1976, **103,** 457–463.

Jesse, M., Klein, B., Hokanson, J., Levine, R., & Gourley, J. Blood pressures in childhood: Initial recording versus one year follow up. Paper presented at American Heart Association Meeting in Miami, Florida, 1976.

Jesse, M. J., Levine, R. S., Hokanson, J., & Gourley, J. Longitudinal study of the first year of life of the blood pressure of offspring of hypertensive, pre-eclamptic and normotensive mothers. Unpublished manuscript, 1975.

Jones, O. Mother-child communication in very young Down's syndrome and normal children. In T. Field et al. (Eds.) *High-risk infants and children: Adult and peer interactions.* New York: Academic Press, 1980.

Kagan, J. *Change and continuity in infancy.* New York: Wiley, 1971.

Kaye, K., & Brazelton, T. B. Mother-infant interaction in the organization of sucking. Paper presented at meeting of the Society for Research in Child Development, Minneapolis, April 1971.

Kilbride, H. W., Johnson, D. L., & Streissguth, A. P. Social class, birth order and newborn experience. *Child Development,* 1977, **48,** 1686–1688.

Klein, B. Genetics and familial aggregation of blood pressure. In G. Oresti & C. R. Kleinst (Eds.), *Hypertension: Determinants, complications and intervention.* New York: Grune & Stratton, 1979.

Klein, B., Hennekens, C. H., Jesse, M. J., Gourley, J. E., & Blumenthal, S. Longitudinal studies of blood pressure in offspring of hypertensive mothers. In P. Oglesby (Ed.) *Epidemiology and control of hypertension.* Miami: Publication Symposia Specialists, 1975.

Klein, B., Jesse, M. J., Hennekens, C. H., Gourley, J. E., & Blumenthal, S. Aggregation of blood pressure in young siblings. *American Journal of Epidemiology,* 1975, **102,** 437.

Kogan, K. L. Interaction systems between preschool aged handicapped or developmentally delayed children and their parents. In T. Field et al. (Eds.), *High-risk infants and children: Adult and peer interactions.* New York: Academic Press, 1980.

Kubicek, L. Mother interactions of twins: An autistic and non-autistic twin. In T. Field et al. (Eds.), *High-risk infants and children: Adult and peer interactions.* New York: Academic Press, 1980.

Lakin, M. Personality factors in mothers of excessively crying (colicky) infants. *Monographs of the Society of Research in Child Development,* 1957, **22,** 1–48.

Lee, Y., Rosner, B., Gould, J., Lowe, E., & Kass, E. H. Familial aggregation of blood pressures of newborn infants and their mothers. *Pediatrics,* 1976, **58,** 722–729.

Levine, R. S., Hennekens, C. H., Briese, F. W., Robertson, E., Cassady, J., Gourley, J., & Gelband, H. A prospective study of blood pressure in newborn twins. In W. E. Nance (Ed.), *Twin research. Part C: Clinical Studies.* New York: Alan R. Liss, 1978.

Levine, R. A., Hennekens, C. H., Gourley, J., Cassady, J., Klein, B., Briese, F. W., Jesse, M. J., & Gelband, H. A prospective study of maternal and infant blood pressure levels. *Clinical Research,* 1978, **26,** 69a.

Levine, R., Hennekens, C. H., Klein, B., Gourley, J., Briese, F. W., Hokanson, J., Gelband, H., & Jesse, M. Tracking correlations of blood pressure in infancy. *Pediatrics,* 1978, **61,** 121–123.

Lewis, H., Brooks, J., & Haviland, J. Hearts and faces: A study of measurement of emotion. In M. Lewis & L. A. Rosenblum (Eds.), *The development of affect.* New York: Plenum Press, 1978.

Lewis, M., & Rosenblum, L. A. (Eds.) *The affect of the infant on its caregiver.* New York: Wiley, 1974.

Lewis, M., Wilson, C. D., & Ban, P. An exploratory study of resting cardiac rate and variability from the last trimester of prenatal life through the first year of postnatal life. *Child Development,* 1970, **31,** 799–811.

Lipton, E. L., Steinschneider, A., & Richmond, J. B. Autonomic function in the neonate: VII. Maturational changes in cardiac control. *Child Development,* 1966, **37,** 1–16.

Martini, M., & Kirkpatrick, J. Interactions between caretakers and infants on the Marquesan Island of Ua Pou. In T. Field, A. Sostek, P. Vietze, & A. Leiderman (Eds.), *Culture and early interactions.* Hillsdale, N.J.: Lawrence Erlbaum, 1981.

Massie, H. N. The early natural history of childhood psychosis: Ten case studies by analysis of family home movies of the infancies of the children. *Journal of Child Psychiatry,* 1978, **17,** 29–45.

McCall, R. B., Kennedy, C. B., & Applebaum, M. I. Magnitude of discrepancy and the distribution of attention in infants. *Child Development,* 1977, **48,** 772–785.

McCall, R. B., & McGhee, P. S. The discrepancy hypothesis of attention and affect in human infants. In I. C. Uzgiris & F. Weizmann (Eds.), *The structuring of experience*. New York: Plenum Press, 1977.

Pawlby, S., & Hall, F. Interaction of infants whose mothers come from disrupted families. In T. Field et al. (Eds.), *High-risk infants and children: Adult and peer interactions*. New York: Academic Press, 1980.

Porges, S. W., Arnold, W. R., & Forbes, E. J. Heart rate variability: An index of attentional responsivity in human newborns. *Developmental Psychology,* 1973, **8**, 85–92.

Sameroff, A. J., Bakow, M. A., McComb, N., & Collins, A. Racial and social class differences in newborns' heart rate. *Infant Behavior and Development,* 1978, **1**, 199–204.

Sandler, H. M., & Vietze, P. M. Obstetric and neonatal outcomes following intervention. In K. Scott, T. Field, & E. Robertson (Eds.), *Teenage parents and their offspring*. New York: Grune & Stratton, 1979.

Schacter, J. Pain, fear, and anger in hypertensives and normotensives. *Psychosomatic Medicine,* 1957, **19**, 71–79.

Schachter, J., Kerr, J. L., Wimberly, F. C., & Lakin, J. M. Heartbeat levels in black and white newborns. *Psychosomatic Medicine,* 1974. **38**, 513–524.

Schaffer, H. R. Cognitive components of the infant's responses to strangeness. In M. Lewis & L. Rosenblum (Eds.), *The origins of fear.* New York: Wiley, 1974.

Sigman, M. The influence of medical neurological and environmental factors on the development of the preterm infant. In S. L. Friedman & M. Sigman (Eds.), *Pre- and post-term birth: Relevance to optimal psychological development*. New York: Academic Press, 1980.

Spielberger, C. D. (Ed.) *Anxiety and behavior.* New York: Academic Press, 1966.

Spielberger, C. D., Gorsuch, R. L., & Lushene, R. E. *The State-Trait Anxiety Inventory.* Palo Alto, Calif.: Consulting Psychologists Press, 1970.

Sroufe, L. A., Waters, E., & Matas, L. Contextual determinants of infant affective response. In M. Lewis & L. Rosenblum (Eds.), *The origins of fear.* New York: Wiley, 1974.

Stern, D. A micro-analysis of mother-infant interaction: Behavior regulating social contact between a mother and her 3½-month-old twins. *Journal of the American Academy of Child Psychiatry,* 1971, **10**, 501–517.

Trevarthen, C. B. The nature of an infant's ecology. Paper presented at the International Society for the Study of Behavioral Development, Guilford, Conn., 1975.

Tronick, E., Als, H., Adamson, L., Wise, S., & Brazelton, T. B. The infant's response to entrapment between contradictory messages in face-to-face interaction. *Journal of Child Psychiatry,* 1978, **17**, 1–13.

Tulkin, S., & Kagan, J. Mother-child interaction in the first few years of life. *Child Development,* 1972, **43**, 31–41.

Waters, E., Matas, L., & Sroufe, I. Infants' reactions to an approaching stranger: Description, validation and functional significance of wariness. *Child Development,* 1975, **46**, 348–356.

Wedell-Monnig, J., & Lumley, J. M. Child deafness and mother-child interaction. *Child Development,* 1980, **51**, 766–774.

Widmayer, S., & Field, T. Effects of Brazelton demonstrations on early interactions of preterm infants and their mothers. *Infant Behavior and Development,* 1980, **3**, 79–89.

Wiesenfeld, A. R., & Klorman, R. The mother's psychophysiological reactions to contrasting affective expressions by her own and an unfamiliar infant. *Developmental Psychology,* 1978, **14**, 294–304.

Zaslow, M., Sostek, A., Vietze, P., Kreiss, L., & Rubinstein, D. Contribution of context to interactions with infants in Fais and the U.S.A. In T. Field et al. (Eds.), *Culture and early interactions*. Hillsdale, N.J.: Lawrence Erlbaum, 1981.

Zinner, S. H., Levy, P. S., & Kass, E. H. Familial aggregation of blood pressures in children. *New England Journal of Medicine,* 1971, **284**, 401.

9

Etiological Considerations in Childhood Hyperactivity

Donald R. Kanter

THE STORY OF FIDGETY PHILIP*
Let me see if Philip can
Be a little gentleman
Let me see if he is able
To sit still for once at the table.
. . . But Philip did not mind
His father who was so kind.
He wiggled and giggled,
And then I declare
Swung backward and forward
And tilted his chair,
Just like any rocking horse;
"Philip, I am getting cross."
See the naughty restless child,
Growing still more rude and wild,
Till his chair falls over quite
Philip screams with all his might,
Catches at the cloth, but then
That makes matters worse again.
Down upon the ground they fall,
Glasses, bread, knives, forks and all.
How Mamma did fret and frown,
When she saw them tumbling down. . . .
And papa made such a face
Philip is in sad disgrace.
Where is Philip? Where is he? . . .

*From Struwwelpeter, Frankfurt: Literariseag Anstalt, 1845.

211

Today, more than 135 years since the writing of this verse by the German physician Heinrich Hoffman, the search for Fidgety Philip has continued, resulting in a rather astounding discovery. We have found that "Fidgety Philips" number in the hundreds of thousands. Brodemus and Swanson (1977-78) report that between 150,000 and 500,000 children in the United States are currently receiving psychoactive medication to alleviate hyperactivity, with estimates of incidence ranging from 5 percent to 10 percent of the school-age population (Shaywitz, Klopper, & Gordon, 1978). The variability of incidence reports may reflect disagreement among investigators concerning criteria in differential diagnosis of this disorder, or heterogeneity of the population. One relevant study, however, indicates that the best predictor of differing diagnosis for the same children is the etiological bias of the diagnostician (Lambert & Grossman, 1964). The hyperactive child has been variously described as overactive, impulsive, aggressive, easily frustrated, and distractible, with a short attention span (Stewart, 1970). In fact these children frequently are distinguished more by a lack of effectiveness in purposeful activities than by high levels of motor activity per se.

The literature is replete with an impressive array of terms to describe the hyperactive child with learning difficulties.[1] These terms, which range from "minimal brain damage" to "psychogenic impulse control disorder," usually reflect the assumed etiological course. Although it has been suggested that some of these labels represent homogeneous subgroups within the heterogeneous group classified as hyperactive, uniform *a priori* operational distinctions are absent from the current literature. No single etiological factor has emerged from the voluminous research devoted to the topic, although numerous hypotheses have been proposed, including minimal brain damage or dysfunction, possibly due to genetic contribution; pre- or perinatal trauma; toxic or infectious insult; pathological environmental factors such as chemical additives in food; radiation; disorganized, chaotic family situations; psychosocial stress; or some interaction of two or more of these factors.

This chapter is a review of the evidence of this diversity of etiological influences, with special focus on the interrelated, interactional, and multivariate nature of factors that seem to manifest themselves via the final common symptomatic pathway of childhood hyperactivity.

This chapter is not an exhaustive review of all the research that has focused on childhood hyperactivity. Rather, it represents an attempt to integrate the various understandings of this phenomenon that have emerged from diverse fields, all of which have found some special reason to be intrigued by the puzzle of childhood hyperactivity.

The chapter begins with a discussion of genetic factors and the related phenomena of minor congenital anomalies. Examples of evidence implicating environmental hazards such as lead poisoning, food additives, and radiation are examined next. The focus is then directed to the historic development and current state of knowledge regarding theories of biochemical imbalance. Finally, a look at the social and cultural context serves to bring together the diversity of factors into a single picture.

GENETIC INFLUENCES

It is difficult to determine the relative roles of genetic and environmental influences in childhood hyperactivity (CHA). It is likely that if a genetic basis for CHA exists, the different clinical phenotypes represent complex interactions of environmental conditions with genetically influenced variables such as intelligence. In spite of these limitations, recent evidence has strongly implicated hereditary factors in the etiology of CHA. Epidemiologic studies have found higher frequency of CHA in boys than in girls, with boy-girl ratios ranging from 4:1 to 6:1 (Cantwell, 1975a). These findings suggest the possibility of an X-linked chromosomal abnormality. Actual examination of chromosomal structures in hyperactive children, however, has not revealed any chromosomal abnormality (Warren, Karduck, Bussaratid, Stewart, & Sly, 1971). Although numerous investigators have noted increased incidence of psychopathology among parents of hyperactive children (Cantwell, 1972, 1975b; Morrison & Stewart, 1971, 1973, 1974), familes of adopted hyperactive children do not have a high prevalence of such disorders (Morrison & Stewart, 1973; Stewart, 1970). While this evidence of pathology in both parent and child may be taken as evidence of a polygenetic etiological basis for a hyperactivity component, an equally plausible explanation is that CHA may be the result of the extreme stress of growing up in a chaotic, disorganized family environment in which the child never knows what to expect next from parental caretakers who may be emotionally unbalanced. Unfortunately, adoptive studies have been confounded by an inability to control for early social traumata; nevertheless, available evidence indicates that genetic factors may be of some etiological importance in childhood hyperactivity (Cantwell, 1975b; Safer, 1973).

Minor physical anomalies. A number of investigators report the high incidence of physical anomalies among children with behavioral difficulties (Durfee, 1973; Rapoport, Quinn, & Lamprecht, 1974; Waldrop & Goering, 1971; Waldrop, Pedersen, & Bell, 1968). The presence of these congenital stigmata in hyperactive children suggests several possible explanations, such as a genetically transmitted defect; a toxic insult during embryonic development that resulted in these minor anomalies and concomitant behavior and learning disorders; or pathogenic intrauterine environments associated with extreme maternal emotional stress, perhaps via altered maternal adrenocortical function. A pertinent study by Stott (1971) reported evidence of the association of increased incidence of congenital anomalies and maternal emotional stress during pregnancy. Another study (Rapoport et al., 1974) found evidence that hyperactive children with high anomaly scores also had altered catecholamine[2] metabolism. It is unclear whether this altered metabolism was due to genetic factors, thought to influence baseline levels, or reflective of a stressful state, also thought to affect this index (Weinshiboum, Kvetnansky, & Axelrod, 1971).

If there is a genetic basis for childhood hyperactivity, what aspect of brain function is affected and how is this alteration genetically transmitted? Wender (1971) proposed a genetically controlled metabolic defect involving the metabolism of catecholamines. According to Wender, hyperactivity and restlessness are determined by one set of genes and short attention span by another set. When both of these sets of genes randomly converge in the same child, the outcome may be hyperactivity.

PRE-, PERI-, AND POSTNATAL TRAUMA

Hyperactivity has been associated with a number of difficulties in pregnancy and delivery (Laufer, Denhoff, & Solomons, 1957), head trauma (Blau, 1936), anoxia at birth (Rosenfeld & Bradley, 1948), and premature birth (Burks, 1960). Other investigators have found evidence suggesting that hyperactivity may be inversely related to birth weight (Harper, Fischer, & Rider, 1959). However, subsequent investigations have found that many of the perinatal factors alluded to occur as often in normal children as in children who become hyperactive (Kinsbourne, 1976; Minde, Webb, & Skyes, 1968; Stewart, Pitts, Craig, & Dieruf, 1966).

A relevant animal study examining the role of suffocation shortly after birth found that monkeys asphyxiated for 15 minutes after birth demonstrated striking similarities to hyperactive children in areas of hyperactivity, lack of coordination, decreased attention span, and impaired impulse control (Sechzan, Faro, & Windle, 1973). While it seems improbable that any substantial number of children is subjected to such an extreme degree of asphyxiation, it is likely that lesser levels of asphyxiation result in similar, although perhaps more subtle, impairments.

Evidence has recently emerged from a number of studies suggesting an interaction between perinatal complications and the caretaking environment. Specifically, children with histories of perinatal trauma who also are raised in economically and/or educationally disadvantaged or unstable families appear to have a higher incidence of learning difficulties than those children with a history of perinatal trauma who are raised in more favorable environments (Broman, 1977; Drillien, 1957; Werner, Bierman, & French, 1971).

Other possible sources of trauma include subteratogenic[3] doses of substances such as aspirin and salicylates (during pregnancy) which have been shown to impair learning ability in animals (Butcher, 1979).

Available evidence, from well-controlled studies, seems to indicate that pre-, peri-, and postnatal stress have not (when examined alone) been associated with an increased incidence of hyperactivity. However, it appears that the subtle effects of these antecedent traumata are perhaps potentiated by environmental stressors associated with unstable families, poor-quality parent-child interactions, and low socioeconomic status. It is important to note that the direction of causality remains obscure in these relationships; an intractable child may be the result or the cause of poor parent-child interactions or family instability. Also, children of low socioeconomic status families are at greater risk of exposure to virtually every type of organic and environmental stressor. The conclusion that emerges most clearly from these studies is the need for a multivariate, contextual approach in future studies of etiological factors.

Lead

Perhaps the best understood toxin that has been related to hyperactivity is lead, a recognized neurotoxin and identified as a substantial health hazard in children. As noted by Silbergeld (1977), clinical reports of lead-exposed children (Waldron & Stöfen, 1974) bear substantial similarities to the constellation of symptoms exhibited by hyperactive chilren. While it is well known that extremely high lead exposure results in frank neuropathy, little is known about the effects of lead exposure at the low end of the spectrum. David, Clark, and Voeller (1972) found evidence indicating elevated (though not toxic) blood lead levels in more than half of a group of hyperactive children, and toxic-level elevation of urine levels (reflective of early exposure) after challenge with a chelating agent.[4] These findings suggest that elevated levels of lead (in the subtoxic range) over an extended period of time may result in hyperactivity. Another pertinent study by de la Burde and Choate (1975) found increased incidence of CHA in children with histories of early lead exposure.

A study of 80 preschool children found an association of cognitive, verbal, and perceptual impairment with elevated body lead levels previously presumed to be in a subtoxic (safe) range (Perino & Ernhart, 1974).

These recent findings concerning the effects of "subclinical" lead exposure to children demand a reconceptualization of this etiologic consideration. Rather than view body lead levels as a static factor that either meets an arbitrary criterion level or not,[5] it seems to be clearly more appropriate to consider lead levels as a continuum of adverse influence. Other important but relatively neglected considerations in addition to the intensity of the trauma are: (1) the stage(s) of development at which the toxic insult occurs; and (2) the presence of coincident and/or subsequent pathological processes (see Chapter Two in this volume).

The available data suggest that lead exposure (perhaps even low-level exposure over a long time) may be a significant factor in the etiology of childhood hyperactivity.

Salicylates

Feingold (1973) has proposed that CHA is induced or exacerbated in many cases by low-molecular-weight chemicals. Included in this category are salicylates, compounds that react in the body with salicylates, and common food additives. Feingold's hypothesis originated from clinical and parental observations but has drawn considerable criticism because of the subjective aspects inherent in such an approach. Subsequent controlled studies have produced conflicting results. In a study that employed a salicylate elimination diet and intermittent food dye "challenges" Weiss, Williams, Margen, Abrams, Caan, Citron, Cox, McKibben, Ogar, and Schultz (1980) found that only 2 of 22 subjects showed significant increases in aversive behaviors in responses to salicylate challenges. A similar study that evaluated parent and teacher ratings, classroom observations, and neuropsychological testing did not support the Feingold hypothesis (Harley, Ray, Tomasi, Eichman, Matthews, Chun, Cleeland, & Traisman 1978).

Other investigators, however, have found evidence which appears to support the role of salicylates in CHA. Using global clinical rating scales based on reports of parents, teachers, and clinicians, Conners, Goyette, Southwick, Lees, and Andrulonis (1976) concluded that salicylate reduction diets may reduce hyperkinetic symptoms. More recently Swanson and Kinsbourne (1980) found evidence indicating that high doses of salicylate food dyes impair hyperactive children's performance on learning tests, while a nonhyperactive control group was unaffected by the food dye challenge.

Although these discrepancies concerning the role of salicylates in CHA—perhaps due to differing criteria for subject inclusion and varied dosage levels of salicylate challenges—are not easily resolved, present data suggest that salicylate compounds may represent another significant causal consideration in childhood hyperactivity.

Radiation

Low-dose radiation from television and fluorescent lighting has recently been implicated in the etiopathology of CHA. A pilot study reported by Ott (1974) suggests that the installation of radiation shields on fluorescent light fixtures in school classrooms resulted in a reduction of hyperactive behaviors in first grade children. A related study on TV radiation also found suggestive evidence that low-dose radiation may play a causal role in hyperactive behavior (Ott, 1973). Ott (1974) postulates that exposure to low-level radiation from various sources such as microwave ovens and telephone microwave relay stations, and the deficiency of certain wavelengths present in natural sunlight, may exert a pathogenic influence by way of a retinal hypothalmic pathway.

Although these initial studies are suggestive, they are seriously flawed by several methodological shortcomings:

1. No control groups were employed.
2. Variables have been confounded—for example, radiation shields have been installed and full spectrum lighting introduced simultaneously.
3. Observations have not been standardized—time lapse photography has been used to rate the occurrence of hyperactivity, rather than established rating scales such as that developed by Conners (1973).
4. Double blind methodologies have not yet been employed.

In view of these considerations, conclusions about the intriguing possibility that low-level radiation may be of etiologic importance in CHA must await controlled investigations.

BIOCHEMICAL IMBALANCE

Since Wender (1971a; Wender, Epstein, Kopin, & Gordon, 1971) proposed that the principal etiological factor of hyperactivity was a biochemical imbalance involving the neurotransmitters dopamine, norepinephrine, and serotonin (most probably a dopamine deficit), a flurry of biochemical research has been conducted to substantiate this hypothesis.

Several historical events have provided a rationale for hypothesizing the involvement of the catecholamines in CHA. The first circumstance to occur in this chain of events was the encephalitis[6] epidemic that followed World War I. A remarkable similarity was noted between accounts of post encephalic behaviors in children and the clinical picture presented by hyperactive children (Ebaugh, 1923). Later findings indicating that encephalitis specifically attacked dopamine-rich areas of the brain further corroborated the association of catecholamines and CHA. Bradley's 1937 report of unexpected beneficial effects of d-amphetamine in refractory children became well documented, along with evidence indicating that d-amphetamine exerted its effects by way of catecholamine pathways (principally dopamine).

Excessive exposure to lead, an event long suspected to be a causal factor in some proportion of hyperactivity cases, was found to deplete dopamine,[7] further implicating dopamine in the pathogenesis of CHA. Furthermore, lead-poisoned laboratory animals exhibit an altered response to d-amphetamine reminiscent of the unexpected response noted in children by Bradley (1937). It was reasoned that hyperactive children were suffering from a dopamine deficit that was corrected (thus allowing normal behavior) by stimulant drugs like d-amphetamine and methylphenidate (Ritalin), which are thought to achieve their effects via catecholamine-mediated neural systems. The apparent calming and organizing effect of stimulant drugs became known as "the paradoxical response."[8] Some clinicians went so far as to use "the paradoxical response" to confirm a diagnosis of hyperactivity with equivocal cases, or to infer organicity despite strident protests from colleagues that such a practice was perhaps circular in nature. Although the effects of psychostimulants in normal children had not been examined (for obvious ethical reasons), it was presumed that hyperactive children's response to stimulants was unusual and reflective of underlying pathology. Very recently a team of investigators at the National Institute of Mental Health conducted the crucial experiments and examined the effects of psychostimulants in normal children (Rapoport, Buchsbaum, Weingartner et al., 1980; Rapoport, Buchsbaum, & Zahn, 1978). Rapoport and coworkers found that normal children and diagnosed hyperactive children were *not* differentially affected by psychostimulant drugs.

The impact of the Rapoport et al. studies upon the dopamine deficit hypothesis appears to be that of another beautiful theory ruined by an ugly fact.

Although inferences of neurochemical imbalance based on stimulant drug responses are no longer warranted, this does not obviate the possibility that catecholamines may be implicated in the etiopathology of childhood hyperactivity.

Dopamine (DA). In a study of cerebrospinal fluid metabolites[9] Shaywitz, Cohen, and Bowers (1977) found evidence suggestive of lower dopamine turnover in minimal brain dysfunction (MBD) children. Furthermore, in a related animal study Shaywitz, Klopper, and Gordon (1978) selectively reduced DA in the rat brain by administering 6-hydroxydopamine[10] and produced rat pups with high activity levels and learning deficits. A study of CSF metabolites by Shetty and Chase (1976) found no differences between hyperactive children and normal controls; however, treatment with d-amphetamine resulted in a significant decrease in the index of dopamine function, which was highly correlated with clinical improvement. These findings do not convincingly demonstrate that DA plays a causal role in the pathogenesis of CHA, but rather suggest that amphetamine achieves its clinical effects via the dopaminergic systems.[11]

Norepinephrine (NE). Another line of investigation concerning the role of catecholamines in CHA has focused on norepinephrine. In a study of urinary metabolites (MHPG) of norepinephrine, Wender, Epstein, Kopin, and Gordon (1971) found no differences between MBD children and normal controls. Other studies of urinary metabolites (Shekim, Dekirmenjian, & Chapel, 1977, 1978) found evidence suggestive of a relationship between CNS norepinephrine and hyperactivity. The role of norepinephrine in hyperactivity was further supported by Rapoport, Lott, Alexander, and Abramson (1970) in a study that found an inverse relationship between norepinephrine and hyperactive behaviors. A later study of Rapoport, Mikkelsen, Ebert, Brown, Weise, and Kopin (1978) found higher levels of norepinephrine in hyperactive children, but norepinephrine indices did not correlate with motor activity or level of arousal.

Serotonin. In a study examining 5-hydroxyindoles (an index of serotonergic[12] function) in whole blood, Wender (1969) found evidence suggestive of depressed serotonin in MBD children as compared to normal controls. However, doubt is case upon the etiological significance of this finding since, as was noted by Wender (1969), depressed 5-hydroxyindole levels have been consistently seen in patients reacting to the stress of hospital admission. This initial finding of depressed 5-hydroxyindole levels was not supported in a subsequent study of urinary concentrations of 5-HIAA by Wender (1971), who found no significant differences between MBD children and normal controls. A noteworthy study by Coleman (1971) on whole blood concentrations of 5-hydroxyindole did, however, support the finding of lower levels in CHA children than in controls. Interestingly, it was noted that during hospitalization two of the children's serotonin levels rose toward normal and the children's hyperactivity lessened; however, when they returned home their serotonin levels returned to prehospitalization (depressed) levels and hyperactivity increased. This finding suggests that altered 5HT levels may occur in response to environmental stress rather than have any primary causal role in childhood hyperactivity.

More recent studies of platelet serotonin in MBD children have also produced equivocal findings. Bhagavan, Coleman, and Coussin (1975) reported lower than normal levels of platelet serotonin in MBD children, which showed appreciable increase in response to pyridoxine hydrochloride (vitamin B_6) administration. In a similar investigation Coleman, Greenberg, Bhagavan, Steinberg, Tippett, and Coussin (1976) selected hyperactive subjects with depressed blood levels and assessed the effects of vitamin B_6 and methylphenidate (Ritalin) on serotonin levels and hyperactive behavior. It was found that the serotonin content of blood rose in response to vitamin B_6 and hyperactivity decreased. Administration of methylphenidate, however, did not affect serotonin levels, though it did result in behavioral improvements in these children. Another study of platelet serotonin by Rapoport, Quinn, Scribanu, and Murphy (1974) using behavioral selection criteria for hyperactive subjects found no significant differences between hyperactive children and normal controls; also, no correlation was found between severity of hyperactivity and serotonin levels. This apparent independence of serotonin levels and behavioral indices also argues against a causal role for serotonin in childhood hyperactivity. In two studies employing a more direct index of serotonin functioning in the brain, no differences were found between MBD and controls in 5 HIAA levels deduced from cerebral spinal fluid (Shaywitz, et al., 1977; Shetty & Chase, 1976).

Summary

An examination of available evidence does not indicate a primary causative role of catecholamines in childhood hyperactivity. Difficulties inherent in many of these studies stem from the limitations of deducing CNS neurotransmitter levels from peripheral markers (blood and urine). For example, central serotonin is estimated to comprise only 1 to 2 percent of the total body pool. One plausible explanation of altered catecholamine levels in childhood hyperactivity is that they represent a clinical correlate of hyperactivity due to pathogenic stress.

STRESS

Psychosocial stress may well be the most ubiquitous etiologic factor in CHA. Although the tendency in the past has been to identify causal influences as either psychogenic or organic, it seems likely that many cases represent subtle and complex interactions between these two sources.

As was so poignantly articulated by Durfee (1973), the subtly impaired child may often be caught in a vicious spiral in which existing difficulties are compounded and exacerbated by social ostracism and the resultant stress, self-evaluation, and negative self-image experienced by these children.

> Needless to say, for a child to develop a negative image of himself it does not take too many experiences of being subjected to class ridicule because he read saw for was or on for no (since he sees the word that way), . . . or running up on a fly ball and having it fall some distance behind him. [p. 313]

Anxiety has been described as the "key commonality in many cases of hyperactive behavior" (Kenny, 1980). It has often been suggested that anxiety is likely to play a contributing and perhaps, in some cases, a primary role in the processes associated with childhood hyperactivity. However, little systematic investigation has been conducted to elucidate the role of this elusive yet probably pervasive factor. A suggestive study by Braud (1978) that focused on anxiety reduction in hyperactive children is pertinent to this issue. Braud employed relaxation training (either the Jacobsen technique or biofeedback training) with hyperactive children and found substantial improvement on indices of relaxation and in concomitant behavior ratings by parents for both techniques.

Familial Influences

It is obviously difficult to attribute a primary causal role to familial factors such as supportiveness and understanding. Nevertheless, these factors seem to play important roles (perhaps via interactional-reciprocal means) in the causal processes of hyperactivity. Several investigators have found evidence suggesting the importance of family supportiveness, understanding (Werner & Smith, 1977), and quality of parent-child interactions (Minde, Weiss, & Mendelson, 1972) in the later adjustment of these children. Studies of parent-child interactions have associated increased maternal involvement (e.g., suggestions, disapproval, encouragement) with impulsivity, inattention, and hyperactivity during problem-solving tasks (Bee, 1967; Campbell, 1973, 1975). A related study by

Cvejic and Kruger (1975) found that mothers of extremely hyperactive children were more frustrated and used more physical punishment than mothers of less hyperactive children. However, the direction of causality is unclear in these relationships. It may be that these children have never adequately established behaviors conducive to effecive problem solving because of constant maternal interference, or because constant feedback on performance (disapproval, encouragement, etc.) creates a debilitating level of anxiety for these children. It is equally plausible that these children elicit maternal interference and concern by their inability to adequately deal with problem solving situations.

CULTURAL FACTORS

Socioeconomic Influences

In previous sections, connections between socioeconomic status (SES), psychological stress, and perinatal traumata have been touched upon briefly. By assuming a different perspective and reexamining these aspects within the broad context of the cultural arena, the interplay and overlap of many of these influences may become more apparent.

The reciprocity of SES and various traumata has been implicated in the pathogenesis of hyperactivity by a number of considerations.

1. The highest incidence of infant death and traumata is found in low SES and disenfranchised minority segments of the population (Birch & Gussow, 1970; Drillien, 1964; Pasamanick, Rogers, & Lilienfeld, 1956).

2. Lower social classes in the United States are concentrated in the inner-city, pre–World War II housing that has been termed "The Urban Lead Belt" (Needleman, 1973). These environments dramatically increase the probability of lead exposure from ingestion of paint, plaster, and contaminated dirt, and of airborne particles from leaded gasoline and industrial emissions.

3. As noted by Sameroff and Chandler (1975) there is an increased incidence of child abuse and neglect among lower-SES and unemployed populations. Children exposed to these conditions may be emotionally stressed beyond their adaptive capacities. Also, subtly compromising sequelae of antecedent traumata may be potentiated by abusive or neglectful circumstances.

While it is certainly not a novel observation it remains a sobering one that children of the poor and disenfranchised are more likely to be assailed by virtually every known noxious circumstance.

DISCUSSION AND CONCLUSIONS

Formulations of etiological influences have generally been cast in the mold of linear models of causality, in which factors are sharply delineated in "black or white" or "present or absent" categories. A phenomenon is typically investigated in relation to a single presumed causal event. In this approach the presumed causal influence, for example lead poisoning, is evaluated in terms of its presence or absence (at a clinically toxic level). If the presumed causal agent is present (to a significant extent) in some cases but not in others, it is assumed that the positive cases represent a homogeneous subgroup within the larger (and now presumably more poorly defined) heterogeneous population.

Often it is presumed that if only this heterogeneous population could be more precisely defined, these homogeneous subsets would then "fall out" and at last clarity of the homogeneous, single causal forces of the phenomenon would become evident. This approach engenders a subtle circularity, reflected in the present confusion of etiological knowledge of childhood hyperactivity. An example may further elucidate this point. Recently it has been postulated that hyperactive children are centrally or autonomically underaroused (Satterfield & Dawson, 1971; Stewart, 1970; Werry, Sprague, Weiss, & Minde, 1970; Zentall, 1975). According to this view, the seemingly aimless overactivity exhibited by these children represents a homeostatic adjustment mechanism that increases proprioceptive input (by way of increasing activity), hence compensating for the underaroused state. Subsequent research addressed to the examination of this hypothesis has employed various indices, for example EEG alpha wave activity, evoked potentials, heart rate, respiration, electropupilograms, and measures of skin conductance. The findings from this body of investigation are that a subset of hyperactive children is underaroused and that another subset is overaroused, while still others exhibit normal levels of arousal. One might reasonably infer, on the basis of this evidence, that hyperactive children are (as one might expect with regard to other variables such as height) normally distributed along the dimension of arousal. However, it has instead been suggested that these variations in arousal represent the presence of homogeneous subgroups within the heterogeneous clinical population imprecisely defined as hyperactive. Furthermore, studies that have then defined subgroups (per this *post hoc* theorizing) according to level of arousal, have found little evidence that these subgroups are indeed homogeneous in any respect other than level of arousal.

Obviously this practice of selectively focusing upon evidence that confirms one's hypothesis, and redefining cases that do not fit as "other" homogeneous subgroups, does little to answer the questions originally posed.

The available evidence seems to strongly suggest the multivariate nature of the etiological elements of childhood hyperactivity. It is very unlikely that CHA is determined simply or that one etiological factor is responsible for causing one "homogeneous" group of children to become hyperactive. It seems much more probable that CHA is *multiply determined* and is the outcome of several pathogenic influences interacting in complex ways. Moreover, each of the etiological influences are probably continua that can adversely affect the child to varying degrees, depending on the intensity of the traumatic event, the stage of development at which it occurs, and the concomitant or subsequent occurrence of other noxious events. The practice of viewing pathogenic factors as discrete phenomena, which are either present or absent (according to some preset criteria), has obscured the elucidation of the subtle but probably important interplay of factors in the processes associated with the occurrence of CHA.

FUTURE DIRECTIONS

In contrast to an inflexible linear model of causality, Sameroff and Chandler (1975) present an organismic or transactional perspective on causal relationships. According to this dynamic conceptualization, reciprocity between continua of reproductive and caretaking casuality must be taken into account to understand the etiopathogenesis of a disorder. Sameroff and Chandler state:

> Transactions between the child and his caretaking environment serve to break or maintain the linkage between earlier trauma and later disorder and must be taken into account if successful predictions are to be made. To gain predictive validity from the continuum of reproductive casuality one must take into account the maintaining environment. Similarly, to gain predictive validity from the continuum of caretaking casuality one must take into account the characteristics of the victimized child [p. 483].

Past investigative approaches have, for the most part, focused sharply, although narrowly, on individual suspected causal events. The result of this approach has been a virtual explosion of knowledge delineating these individual evidential threads. Other evidence from contextual-interactive studies clearly suggests that these individual influences are inextricably interwoven into complex processes that form the phenomenological fabric of childhood hyperactivity. Studies of the interrelationships of these individual influential "threads" offer the greatest potential for understanding the etiological considerations of childhood hyperactivity.

NOTES

1. It is noteworthy that the most recent edition of the *Diagnostic and Statistical Manual* (3rd ed.; American Psychiatric Association, 1980) has changed the term used to describe this disorder from "hyperkinetic reaction of childhood" to "attention deficit disorder." However, at the present time there is no universally agreed-upon term to describe these children. For example, the World Health Organization uses the term "hyperkinetic syndrome of childhood" in its International Classification of Diseases. The term that seems to appear most frequently in the literature is "hyperactivity." In the present text the term "hyperactivity" will be used in general discussions of the disorder and the terminology used in the original article will be used when describing specific research findings.

2. Catecholamines are a group of chemical messengers (neurotransmitters) that are present in the brain and are thought to mediate the orchestration of learning processes and physical movement.

3. The term teratogen has traditionally referred to any chemical substance that may induce physical abnormalities in fetal development if ingested during pregnancy. Recent work in this area indicates that very low levels of many compounds do not result in physical anomalies of the fetus but may, however, cause impairment of mental functioning in areas such as learning. This low-level exposure is referred to as subteratogenic.

4. Chelating agents are chemical compounds that leach lead deposits from long-term body stores, for example in bones, and in doing so allow assessment of lead exposure that occurred in the past. In contrast, assessment of blood and urine indices without the use of a chelating agent reflects only very recent exposure to lead. See Rutter (1980) for a comprehensive review of lead poisoning in children and relevant indices of this phenomenon.

5. It has been argued that because of the difficulty in diagnosing lead poisoning in the early stages, most cases only come to attention when they have reached a crisis level; therefore since only these extreme cases have been used to set the criteria for danger levels, the resultant criteria for toxicity may be too high. See David, Hoffman, and Koltun (1978) for a more thorough discussion of this issue.

6. Von Economo's encephalitis, a viral disease causing inflammation of the brain, swept the world during World War I.

7. A confluence of evidence has implicated the neurotransmitter dopamine in the neurochemical processes associated with hyperactivity. In addition to encephalitis-related evidence, lead poisoning has been associated with both dopamine depletion and hyperactivity. Drugs that specifically reduce available dopamine (6-hydroxydopamine) in the brain have been employed to create an animal model of hyperactivity. Drugs that increase available dopamine in the brain (amphetamine and methylphenidate) have been successfully used in a majority of cases to treat childhood hyperactivity.

8. This phenomenon was termed "paradoxical" because it seemed counterintuitive that a stimulant drug should have a calming effect on a large proportion of hyperactive children.

9. Various markers that are present in cerebrospinal fluid, blood, and urine are used as indices of neurotransmitter activity in the brain.

10. The drug 6-hydroxydopamine (6HD) selectively reduces available dopamine in the brain. As such, 6HD provides a convenient tool to test the "reduced dopamine" explanation of hyperactivity.

11. "Dopaminergic" refers to the neural systems mediated by the neurotransmitter dopamine.

12. "Serotonergic" refers to the neural systems mediated by the neurotransmitter serotonin.

REFERENCES

American Psychiatric Association. *Diagnostic and statistical manual of mental disorders* (3rd ed.). Washington, D.C.: American Psychiatric Association, 1980.

Bee, Helen L. Parent-child interaction and distractibility in 9-year-old children. *Merrill-Palmer Quarterly,* 1967, **13**, 175–190.

Bhagavan, H. N., Coleman, M., & Coussin, D. B. The effect of pyridoxine hydrochloride on blood serotonin and pyridoxal phosphate contents in hyperactive children. *Pediatrics,* 1975, **55**, 3.

Birch, H., & Gussow, G. D. *Disadvantaged children.* New York: Grune & Stratton, 1970.

Blau, A. Mental changes following head trauma in children. *Archives of Neurology and Psychiatry,* 1936, **35**, 723–769.

Bradley, C. The behavior of children receiving benzedrine. *American Journal of Psychiatry,* 1937, **94**, 577–585.

Braud, L. W. The effects of frontal EMG biofeedback and progressive relaxation upon hyperactivity and its behavioral concomitants. *Biofeedback and Self Regulation,* 1978, **3,** 69–89.

Brodemus, J., & Swanson, J. The paradoxical effect of stimulants upon hyperactive children. *Drug Forum,* 1977–78, **2,** 117–126.

Broman, S. H. Early development and family characteristics of low achievers. Paper presented at the 14th International Conference of the Association for Children with Learning Disabilities, Washington, D.C., March 1977.

Burks, H. The hyperkinetic child. *Exceptional Children,* 1960, **27,** 18–26.

Butcher, R. Behavioral teratology. Paper presented at the University of Cincinnati Research Seminar, October 14, 1979.

Campbell, S. B. Mother-child interaction in relective, impulsive and hyperactive children. *Developmental Psychology,* 1973, **8,** 341–349.

Campbell, S. B. Mother-child interaction: A comparison of hyperactive, learning disabled and normal boys. *American Journal of Orthopsychiatry,* 1975, **45,** 51–57.

Cantwell, D. P. Psychiatric illness in the families of hyperactive children. *Archives of General Psychiatry,* 1972, **27,** 414–417.

Cantwell, D. Genetic studies of hyperactive children: Psychiatric illness in biological and adopting parents. In R. Fieve, D. Rosenthal, and H. Brill (Eds.) *Genetic research in psychiatry.* Baltimore: Johns Hopkins University Press, 1975.(a)

Cantwell, D. P. *The hyperactive child: Diagnosis, management and current research.* New York: Spectrum, 1975.(b)

Coleman, M. Serotonin concentrations in whole blood of hyperactive children. *Pediatrics,* 1971, **78,** 985–990.

Coleman, M., Greenberg, A., Bhagavan, H., Steinberg, G., Tippett, J., & Coussin, D. The role of whole blood serotonin levels in monitoring vitamin B_6 and drug therapy in hyperactive children. *Monograph of Neural Science,* 1976, **3,** 133–136.

Conners, C. K. Psychological assessment of children with minimal brain dysfunction. *Annals of New York Academy of Science,* 1973, **205,** 283.

Conners, C. K., Goyette, C. H., Southwick, D. A., Lees, J. M., & Andrulonis, P. A. Food additives and hyperkinesis: A controlled double-blind experiment. *Pediatrics,* 1976, **58,** 154–166.

Cvejic, H., & Kruger, M. Stimulant effects on cooperation and social interaction between hyperactive children and their mothers. *Journal of Child Psychology and Psychiatry,* 1978, **19,** 13–22.

David, D., Clark, J., & Voeller, K. Lead and hyperactivity. *Lancet,* October 28, 1972, 900–903.

David, O. J., Hoffman, S., & Koltun, A. Threshold levels and lead toxicity. *Psychopharmacology Bulletin,* 1978, **14,** 50–53.

de la Burde, B., & Choate, M. S. Early asymptomatic lead exposure and development at school age. *Pediatrics,* 1975, **87,** 638–642.

Drillien, C. M. *The growth and development of the prematurely born infant.* Edinburgh and London: E. S. Livingstone, 1964.

Durfee, K. E. Crooked ears and the bad boy syndrome: Asymmetry as an indicator of minimal brain dysfunction. *Bulletin of the Menninger Clinic,* 1973, **38,** 305–316.

Ebaugh, F. Neuropsychiatric sequelae of acute epidemic encephalitis in children. *American Journal of Diseases of Children,* 1923, **25,** 89–97.

Feingold, B. F. Food additives and child development (signed editorial). *Hospital Practice,* 1973, 11.

Harley, J. P., Ray, R. S., Tomasi, L., Eichman, P. L., Matthews, C. G., Chun, R., Cleeland, S., & Traisman, E. Hyperkinesis and food additives: Testing the Feingold hypothesis. *Pediatrics,* 1978, **61,** 818–828.

Harper, P. A., Fischer, L. V., & Rider, R. V. Neurological and intellectual states of prematures at three to five years of age. *Journal of Pediatrics,* 1959, **55,** 679–690.

Kenny, T. J. Hyperactivity. In H. E. Rie & E. D. Rie (Eds.), *Minimal brain dysfunction.* New York: Wiley, 1980.

226   Child Health Psychology

Kinsbourne, M. Definition and differential diagnosis of learning disabilities. Paper presented at the meeting of the International Neuropsychology Society, Toronto, February 1976.

Lambert, N., & Grossman, H. *Problems in determining the etiology of learning and behavior problems.* Sacramento: California State Department of Education, 1964.

Laufer, M. W., Denhoff, E., & Solomons, G. Hyperkinetic impulse disorder in children's behavior problems. *Psychosomatic Medicine,* 1957, **50,** 38–49.

Minde, K., Webb, G., & Sykes, D. Studies on the hyperactive child. VI: Prenatal and perinatal factors associated with hyperactivity. *Developmental Medicine and Child Neurology,* 1968, **10,** 355–363.

Minde, K., Weiss, G., & Mendelson, N. A five year follow-up study of 92 hyperactive school children. *Journal of the American Academy of Child Psychiatry,* 1972, **11,** 595–610.

Morrison, J. R., & Stewart, M. A. A family study of the hyperactive child syndrome. *Biological Psychiatry,* 1971, **3,** 189–195.

Morrison, J. R., & Stewart, M. A. Evidence for a polygenetic inheritance in the hyperactive child syndrome. *American Journal of Psychiatry,* 1973, **130,** 791–792.

Morrison, J. R., & Stewart, M. A. Bilateral inheritance as evidence for polygenicity in the hyperactive child syndrome. *Journal of Nervous and Mental Disease,* 1974, **158,** 226–228.

Needleman, H. L. Lead poisoning in children: Neurologic implications of widespread subclinical intoxication. In W. Walzer & P. H. Wolff (Eds.), *Minimal cerebral dysfunction in children.* New York: Grune & Stratton, 1973.

Ott, J. N. *Health and light.* New York: Devin-Adair, 1973.

Ott, J. N. The eyes' dual function. *Eye, Ear, Nose and Throat Monthly,* 1974, **53,** 42–60.

Pasamanick, B., Rogers, M., & Lilienfeld, A. Pregnancy experience and the development of behavior disorder in children. *American Journal of Psychiatry,* 1956, **112,** 613–619.

Perino, J., & Ernhart, C. B. The relation of subclinical lead level to cognitive and sensorimotor impairment in black preschoolers. *Journal of Learning Disabilities,* 1974, **7,** 26–30.

Rapoport, J. L., Buchsbaum, M. S., Weingartner, H., et al. Dextroamphetamine: Cognitive and behavioral effects in normal and hyperactive boys and normal adult males. *Psychopharmacology Bulletin,* 1980, **16,** 21–23.

Rapoport, J., Buchsbaum, M., & Zahn, T. Dextroamphetamine: Cognitive and behavioral effects in normal prepubertal boys. *Science,* 1978, **199,** 560–563.

Rapoport, J., Lott, I., Alexander, D., & Abramson, A. Urinary noradrenaline and playroom behavior in hyperactive boys. *Lancet,* 1970, 1141.

Rapoport, J. L., Mikkelsen, E. J., Ebert, M. H. Brown, G. L., Weise, V. K., & Kopin, I. J. *Journal of Nervous and Mental Disease,* 1978, **166,** 731–737.

Rapoport, J. L., Quinn, P. O., & Lamprecht, F. Minor physical anomalies and plasma dopamine-beta-hydroxylase activity in hyperactive boys. *American Journal of Psychiatry,* 1974, **134,** 386–390.

Rapoport, J. L., Quinn, P. Q., Scribanu, N., & Murphy, D. L. Platelet serotonin of hyperactive school age boys. *British Journal of Psychiatry,* 1974, **125,** 138–140.

Rosenfeld, G. B., & Bradley, C. Childhood behavior sequelae of asphyxia in infancy: With special reference to pertussis and asphyxia neonatorum. *Pediatrics,* 1948, **2,** 74–84.

Rutter, M. Raised lead levels and impaired cognitive-behavioral functioning: A review of the evidence. *Developmental Medicine and Child Neurology,* 1980, **22,** (supplement), 1–26.

Safer, D. A familial factor in minimal brain dysfunction. *Behavioral Genetics,* 1973, **3,** 175–186.

Sameroff, A., & Chandler, M. J. Reproductive risk and the continuum of caretaking casuality. In F. D. Horowitz (Ed.), *Review of child development research,* Vol. 4. Chicago: University of Chicago Press, 1975.

Satterfield, J., & Dawson, J. Electrodermal correlates of hyperactivity in children. *Psychophysiology,* 1971, **8,** 191–197.

Sechzen, J. A., Faro, M. D., & Windle W. F. Studies of monkeys asphyxiated at birth: Implications for minimal cerebral dysfunction. In S. Walzer & P. H. Wolf (Eds.), *Minimal cerebral dysfunction in children.* New York: Grune & Stratton, 1973.

Shaywitz, B. A., Cohen, D. J., & Bowers, M. B. CSF monoamine metabolites in children with minimal brain dysfunction: Evidence for alternative of brain dopamine. *Pediatrics,* 1977, **90,** 67–71.

Shaywitz, B. A., Klopper, J. H., & Gordon, J. W. Methylphenidate in 6-hydroxydopamine treated developing rat pups. *Archives of Neurology,* 1978, **35,** 463–469.

Shekim, W. O., Dekirmenjian, H., & Chapel, J. L. Urinary catecholamine metabolites in hyperkinetic boys treated with d-amphetamine. *American Journal of Psychiatry,* 1977, **134,** 1276–1279.

Shekim, W. O., Dekirmenjian, H., & Chapel, J. L. Urinary MHPG excretion in the hyperactive child syndrome and the effects of dextroamphetamine. *Psychopharmacology Bulletin,* 1978, **14,** 42–44.

Shetty, T., & Chase, T. M. Central monoamines and hyperkinesis of childhood. *Neurology,* 1976, **26,** 1000–1002.

Silbergeld, E. K. Neuropharmacology of hyperkinesis. *Current Developments in Psychopharmacology,* 1977, **4,** 181–214.

Stewart, M. A. Hyperactive children. *Scientific American,* 1970, **222,** 94–98.

Stewart, M. A., Pitts, F. N., Craig, A. G., & Dieruf, W. The hyperactive child syndrome. *American Journal of Orthopsychiatry,* 1966, **36,** 861–867.

Stott, D. H. The child's hazards in utero. In J. G. Howells (Ed.), *Modern perspectives in international child psychiatry.* New York: Brunner/Mazel, 1971.

Swanson, J. M., & Kinsbourne, M. Food dyes impair performance of hyperactive children on a laboratory learning test. *Science,* 1980, **207,** 1485–1486.

Waldron, H. A., & Stöfen, D. *Subclinical lead poisoning.* New York: Academic Press, 1974.

Waldrop, M. F., & Goering, J. D. Hyperactivity and minor physical anomalies in elementary school children. *American Journal of Orthopsychiatry,* 1971, **41,** 602–607.

Waldrop, M. F., Pedersen, F. A., & Bell, R. Q. Minor physical anomalies and behavior in preschool children. *Child Development,* 1968, **39,** 391–400.

Warren, R., Kardurk, W., Bussaratid, S., Stewart, M., & Sly, W. The hyperactive child syndrome. *Archives of General Psychiatry,* 1971, **24,** 161–162.

Weiss, B., Williams, J. H., Margen, S., Abrams, B., Caan, B., Citron, L. J., Cox, C., McKibben, J., Ogar, D., & Schultz, S. Behavioral responses to artificial food colors. *Science,* 1980, **207,** 1487–1488.

Weinshiboum, R. M., Kvetnansky, R., & Axelrod, J. Elevation of serum dopamine-B-hydroxylase activity with forced immobilization. *Nature,* 1971, **230,** 287–288.

Wender, P. H. Platelet-serotonin level in children with "minimal brain dysfunction." *Lancet,* November 8, 1969, 1012.

Wender, P. H. *Minimal brain dysfunction in children.* New York: Wiley-Interscience, 1971.

Wender, P. H., Epstein, R. S., Kopin, I. J., & Gordon, E. K. Urinary monoamine metabolites in children with minimal brain dysfunction. *American Journal of Psychiatry,* 1971, **127,** 1411–1415.

Werner, E. E., Bierman, J. M., & French, F. E. *The children of Kauai: A longitudinal study from the prenatal period to age ten.* Honolulu: University Press of Hawaii, 1971.

Werner, E. E., & Smith, R. S. *Kauai's children come of age.* Honolulu: University Press of Hawaii, 1977.

Werry, J. S., Sprague, R. L., Weiss, G., & Minde, K. Some clinical and laboratory studies of psychotropic drugs in children: An overview. In W. L. Smith (Ed.), *Drugs and cortical function.* Springfield, IL: Charles C. Thomas, 1970.

Zentall, S. G. Optimal stimulation as a theoretical basis of hyperactivity. *American Journal of Orthopsychiatry,* 1975, **45,** 549–563.

10

Mental Health Screening in the Public Schools: Steps Toward Prevention*

Frank Addrisi
and
Walter S. Handy, Jr.

CONSIDERATIONS IN WRITING THIS CHAPTER

In 1972 the Social Skills Development Program (SSDP) began providing systematic early identification and early secondary intervention services to primary grade children within several schools in the Cincinnati, Ohio, public school system. In 1977 it added a physical health component to its existing mental health system (Handy & Pedro-Carroll, 1980). The program's goal is to prevent later, more serious dysfunction and to promote social competence through the identification and intervention services it provides. Several key concepts that are essential in understanding a prevention program such as the SSDP—prevention, systematic mass screening, and social competence training—have proven crucial in the successful functioning of the SSDP's school-based prevention program. We believe they are crucial to the operation of any successful school-based prevention program. For this reason these three concepts are the focus for three of this chapter's four major subheadings.

While writing this chapter, one fact seemed inescapable—that we are part of a program that has been operating in the public school system for the past eight years. It seemed to us that our unique contribution lay in our daily experience with managing the SSDP over the past several years.

That experience was multifaceted and incorporated numerous activities. For the purposes of illustration, we list here several of the more salient components of our experience.

*The order of authorship was determined by the flip of a coin. This chapter was prepared under the partial support of HEW Grant no. 11-P-90468/5-03 and LEAA Grant no. 80-JJ-C03-0070.

We prepared two federal grants each year, with the attending routine progress and fiscal reporting required each grant year. We kept our fingers on the pulses of ever-changing political climates within a large city government to maintain a local funding base. Since the SSDP is a guest in its host's setting, the public school, we strove to be sensitive to our host's many needs, apart from the provision of service to children. We also attempted to maintain a vivid and positive image in the eyes of a myriad of local community groups representing a variety of vested interests. Among these are "prolife" and "prochoice," liberal and conservative, and black and white groups, as well as a diversity of cultural and economic subgroups. Also included in our experience base was the challenge of helping parents to obtain numerous services needed for their families without usurping their parental responsibilities, and therefore, interfering with their ability to use the health service network in the future. Finally, we strove to carefully wind our way through a maze of paperwork and other requirements of three large bureaucratic systems: the city government, the school system, and the health department. Tasks such as these confront any program seeking to delivery prevention services in a school system. It has been our experience— and we have also been witness to countless programs across the nation that, because they failed to lay long-range plans for confronting these issues, were laid to rest in their infancy.

In keeping with our desire to ground conceptual presentations firmly in the SSDP's experience, we do not intend to present lengthy reviews of various conceptual issues. Instead, it will be our goal to present the fundamental issues involved in mental health screening and subsequent intervention in a public school system. We will endeavor to cite recent literature for those readers who wish to pursue conceptual issues further.

In developing a framework for writing this chapter, the authors also wish to express a value for regarding the child as a whole being. We feel that the use of such dichotomous variables as physical versus psychosocial health foster divisiveness and produce gaps in research and in-service delivery programming.

We will also not attempt an extensive review of issues regarding prevention. Such discussion is presented elsewhere (e.g., Albee, 1979; Albee & Joffee, 1975; Caplan, 1964; Cowen, 1973).

Finally, while we strongly believe in the value of preventive efforts, we also value individual choice in adopting preventive health behaviors. We believe the system can facilitate the adoption of preventive health behaviors through education and consultation efforts. We view these as methods of persuasion and influence and not coercion.

PREVENTION VERSUS REMEDIATION

The history of man's preventive activities is as old as the history of man itself. Undoubtedly, many of man's early ritualistic behaviors were attempts to appease the poorly understood forces of nature, thereby to prevent blight, famine, and other natural catastrophes. Although such attempts may have seemed crude by today's standards, and were based on a primitive and often erroneous understanding of natural forces, they were nonetheless attempts at prevention.

The most frequently cited scientifically grounded prevention effort was Lord Snow's stemming of the cholera epidemic in England in the late 1800s. Lord Snow, without an understanding of the etiology of cholera, reasoned by observation that people who obtained water from a particular well inevitably contracted cholera. His preventive tactic, based on his observational data, was to shut down the well in question.

Caplan (1964) provided what seems to be the most frequently used schema for the conceptualization of preventive activities. He described preventive activities as being primary, secondary, or tertiary. Primary prevention includes those activities that seek to reduce the incidence of a given disorder. These activities are typically targeted at a "high-risk" population and are designed to forestall the occurrence of a disorder or, using educative methods, to promote growth. It is important to note that although a population may be at risk for contracting a disease, in order to qualify as a primary prevention activity the activity must target a population that has *not yet* contracted the disease.

Secondary prevention activities seek to reduce the prevalence of a disorder, and are targeted at a population which has contracted a disorder. They are designed to shorten the disorder's duration and curtail harmful aftereffects. Central to secondary prevention is the concept of early identification, since the earlier a disease is detected in its development, the more favorable will be the prognosis (Cowen, Gardner, & Zax, 1967).

Tertiary prevention activities have as their goal the reduction of impairment caused by a disorder. Tertiary activities are usually targeted at populations with chronic or irreversible disorders, and they seek to keep dysfunction to a minimum or prevent it from worsening. These activities may be considered rehabilitative inasmuch as their focus is on maintaining the individual as a productive member of society although there usually has been noticeable dysfunction. It can be argued that psychotherapy, with the possible exception of crisis intervention, is a tertiary activity.

While there have been many outspoken proponents of primary prevention (Caplan, 1961a,b, 1964; Klein & Goldston, 1977), there can be little doubt that the major focus of the energy in the mental health field has been in tertiary prevention. The percentage of the general population affected directly by mental health problems coupled with the shortage of trained professionals was highlighted in a report of the Joint Commission on Mental Illness and Health as early as 1961, and has been further elaborated by others (Albee, 1963). This report helped to enable passage of PL94-63, the Community Mental Health Center Act of 1964, which established community mental health centers that were to serve geographic areas across the nation according to federal regulations that determined size and boundaries. Among the philosophical underpinnings of this act was the recognition that mental health problems should be treated within, and not outside, the community (for example, in the state hospital), and further, that communities should become increasingly more aware of and involved with their own mental health issues (Bloom, 1968). The original act, of 1963, mandated that community mental health centers provide five major services. One of these, "consultation and education," was the service that best epitomized a preventive orientation. However, a 1974 survey of about 400 federally funded mental health centers revealed that only about 5.2 percent of staff time was devoted to this activity (Goldston, 1977). Furthermore, there is evidence that providing mental health service where none previously existed stimulates an increase in service demand rather than reducing existing demand (Gelfand, 1977; Joint Commission on Mental Health of Children, 1970). Cowen (1973), in a review looking closely at this dilemma, proffered the observation that the sum of the activities of a profession would reveal its actual conceptual focus. The data offered by Goldston (1977) is interesting in the light of Cowen's comment, and would certainly suggest that the *behavior* of mental health workers does not reflect a commitment to prevention activities.

While undoubtedly a number of factors contribute to the limited focus on prevention activities among mental health workers, we believe that the traditional graduate school education and the lack of both conceptual clarity about and empirical support for prevention activities are major contributors. The traditional emphasis in the graduate training of psychiatrists, psychologists, and social workers is on providing treatment for individuals identified as "disordered." This clearly places the advanced training historically offered by these disciplines in the arena of tertiary and secondary prevention, or in what Cowen (1977) has labeled a "casualty-repair orientation." So long as we continue to focus our training on "casualty-repair," there is little reason to believe that the vast majority of mental health professionals will adopt an alternative orientation.

The second problem is even more plaguing than the first. Here we must agree with Cowen's (1977) observation that mental health workers are often imprecise in labeling their programs as primary or secondary prevention and that, furthermore, there are very few empirically documented examples of primary prevention programs with a substantiated positive outcome for their participants. We believe that the reasons for this include interventions that are vague in their applications and often have no clear relationship to a theoretical base (Peterson, Hartmann, & Gelfand, 1980); programs with vague, unclear objectives or, as is often the case, no objectives at all; and, finally, programs that are not carefully evaluated, or for which evaluation is an afterthought (applied *post hoc*), often using a dependent measure with little relevance to the program goals. All of these shortcomings have as a common element a lack of precision and ample forethought in program design such that program staff are not clear regarding what is to be accomplished with what group of people, or what the theoretical basis is for believing that the program will work. This is an unfortunate state of affairs, which others have suggested excellent strategies for overcoming (Bloom, 1968). Finally, there simply are no good examples to show that primary prevention programming has lived up to its original expectations in terms of savings in either human suffering or economic cost.

With the aforementioned in mind, we would like to argue the merits of early secondary prevention as indeed "a step toward prevention." Compared to primary prevention, early secondary prevention has two advantages to be considered: the conceptual appropriateness of a school-based population for a preventive focus, and the accessibility of a school-based population for preventive programming.

The Appropriateness of Targeting Prevention Activities for Primary Grade Children

We are neither the first nor the only ones to advocate the appropriateness of prevention activities targeted at young, school-age children. Cowen et al. (1967) concluded that both the family and school were prime targets for preventive endeavors. The Joint Commission on Mental Health of Children (1970) suggested that "schools have a tremendous potential for enhancing the mental health of all children who attend them, preventing the development of serious emotional disorders, and improving the condition of those children who are already suffering from such difficulties [p. 383]." They go on to point out that many children experience difficulty in making the transition from home to school, a transition that is important in shaping the child's adjustment in general but especially to school. If this transition is not managed effectively, it can have a cumulative effect on the child's overall development.

Although we would agree with Cowen et al. (1967) that the family is an appropriate target for prevention activities, whole families are often more difficult to involve in preventive activities than are schoolchildren, and it is more costly to structure effective programs for the former than for the latter. Further, effective involvement with families requires an understanding of the complex dynamics that usually accompany a family's functioning as a unit. It is often difficult for a professional not experienced in family work to wade through this complexity in an effective way. It would be more difficult, if not impossible, for a paraprofessional to do so without extensive and expensive training. Obviously one could rely on trained family therapists, but this increases cost and raises the problem of human resource shortage.

In addition to these reasons of outreach, cost, and complexity of interventions, there is the additional consideration that adjusting to school is, *by itself*, a serious challenge for many children. Indeed, as Glidewell and Swallow (1969) point out, school maladaptation may affect as many as 30 percent of all school children. With so many affected negatively in ways that are cumulative, we must argue strenuously for the appropriateness of school-based prevention.

Early Secondary Prevention: The Practical Advantage

One major difficulty faced by school-based prevention programs is the "squeaky wheel phenomenon"—in less catchy phraseology, the expectation that the children who will be provided services first will be those identified by teachers and principals.

Three additional considerations result from this phenomenon. First, children identified as a priority by school staff are apt to be seriously disturbed and severely disruptive children whose behavioral problems might be identified as "acting out." Reliance on the traditional method of identification and referral will very likely result in a situaton where school staff will overlook the child who sits passively or in a withdrawn fashion. This child, who is least likely to be perceived as disruptive, may need services to the same extent as the acting-out child, however.

Second, since it is almost always the case that service needs far outstrip service resources, we would argue that limited resources will have a better payoff if applied to the moderately maladaptive child than to the seriously maladaptive child. Finally, a major practical advantage of an early secondary prevention program compared to a primary preventive program is that it does deal with children who, despite some controversy, are likely to be viewed by school staff as needing services. In the SSDP we have found this to be extremely important in securing and cementing a positive relationship with school staff. Although a controversy often exists regarding the specific children to be seen, and in what order, it is less problematic, we believe, in an early secondary prevention program than it might be in a primary prevention program. The difficulty that often becomes pronounced in primary prevention programs centers around complaints by school staff that such programs fail to make their lives easier because they do not deal directly with children who are clearly disruptive and consume a lot of teachers' time and energy.

A second potential problem lies in the school staff's expectation that results will be immediately forthcoming. School staff are often unwilling to accept on faith that two or three years from the initiation of the intervention a child will not be a behavior problem. Teaching, especially in inner city schools, is a demanding, lonely, and stressful job, and teachers expect help immediately, not in three years (Sarason, Levine, Goldenberg, Cherlin, & Bennett, 1966). The SSDP's experience, not unlike that of similar programs (Cowen, Trost, Lorion, Dorr, Izzo, & Isaacson, 1975), has been that observable change does occur in children within a given school year and that teachers respond very positively to these results (Kirschenbaum, Marsh, & DeVoge, 1979). Again, the practical advantage of this situation must be stressed. The teacher's expectations are often met and this positively influences the relationship between SSDP staff and school staff. The result of this positive impact is that teachers become more willing to collaborate in an intervention plan with the prevention staff.

A final issue regarding school-based prevention programs is that of cultural diversity. It would be far easier if the role of cultural diversity were an issue limited just to the children we serve; alas, it becomes manifest in at least a three-way interaction involving the children served, the school staff, and the program staff. As the report of the Joint Commission on Mental Health of Children (1970) clearly pointed out, poverty and being a member of a minority group pose special problems for children in terms of physical and mental health, availability of services of nearly all kinds, racism, and adaptation to the school environment. If a particular school represents a social institution complete with a culture of its own, then the culture of the school produces attitudinal and behavioral expectations to which elementary-grade children are expected to conform. In many cases the child has been acculturated to a very different set of values and adaptive behaviors than those that prevail in the typical middle-class school (Joint Commission on Mental Health of Children, 1970). Many children faced with the task of modifying several years of cultural adaptation in order to fit into this new environment experience potentially debilitating conflict. The potential conflict the child experiences may be eased or intensified by the school staff's sensitivity to the cultural incongruence facing many children. For many children there is no underlying "personality flaw" or inherent weakness in their development thus far. Acculturation to the school setting becomes a task which they may be doomed to fail, due to the often uncompromising dissonance between the cultural expectations of the school staff and those of their families and neighbors. Their school years often become thoroughly negative experiences, and the conflict produced by this dissonance may accumulate until it reaches a pitch where children (usually by now teenagers) either drop out of school or experience such conflict with the school staff that they are expelled.

What becomes crucial now is that prevention specialists (with their own cultural expectations) have some degree of understanding and acceptance of the cultural background of both the child and the school staff. We have found in the SSDP, for instance, that while "gutsiness" was conceptualized by Gesten (1976) as an example of competence, it correlates directly with "acting out" in the view of many Cincinnati schoolteachers. The SSDP staff, however, tend to view "gutsiness," as did Gesten, as an appropriate behavior and as a skill to be taught and reinforced. This poses a dilemma for SSDP staff with respect to rewarding gutsiness, which is almost assuredly an appropriate skill in the neighborhoods of most low-income children but may be seen as acting out by school staff when displayed within the school setting. The problem then becomes one of rewarding gutsiness in the child while simultaneously teaching the child to discriminate between environments in which it is differentially appropriate. Obviously, it is not sufficient to treat only the child in these situations but also to work with teachers in helping them understand and be sensitive to cultural diversity (Handy & Pedro-Carroll, 1980).

MASS SCREENING

Mass screening is often misunderstood, and more often than not has a negative connotation. Often it seems to call up fantasies of herding children like cattle through some impersonal, ineffectual process. Undoubtedly there have been and are still occasions where reality has approximated this fantasy. Even in these cases one will usually find an inadequate, erroneous understanding of the concept on the part of the parties responsible for conducting the screening program. What then is mass screening and, more important, what does it seek to achieve? What would constitute a good mass screening program?

Screening is an activity that inspects a group of individuals for purposes of assignation to two or more subgroups. Mass screening means that the screening activity is applied to virtually all members of a large group. While the term "screening" does not by itself usually carry a negative connotation, when one adds the word "mass" negative connotations emerge. The basis for this effect appears to lie in an association with inferiority ("since it involves such large numbers, it can't be any good"); also, to be identified as "different" often carries the implication that one is abnormal or imperfect (Hodge, Struckmann, & Trost, 1975). The label "impersonal" conveys the sense that "since the group is so large, I will be just another face in the crowd, and if so, my *essence* cannot be known." Both of these assumptions are logically fallacious. First, because an activity is large-scale does not mean it is inferior; conversely, there are many small-scale activities that are of decidedly poor quality. Second, there are many activities for which an intimate knowledge of the participants is unnecessary to accomplish the stated goal.

Recast within the framework of a secondary prevention program, mass screening may be defined as an activity that systematically inspects a large number of individuals to identify those individuals who are showing early signs of a disorder. In the SSDP's case, screening identifies those children who exhibit a deficit in social skills or who reveal early signs of difficulty in adapting to school. This is not unlike inspection in order to assign the individual to one of two groups, with the further refinement that additional, more intensive inspection occurs at a later point.

Before proceeding to a more detailed description of the SSDP's screening process and considerations in undertaking any screening process, there are two conceptual issues that warrant further exploration. These issues involve the ultimate purpose of a screening program and the relationship between screening assessment and intervention.

It must be firmly stressed that, conceptually, screening is *not* designed to be a terminal activity. Screening should never be undertaken simply to identify. Once identification has occurred, there *should* always be some action that follows. We emphasize the "should" because it is for overlooking this emphasis that many programs have been criticized. Applied to school-based programs, this translates into the principle that screening should only occur to head off or mitigate a disorder. Screening, thèrefore, should be applied only in cases where the disorder is detectable and treatable. It might also be argued that screening should only be undertaken for disorders that, if left untreated, would result in chronic handicapping conditions. There is ample evidence that it is possible to detect children in the primary grades who are exhibiting early signs of disorders that, if left untreated, will become progressively more serious (Cowen, Peder-son, Babigian, Izzo, & Trost, 1973). If this were not the case there would be little reason to screen and treat, since it would not make a substantial difference and would make even less sense from a cost standpoint. However, in cases where not providing service does appear to result in progressive deterioration, a screening method would be desirable which erred in the direction of identifying some false positives while minimizing the miss or false negative rate. Under these conditions, screened children would be assessed (not screened since this has occurred already) to determine if they were correctly identified. If they were, assessment procedures would delineate the nature of the difficulty and form the basis for an intervention plan. We must stress that, in our view, screening is not equivalent to assessment. Screening activities merely categorize children into two groups: those that appear to be adapting and those who are having difficulty doing so. Once this gross categorization has been accomplished, it is necessary to assess each child in the latter group in order to delineate clearly and accurately the nature of the adaptation difficulty, if there is one. Although the SSDP favors a behavioral assessment for several reasons, the key issue is that once screening has taken place, assessment of some type is a necessary although not sufficient condition for successful intervention.

There are a number of ways to screen primary grade children for early signs of behavioral maladaptation: days absent, grade point average, various teacher ratings, various scales administered to the child, achievement test scores, peer nominations, various forms of behavior observation, parent ratings, and so forth. In an attempt to critically evaluate the relative efficacy of some 24 indices used to identify maladaptive children, researchers (Cowen et al., 1973) concluded that the single best predictor was peer sociometric ratings. We feel, however, that use of peer sociometric data presents practical difficulties sufficient to deter implementation, and that other methods of identification are more practical.

The SSDP has relied on various forms of teacher identification, on the assumption that the classroom teacher knows best how well a child is functioning. This is especially true if a structured method is used to secure the teacher's impressions. Over its eight-year history, the SSDP has used two methods, each of which offers its own advantages.

The AML. One method employs the use of the AML, an 11-item questionnaire developed by the Primary Mental Health Project (PMHP) under the direction of Emory Cowen (Beach, Cowen, Zax, Laird, Trost, & Izzo, 1968; Cowen et al., 1973). The questionnaire contains five items that identify acting-out children (A), five items that identify shy-moody-withdrawn children (M), and one item that identifies children with learning problems (L). Over the years PMHP has gathered extensive data on the reliability and validity of this instrument, as well as extensive normative data. Teachers are asked to complete the AML on every child in their classrooms. Once completed the AML is scored and, using normative data as a guide, children are identified or "screened in" using a combination of their subscale and total scale scores. Although the SSDP has found the AML to be a very effective screening tool (Kirschenbaum et al., 1977), teachers have raised complaints about having to complete an AML on some 30 to 45 children in each class. Complaints from teachers about the amount of time they were required to spend completing AMLs made us concerned that this would lead teachers to complete AMLs hurriedly or in other undesirable ways. In addition, the AML focuses exclusively on children's problems and not on their strengths, skills, or competencies. For these reasons some thought was given to an alternative screening procedure that was equally reliable.

The social competence interview. Because of the cited disadvantages of the AML, the SSDP developed the social competence interview. This method is less time-consuming for teachers and also requires that a teacher focus on and identify not only maladaptive behavior but also skills and competencies. The procedure requires that an SSDP staff member meet with a teacher and explain to the teacher the meaning of the competence construct. This is accomplished by explaining both the definition of competence in an abstract way and by citing specific behaviors as examples of high and low competence. Specific examples cited are, for instance, self-care behavior, assertive versus subassertive versus aggressive behavior, impulsivity, communication skills, and self-esteem. Once teachers understand the concept and can apply it specifically, they are asked to rank order the five children that they see as least competent in their classrooms and the three children seen as most competent. They then cite specific behaviors in these eight children that are deemed to be examples of high and low competence and led to the respective rank orderings. We have found this method to correspond closely to AML ratings, with low competent children falling in the screened-in range on the AML and high competent children tending to fall outside of the screened-in range. Teachers report that this is a less demanding task and more enjoyable than struggling through AML after AML. Although the task does not require less time, there appears to be a distinctly perceived difference in terms of enjoyment versus drudgery. In addition, teachers are required to consider the skills that the screened-in children possess as well as their deficits.

It is important to note that systematic screening is not the same as a traditional reliance on referrals. Kirschenbaum et al. (1977) found that systematic screening identified 1.5 times as many children than would have been identified through a traditional referral process. Also, a referral process, as stated previously, functions reasonably well in identifying the acting-out child, but is very likely to overlook the shy, withdrawn child who sits quietly and does not disrupt the classroom or otherwise menace the teacher or other children.

A final note: neither the AML nor the social competence interview require administration by a trained professional. The AML is straightforward, with instructions printed on the top of the questionnaire. The social competence interview is a bit more complex, inasmuch as it might be potentially influenced by instructional set. We have found it necessary to conduct four to six hours of training with our paraprofessional staff in order to achieve a satisfactory level of standardization of administration across staff. This involves about two to three hours of didactic training in the social competence construct and its expression in specific behaviors. Beyond this, another two to three hours of *in vivo* supervised administration is required for the paraprofessionals to achieve a satisfactory level of performance.

The potential savings in cost using paraprofessional rather than professional staff to conduct screening are substantial. For instance, two paraprofessional staff working part-time, after training and some experience, can screen as many children as one full-time professional staff member. Assume conservatively that the paraprofessional earns half as much as the professional on an hourly basis. This difference in hourly pay coupled with the part-time versus full-time status will result in a savings of about 50 percent of the professional's salary. In addition, the part-time paraprofessional can be hired for nine months, whereas it is rare for a professional to be willing to work on such a basis. This will result in an additional savings, which, combined with the pay difference, comes to about a 65 percent savings in salary. Finally, full-time employees must be paid fringe benefits, whereas part-time employees are usually not. Today most fringe packages run to 22 to 28 percent of an employee's salary. Adding the savings in fringe monies to the previous savings brings the total savings to about 72 percent of the professional's salary. In other words, to accomplish the same task, two half-time paraprofessionals will cost about 72 percent less than one full-time professional. In this age of shrinking budgets and increased demand for accountability, this savings can become substantial when reporting unit costs or cost-effectiveness figures to grantors or politicians controlling the purse strings.

INTERVENTIONS: SOCIAL SKILLS TRAINING
REPLACES COUNSELING

In conducting the Social Skills Development Program, we continued a tradition that emphasizes the development of competence and social skills (Cowen et al., 1967; Cowen, Dorr, & Orgel, 1971; Foster & Ritchey, 1979; White, 1959; Zigler & Trickett, 1978), rather than embracing the more traditional psychopathological conceptualizations of cure, rehabilitiaton, and sickness. Two broad concerns guide our preference. First, our wish is to minimize the stigma (Goffman, 1963) attributed to children identified by our mass screening procedures. Second, our preference is for viewing inappropriate behaviors from a framework of competence rather than sickness or deviation.

Researchers (Peterson, Hartman, & Gelfand, 1980) have for some time been aware of the potential dangers inherent in implementing early intervention programs. One of the primary dangers lies in the process of identification of and intervention with high-risk children: such identification and intervention activities may unintentionally label and stigmatize the child. Typical identification procedures have involved obtaining the assistance of local staff to complete rating scales and to meet with the early intervention staff for consultation. Early identification procedures have targeted children who often had not been previously identified as problem children or even potential problem children. Once they are so identified by their teachers and peers, the development of additional problems may be an unfortunate by-product of early identification activities (Gemunder & Handy, 1980). Our preference is, therefore, to identify these children as manifesting deficits in social skills rather than as sick or maladjusted children. The risk of unintentional labeling is reduced further by casting a deficit in social skills as emerging from a difficulty in adapting to a difference between the home culture and that of the school.

Our second reason for preferring a skills- or competence-based conceptual model lies within a comparison of the connotations of the terms "skills deficit" versus "psychopathological disorder." The former more easily allows an educational approach to interventions, while the latter requires an application of the assumptions of a restorative model. Among the school staff this language system makes a difference: an educational approach connotes optimism and change, whereas a restorative approach usually connotes pessimism and illness management. An additional advantage to viewing children within a preventive, educational model lies in the ease of shifting between the types of prevention (primary, secondary, and tertiary). While all children may be veiwed within the above language structure, the behaviors manifested by the children may be viewed as skill repertoires, and the intervention may take the form of assisting the children in both unlearning socially inappropriate behaviors and learning and strengthening socially appropriate behaviors.

As has been argued elsewhere (Cowen, 1973), the SSDP has relied heavily on paraprofessionals as change agents. It has been demonstrated in a recent literature review that paraprofessionals function as effective change agents (Durlak, 1979). However, paraprofessional helping agents must be selected, trained, and supervised if they are to be maximally effective. Specific suggestions for the conduct of these three activities will be outlined for the reader's consideration.

Selection may be the most important of the above activities. Whatever extra effort and care is expended in the selection process will pay dividends later in quality services, fewer personnel problems, and fewer crises in the schools for the professional to devote his or her time and energy to resolving. A modified version of the attributes suggested elsewhere have proven vital to the SSDP's selection process (Cowen et al., 1973; Sandler, 1972). These characteristics are:

- *Empathy for children.* Shows an ability to empathize with children.
- *Personal warmth.* Seems personally warm, as opposed to rigid, aloof, or distant.
- *Sensitivity to cultural differences.* Shows an understanding that culture influences one's view of the appropriateness of a given behavior.
- *Sensitivity to individual differences.* Is accepting of individual differences among people.
- *Ability to work with others.* Gives evidence of ability to work cooperatively with others.
- *Ability to function independently.* Seems capable of acting independently when required by the situation.
- *Ability to adapt to new situations.* Appears capable of adapting to new situations and new roles.
- *Sound personal adjustment.* Appears to be well adjusted and free of any but minor personal problems.
- *Ability to adapt to new learning experiences.* Is open and oriented to new learning experiences.
- *Ability to engage in active listening.* Incorporates into conversations the meaning of what others say.
- *Energy level and enthusiasm toward project.* Is enthusiastic, eager, and interested in working in this type of setting.

In our own selection interview, some characteristics are assessed directly with structured questions (ability to work with others, empathy for children), while others are assessed through attention to the interview process itself (personal warmth, ability to engage in active listening). We also use a team interview, which includes a senior child aide, a professional who would directly supervise the aide once hired, and a senior member of the core program staff. This procedure has provided a more diverse view of the candidate than would be possible with a smaller and less heterogeneous group of interviewers. We also use a simple seven-point rating scale for each characteristic. Each of the three interviewers independently rates a candidate on each of the characteristics and jots down comments as necessary. After each interview the ratings and comments are discussed and a decision is made about hiring the applicant.

Training is the next task that must be accomplished. Our goal in training the aides is to provide them with a common language and foundation on which to base ongoing supervision. Training is not a replacement for clinical supervision but only provides a diverse group of people with a common starting point. Over the past three years, we have developed training seminars dealing with the following topic areas:

Session 1. (a) Overview of training goals
            (b) Getting acquainted
            (c) Orientation to SSDP and public school system
Session 2. (a) Communication skills/Active listening
            (b) Cultural and racial awareness
Session 3. (a) Screening model
            (b) Social competence/Social skills model
Session 4   (a) Developmental issues/Assessment
            (b) Developing an intervention plan
Session 5. Intervention techniques
Session 6. (a) Charting
            (b) Referral resources
            (c) Summary/Review

We have found that, after the initial training thrust, regular monthly meetings of all the aides helps to maintain enthusiasm among the group and provides an adjunct to regular supervision. Ongoing supervision is provided on a routine basis by master's-level staff once training has been completed.

As was documented earlier, not only does use of paraprofessional staff greatly extend the resources of the professional staff, but it does so in a highly cost-effective manner. An additional savings results from our experience that professionals tend to spend more time in meetings than do paraprofessionals. We will not pose reasons for this, since professional staff tend to decry having to attend many meetings. Nonetheless, we have found that professionals tend to meet prior to implementing an action decision, while paraprofessionals tend to simply act. As a result, paraprofessionals produce higher rates of time spent in direct service than professionals, another reason why use of paraprofessionals reduces administrative overhead costs and yields budget figures that are more cost-effective.

SPECIAL CONCERNS

It would behoove aspiring prevention specialists desirous of displaying their wares in a school setting to be aware of the following potential troublespots: first, the preference on the part of school staff for remedial rather than prevention services; second, the belief on the part of school staff and special program staff alike that each knows exclusively how best to bring about change in the social skills deficits of identified children; third, the likelihood that school staff will often feel overwhelmed by the regular demands of their jobs and therefore may view additional demands on their time as unwanted intrusions; fourth, the likelihood that a special program will often be perceived as embodying implicit, and sometimes explicit, assumptions that if the school staff were doing their jobs, special programming would not be necessary; fifth, the corresponding view held by school staff that they are being singled out by outsiders both because they are viewed as somehow not doing their jobs and because the outsiders do not understand the system; and last, the acknowledgment by both the prevention staff and the school staff that special programming is just that, special: special programs are likely to be short-lived, while school staff have to live with both the educational and geographic communities and the remnants of special programs.

These issues, taken individually or collectively, represent potentially problematic variations in the expectations of the school staff and prevention staff. Because of their importance, three of these issues have been selected for further discussion here.

It is clear to even the casual observer that school teachers have their hands full in attempting to both impart academic knowledge and socialize their classroom pupils. The classroom setting has, however, been long regarded as the province of the classroom teacher, and within that setting the teacher may often be called upon to attend to the disruptive and problematic child rather than to the children who do not call attention to themselves. That is, the teacher is forced into a nonproductive cycle of attending to the disruptive child in order to be able to teach the class but then having insufficient time left to do so adequately. Classroom teachers are also often rated on their ability to control their classes.

Control issues are often more salient with the severely disruptive child than with the passive or minimally disruptive child. Thus if additional help is available to classroom teachers, their preference may be for remedial (secondary or tertiary) interventions. Many teachers even prefer to have such pupils permanently removed from their classes. It is little wonder, then, that teachers often regard primary or early secondary prevention programs as at best superfluous and at worst a waste of their time. Anecdotal evidence suggests that the SSDP's early identification and intervention efforts were best received initially by teachers who had seen the program work or who had been told by peers that it worked, that is, when the program was seen as meeting the needs of school staff in working with problematic children.

The second and third issues for discussion here are the longer-term impact of special programming on the school community and the perceived devaluation of school staff by the presence of special programming. For some time teachers have been expected by society fo fulfill complex socialization and instructional functions. In addition, administrative functions directly and indirectly connected with instruction have increased dramatically. Faced with such expanding and complex responsibilities, teachers have, in recent years, been assisted by a spate of special programs. Programs such as the Social Skills Development Program that focus on, for instance, effective education have received considerable attention over the past few years (Allen, Chinsky, Larcen, Lochman, & Selinger, 1976; Spivack & Shure, 1974). While few would argue against the value of this type of special programming, a relatively small number of such programs (Gesten, Flores de Apodaca, Rains, Weissberg, & Cowen, 1979) have been institutionalized. As a direct result of the failure of such programs to be institutionalized, they are still viewed as "special programming," and occasionally as a nuisance. Often, after having offered services to which the community grows accustomed, they leave abruptly, due to funding cutbacks or for a variety of other reasons. It is then the job of the school staff to explain to the community why the service is no longer available. This may be a difficult task, since the distinction between regular and special programming is clear to school staff but is not always a distinction made by the community. For many parents the distinction between special and regular programs is irrelevant; the school is the school. Even if the distinction is made, it is easier to direct one's frustrations and disappointments at the local school down the block than at a vague entity called "the administration."

As was alluded to earlier in the text, an early intervention program will be effective to the extent that differential expectations between the major protagonists are reduced or at least recognized. More than likely, both the school staff and the program staff bring valid observations to their interactions. Problems arise and become impediments to service when differing opinions are not discussed or negotiated and compromises are not reached. Most often it is the intended clients, the children at risk, that suffer from such failure to communicate. These children are placed in the position of negotiating between countervailing factions, and attempting to do so with communication skills that are acknowledged by all parties as ineffective.

The Social Skills Development Program has managed to minimize these difficulties by maintaining ongoing communications with school staff. Inappropriate behaviors that are particularly troublesome to the classroom teacher are often the content of ongoing consultation between the teacher and program staff. An attempt is made to focus the SSDP interventions on behavioral goals that both enhance prosocial behaviors and minimize the frequency and severity of inappropriate behaviors.

In addition, the SSDP alleviates the problem of being viewed with suspicion as "outsiders" by housing its staff in office space within the school to which it will deliver services during the school year. SSDP staff are thus available to school staff to assist in handling difficult classroom situations and to assist the teachers, at their request, in general classroom management techniques. These office arrangements also help to foster ongoing communication.

RECOGNITION OF CULTURAL COMPETENCE AS A PART OF INTERVENTION EFFORTS

Competence conceptualizations of behaviors often alter the value-laden thinking that infects the traditional problem-oriented literature. The "deficit hypothesis" is a primary example of such value-laden thought as applied to ethnic minorities. The "deficit hypothesis" involves the presumption that any differences found in comparisons of ethnic minority samples and Caucasian samples must be attributed to a central, if not genetic, flaw or "deficit" in the ethnic minority population. Such presumptions totally ignore the pluralistic contributions of cultural relativism. That is, "deficit hypothesis" thinking fails to take into consideration the fact that differences found between such samples must be interpreted in the total cultures (physical, social, cognitive, and so forth) of the respective populations. A shift from problem-oriented approaches to competence approaches does not ensure the application of pluralistic or culturally relevant conceptualizations and interventions, but it does seem to change the focus to the strengths of the minority population, and thereby make consideration of the relevant cultural background of the subjects of the investigation or intervention more likely. However, unless specific attention is paid to issues of cultural values and practices, a competence approach with children may also ignore these variables.

Within the school setting, then, attention is paid to subcultural norms operating within the local ethnic and geographic communities. When children and teachers from different communities meet and interact with each other, difficulties in expectations and communications often arise. It may be said that the development of adaptability in novel social situations represents but one among a number of important developmental tasks. Many teachers and children, however, find such multicultural social transitions outside of their adaptive capacity. By focusing explicitly on such transitions, the SSDP fosters awareness and expression of cultural differences within the total school population.

It is our belief that a substantial proportion of the behaviors that lead a child to be regarded as maladapting to a school environment are behaviors that are deemed socially inappropriate in other (home or community, or both) settings. Thus instead of regarding the child's behaviors as bad, we would propose, these behaviors should be regarded within a cultural competence framework. Within this framework such behaviors should be examined for their functional utility in nonschool settings; if they are found to be "appropriate," explicit attempts would be made to point out to the child the differences between the behavioral expectations of the home or community setting and the related behavioral expectations of the school setting. Alternative approaches to the "problem situation" in school would then be evolved and taught to the child.

Further, we believe that the construct of "culture," especially group norms, helps to explain some observed differences in the matching of behavior to situations. Following the definition proposed by Banks (1979), culture is "behavior patterns, symbols, institutions, values and other human-made components of society [p. 338]."

That Putallaz and Gottman (1982) have included awareness of group norms, and by extension cultural norms, in their definition of social competence is further justification for our thrust to acculturate discussions of social competence training. Banks (1979) and many others (Cheek, 1976; Gibbs, 1974; Handy, Rawlings, & Jackson, 1979; Handy & Pedro-Carroll, 1979; Hayles, 1977; Obidinski, 1978; Olmedo, 1979) have argued that there are many sub- or microcultures within this country's macroculture, each with its own distinctive behavioral group norms, values, and expectations. A child's lack of knowledge of the behavioral implementation of such diverse group norms increases the likelihood that she or he will fail to form the friendship patterns that are important both to school adjustment and later life. Similarly, if children are unaware of a teacher's expectations for their behavior, they are at risk of not conforming to those expectations and thus of being labeled "problem children." Teachers' failure to make explicit their expectations of appropriate classroom behavior is even more likely to result in children being viewed as "maladaptive" when there are marked discrepancies between home-community and school expectations. Mutually rewarding social interactions require that the child be knowledgeable and capable of behaving in ways that are appropriate in each setting. Divergent cultural norms and values often mean that different behaviors will be seen as appropriate in ostensibly similar settings. Accordingly, the concept of cultural competence (Ogbu, 1981) and, more specifically, the concept of multicultural competence warrant further consideration by others.

CONCLUSIONS AND FUTURE DIRECTIONS

Within this chapter we have touched upon our approach to writing this manuscript and then proceeded to discuss issues of prevention versus remediation, mass screening, our approach to social skills intervention, special concerns, and last, the expanding role of cultural considerations within the provision of social competence training. The experience of offering early identification and intervention services within school settings has obviously had its complexities. Such intricacies notwithstanding, the authors find such programming both personally and professionally rewarding.

In our estimation, for both fiscal and conceptual reasons such early, school-based intervention models represent extremely viable alternatives for future child health programming. To promote awareness and serious consideration of such programming, the Social Skills Development Program and the Primary Mental Health Project (PMHP) (Cowen, Dorr, Izzo, Madonia, & Trost, 1971; Zax & Cowen, 1967) have recently entered into a cooperative agreement to disseminate the model. Dissemination activities include the hosting of national training workshops and internship experiences, program consultations, and, most recently, consultations with state-level departments of education, mental health, and health. The goal of such consultations is ultimately to promote institutionalization of this school-based early intervention model, initially in the form of one or more pilot projects in each state. The rationale (Swift, 1980; Tableman, 1980) and implementation of such efforts (Cowen, 1980; Cowen, Davidson, & Gesten, 1980; Cowen, Gesten, & Weissberg, 1980; Cowen, Spinell, Wright, & Weissberg, 1982) have been well documented. According to recent communications (Cowen, 1981), the state of California has enacted a law to support the development of PMHP-type programs within that state. The passage of this law is a legislative first and makes possible the establishment of a network of active PMHP-type programs in California. Thus we end this chapter with a firm faith in the future of this model, and an invitation to readers to review the evidence of our experience as well as the prolific evidence of the experiences of many others and, if convinced of the potency of this model, to search for ways to implement such models on their own turf.

EDITORS' NOTE

We trust that readers will not find it difficult to extend the ideas contained in this chapter (early mass screening and prevention and the use of paraprofessionals in a school-based program) to problems that appear more obviously "medical" or illness-related. Neither the editors nor the chapter authors endorse a dualistic perspective. Therefore, the case for prevention of psychological and social dysfunctions is also the case for prevention of organic disorders. Further, as noted in Chapter Two, social competence and health competence may be closely intertwined.

REFERENCES

Albee, G. W. American psychology in the sixties. *American Psychologist,* 1963, **18,** 90–95.
Albee, G. W. Primary prevention. *Canada's Mental Health,* 1979, **27,** 5–9.

Albee, G. W., & Joffee, J. M. (Eds.) *The primary prevention of psychopathology: The issues.* Hanover, N.H.: University Press of New England, 1975.

Allen, G. J., Chinsky, J. M., Larcen, S. W., Lochman, J. E., & Selinger, H. V. *Community psychology and the schools: A behaviorally oriented multi-level preventive approach.* Hillsdale, N.J.: Lawrence Erlbaum, 1976.

Banks, J. A. Shaping the future of multicultural education. *Journal of Negro Education,* 1979, **48,** 337–352.

Beach, D. R., Cowen, E. L., Zax, M., Laird, J. D., Trost, M. A., & Izzo, L. D. Objectification of a screening procedure for early detection of emotional disorder. *Child Development,* 1968, **39,** 1177–1188.

Bloom, B. L. The evaluation of primary prevention programs. In L. M. Roberts, N. S. Greenfield, & M. H. Miller (Eds.), *Comprehensive mental health: The challenge of evaluation.* Madison, Wis.: University of Wisconsin Press, 1968.

Campbell, D. T., & Stanley, J. C. *Experimental and quasi-experimental designs for research.* Chicago: Rand McNally, 1963.

Caplan, G. *An approach to community mental health.* New York: Grune & Stratton, 1961. (a)

Caplan, G. (Ed.) *Prevention of mental disorders in children.* New York: Basic Books, 1961. (b)

Caplan, G. *Principles of preventive psychiatry.* New York: Basic Books, 1964.

Cheek, D. *Assertive black . . . puzzled white.* San Luis Obispo, Calif.: Impact Publishers, 1976.

Cowen, E. L. The effectiveness of secondary prevention programs using nonprofessionals in the school setting. *Proceedings, 76th Annual Convention, APA,* 1968, **2,** 705–706.

Cowen, E. L. Social and community interventions. *Annual Review of Psychology,* 1973, **24,** 423–472.

Cowen, E. L. Primary prevention misunderstood. *Social Policy,* 1977, **7,** 20–27.

Cowen, E. L. The primary mental health project: Yesterday, today and tomorrow. *Journal of Special Education,* 1980, **14,** 133–154.

Cowen, E. L., Davidson, E., & Gesten, E. L. Program dissemination and the modification of delivery practices in school mental health. *Professional Psychology,* 1980, **11,** 36–47.

Cowen, E. L., Dorr, D., Izzo, L. D., Madonia, A., & Trost, M. A. The primary mental health project: A new way of conceptualizing and delivering school mental health services. *Psychology in the Schools,* 1971, **8,** 216–225.

Cowen, E. L., Dorr, D., & Orgel, A. R. Interrelations among screening measures for early detection of school dysfunction. *Psychology in the Schools,* 1971, **5,** 135–139.

Cowen, E. L., Dorr, D., & Pokracki, F. Selection of non-professional child-aides for a school mental health project. *Community Mental Health Journal,* 1972, **8,** 220–226.

Cowen, E. L., Gardner, E. A., & Zax, M. (Eds.) *Emergent approaches to mental health problems.* New York: Appleton-Century-Crofts, 1967.

Cowen, E. L., Gesten, E. L., & Weissberg, R. P. An interrelated network of preventively oriented school based mental health approaches. In R. H. Price & P. Politzer (Eds.), *Evaluation and action in the community context.* New York: Academic Press, 1980.

Cowen, E. L., Pederson, A., Babigian, H., Izzo, L. D., & Trost, M. A. Long-term follow-up of early detected vulnerable children. *Journal of Consulting and Clinical Psychology,* 1973, **41,** 438–446.

Cowen, E. L., Spinell, A., Wright, S., & Weissberg, R. P. Continuing dissemination of a school-based mental health program. Unpublished manuscript, 1982.

Cowen, E. L., Trost, M. A., Lorion, R. P., Dorr, D., Izzo, L. D., & Isaacson, R. V. *New ways in school mental health: Early detection and prevention of school maladapatation.* New York: Human Sciences Press, 1975.

Durlak, J. Comparative effectiveness of paraprofessional and professional helpers. *Psychological Bulletin,* 1979, **86,** 80–92.

Foster, S. L., & Ritchey, W. L. Issues in the assessment of social competence in children. *Journal of Applied Behavior Analysis,* 1979, **12,** 625–638.

Gelfand, D. M. Prevention: Why must we change our priorities? Presentation to the Association for the Advancement of Behavior Therapy, Atlanta, December 1977.

Gemunder, C., & Handy, W. S. Generalized expectancies for problem-solving: An analysis of their implications for elementary grade inner-city children. Paper presented at the Annual Convention of the American Psychological Association, Montreal, 1980.

Gesten, E. A health resources inventory: The development of a measure of the personal and social competency of elementary school-aged children. Unpublished Ph.D. dissertation, University of Rochester, 1974.

Gesten, E. L. Health resources inventory: The development of a measure of the personal and social competency of primary-grade children. *Journal of Consulting and Clinical Psychology,* 1976, **44,** 775–786.

Gesten, E. L., Flores de Apodaca, R., Rains, M. H., Weissberg, R. P., & Cowen, E. L. Promoting peer related social competence in young children. In M. W. Kent & J. E. Rolf (Eds.), *Primary prevention of psychopathology.* Vol. 3. *Promoting social competence and coping in children.* Hanover, N.H.: University Press of New England, 1979.

Gibbs, J. T. Patterns of adaptation among black students at a predominantly white university: Selected case studies. *American Journal of Orthopsychiatry,* 1974, **44,** 728–739.

Glidewell, J. C., & Swallow, C. S. *The prevalance of maladjustment in elementary schools: A report prepared for the Joint Commission on the Mental Health of Children.* Chicago: University of Chicago Press, 1969.

Goffman, E. *Stigma.* Englewood Cliffs, N.J.: Prentice-Hall, 1963.

Goldston, S. E. Primary prevention: A view from the federal level. In G. W. Albee & J. M. Joffee (Ed.), *Primary prevention of psychopathology,* Vol. 1. Hanover, N.H.: University Press of New England, 1977.

Handy, W., & Pedro-Carroll, J. Prescriptive early intervention with culturally diverse populations: Some initial observations. Paper presented at the annual convention of the American Psychological Association, New York 1979.

Handy, W., & Pedro-Carroll, J. Holistic health program for low-income children. *Urban Health,* 1980, **9,** 46–48.

Handy, W. S., Rawlings, E., & Jackson, G. G. A cultural competence approach to conducting psychotherapy with ethnic minorities. Advanced workshop conducted at the National Convention of the American Psychological Association, New York, 1979.

Hayles, R. The future and black values. Paper presented at the 10th annual convention of the Association of Black Psychologists, August 1977.

Hodge, J. L., Struckmann, T. E., & Trost, L. D. *Cultural bases of racism and group oppression.* Berkeley, Calif.: Two Riders Press, 1975.

Jackson, G. G. The African genesis of the black perspective in helping. *Professional Psychology,* 1976, **7,** 292–308.

Joint Commission on Mental Health of Children. *Crisis in child mental health: Challenge for the 1970's.* New York: Harper & Row, 1970.

Kirschenbaum, D. S., Marsh, M., & DeVoge, J. B. The effectiveness of a mass screening procedure in an early intervention program. *Psychology in the Schools,* 1977, **14,** 400–406.

Kirschenbaum, D. S., Marsh, M., & DeVoge, J. B. Multimodal evaluation of therapy versus consultation components in a larger inner-city early intervention program. *American Journal of Community Psychology,* 1979, **8,** 587–601.

Klein, D., & Goldston, S. E. *Primary prevention: An idea whose time has come.* DHEW publication No. (ADM) 77-447, 1977.

Obidinski, E. Methodological consideration in the definition of ethnicity. *Ethnicity,* 1978, **5,** 213–228.

Ogbu, J. W. Origins of human competence: A cultural-ecological perspective. *Child Development,* 1981, **52,** 413–429.

Olmedo, E. L. Acculturation: A psychometric perspective. *American Psychologist,* 1979, **34,** 1061–1070.

Peterson, L., Hartmann, D. P., & Gelfand, D. M. Prevention of child behavior disorders: A lifestyle change for child psychologists. In P. O. Davidson & S. M. Davidson (Eds.), *Behavioral medicine: Changing health lifestyles.* New York: Brunner/Mazel, 1980.

Putallaz, M., & Gottman, J. Conceptualizing social competence in children. In P. Karoly & J. J. Steffen (Eds.), *Improving children's competencies.* Lexington, Mass.: Lexington Books, 1982.

Sandler, I. N. Characteristics of women working as child-aides in a school-based preventive mental health program. *Journal of Consulting and Clinical Psychology,* 1972, **36,** 56–61.

Sarason, S. B., Levine, M., Goldenberg, I., Cherlin, D., & Bennett, E. M. *Psychology in community settings.* New York: Wiley, 1966.

Spivack, G., & Shure, M. *Social adjustment of young children.* San Francisco: Jossey-Bass, 1974.

Sue, D. W., & Sue, D. Barriers to effective cross-cultural counseling. *Journal of Counseling Psychology,* 1977, **24,** 420–429.

Sue, S. Community mental health services to minority groups: Some optimism, some pessimism. *American Psychologist,* 1977, **32,** 616–624.

Swift, C. F. Prevention: Policy and practice. In R. H. Price, R. F. Ketterer, B. C. Bader, & J. Monahan (Eds), *Prevention in mental health: Research, policy and practice.* Beverly Hills, Calif.: Sage, 1980.

Tableman, B. Prevention activities at the state level. In R. H. Price, R. F. Ketterer, B. C. Bader, & J. Monahan (Eds.), *Prevention in mental health: Research, policy, and practice.* Beverly Hills, Calif.: Sage, 1980.

White, R. C. Motivation reconsidered: The concept of competence. *Psychological Reveiw,* 1959, **66,** 297–333.

Zax, M., & Cowen, E. L. Early identification and prevention of emotional disturbance in a public school. In E. L. Cowen, E. A. Gardner, & M. Zax (Eds.), *Emergent approaches to mental health problems.* New York: Appleton-Century-Crofts, 1967.

Zigler, E., & Trickett, P. K. I. Q., social competence, and evaluation of early education programs. *American Psychologist,* 1978, **33,** 789–798.

Author Index

Subject Index

About the Editors and Contributors

THE EDITORS

Paul Karoly (Ph.D., University of Rochester) is currently Professor and Director of Clinical Training at Arizona State University. His research and professional interests include self-regulation and self-control in children and adults, health psychology, and experimental personality and psychopathology. Dr. Karoly is on the editorial boards of several professional journals including the *Journal of Consulting and Clinical Psychology, Journal of Personality and Social Psychology, Behavior Therapy* and *Behavioral Assessment*. He is the co-editor (with J. J. Steffen) of *Improving the Long-term Effects of Psychotherapy, Self-management and Behavior Change* (with F. H. Kanfer), and a series subtitled "Advances in Child Behavior Analysis and Therapy," the inaugural volumes of which were published in 1982.

John J. Steffen (Ph.D., Rutgers, the State University) is currently Associate Professor and Director of Clinical Training at the University of Cincinnati. He is actively involved in research on interpersonal communication and on the development of social relationships in children and adults. He is co-editor (with P. Karoly) of *Improving the Long-term Effects of Psychotherapy* and the "Advances in Child Behavior Analysis and Therapy" series and serves as a member of the editorial board of the *Journal of Communicaton Therapy*.

Donald J. O'Grady (Ph.D., University of Cincinnati) is currently Associate Professor of Clinical Pediatrics at the University of Cincinnati College of Medicine and Director, Psychology Department, Children's Hospital Medical Center. Dr. O'Grady, who is a Diplomate of the American Board of Examiners in Professional Psychology, has been involved in pediatrics research since 1968. His areas of interest include PKU, developmental disabilities, and symptom relief in cancer, hemophilia, cystic fibrosis, and sickle cell anemia.

THE CONTRIBUTORS

Frank Addrisi (Ph.D., 1978, University of Cincinnati) is currently at the Department of Psychological Services, Wyoming State Hospital. He is involved in the application of learning principles to the treatment of physical symptoms.

John Gerald Beales (Ph.D., 1972, University of Wales) is in the Department of Rheumatology, University of Manchester (England) Medical School. He is presently studying children with chronic joint disease to examine the possible relationship between their pain experience (and their emotional distress) and their beliefs about illness as well as their fantasies about the visual appearance of the internal pathology associated with the disease process.

Edward R. Christophersen (Ph.D., 1970, University of Kansas) has an active practice in behavioral pediatrics and is on the staff of the University of Kansas Medical Center (Kansas City). His research interests include behavioral analysis and intervention with behavior-disordered children, burn trauma, and children's compliance with acute and chronic disease treatment regimens.

Suzanne Craft (B.A., 1976, University of Virginia) is a Ph.D. candidate at the University of Texas at Austin. She is currently interested in clinical neuropsychology with special emphasis on hemispheric lateralization.

Dennis Drotar (Ph.D., 1970, University of Iowa) is currently at Rainbow Babies and Children's Hospital and the Case Western Reserve University School of Medicine. He is a pediatric psychologist specializing in health care consultation and the psychological aspects of chronic illness in children.

Tiffany Field (Ph.D., 1976, University of Massachusetts) is affiliated with the Mailman Center for Child Development at the University of Miami Medical School. Her current research interests include affective development and social skills acquisition in normal and high-risk infants and children.

Charles J. Golden (Ph.D., 1975, University of Hawaii) is currently at the University of Nebraska Medical School. Dr. Golden's research efforts have focused upon validation of the adult and children's verions of the Luria-Nebraska neuropsychological batteries, on the neurological basis of psychiatric disorders, and on the interrelationships between neuropsychological assessment devices.

Walter S. Handy, Jr. (Ph.D., 1976, University of Connecticut) is director of the Social Skills Development Program at the Cincinnati Health Department. His interests include the school-based early identification of and intervention in child psychopathology and elaboration of the concept of social competence in children, with special reference to racial and cultural factors.

Mary Kay Jordan (M.A., 1981, University of Cincinnati) is a doctoral student in the Department of Psychology at the University of Cincinnati and a research assistant at the Children's Hospital Research Foundation. She has participated in research on inborn errors of metabolism as part of an interdisciplinary team.

She has been specializing in assessing intellectual and psychological performance of children over extended periods.

Donald R. Kanter (Ph.D., 1982, University of Cincinnati) is currently at the Veteran's Administration Medical Center, Psychiatry Research Service, in Cincinnati, Ohio. In addition to long-standing interests in childhood psychopathology, he is currently involved in interdisciplinary research on the psychobiology of schizophrenia.

Marc S. Lewis (Ph.D., 1973, University of Cincinnati) is assistant professor of clinical and community psychology at the University of Texas at Austin. His current interests are the epidemiology of schizophrenia and mathematical approaches to disease processes.

Greta N. Wilkening (Psy. D., 1980, University of Denver) is currently instructor in pediatrics and neurology at the University of Colorado Health Sciences Center and is affiliated with The Children's Hospital in Denver. Her research interests include the neuropsychological sequelae of CNS prophylaxis for the treatment of acute lymphocytic leukemia and the continued development and standardization of the Luria-Nebraska neuropsychological battery for children.

Pergamon General Psychology Series

Editors: Arnold P. Goldstein, Syracuse University
Leonard Krasner, SUNY at Stony Brook